Rapid
Paediatrics
and
Child Health

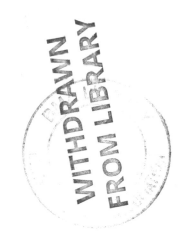

Rapid Paediatrics and Child Health

Helen A. Brough
Clinical Lecturer in Paediatric Allergy and SpR Paediatrics and Child Health

Ram Nataraja
SpR Paediatric Surgery

Second Edition

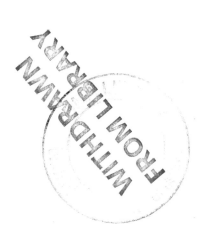

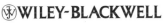

WILEY-BLACKWELL
A John Wiley & Sons, Ltd., Publication

This edition first published 2010, © 2010 by Helen A. Brough and Ram Nataraja.

Previous edition: 2004.

Blackwell Publishing was acquired by John Wiley & Sons in February 2007. Blackwells publishing program has been merged with Wileys global Scientific, Technical and Medical business to form Wiley-Blackwell.

Registered office: John Wiley & Sons Ltd, The Atrium, Southern Gate, Chichester, West Sussex, PO19 8SQ, UK

Editorial offices: 9600 Garsington Road, Oxford, OX4 2DQ, UK
The Atrium, Southern Gate, Chichester, West Sussex, PO19 8SQ, UK
111 River Street, Hoboken, NJ 07030-5774, USA

For details of our global editorial offices, for customer services and for information about how to apply for permission to reuse the copyright material in this book please see our website at www.wiley.com/wiley-blackwell

Library of Congress Cataloging-in-Publication Data
Brough, Helen.
  Rapid paediatrics and child health / Helen Brough, Ram Nataraja. – 2nd ed.
    p. ; cm. – (Rapid series)
  Rev. ed. of: Rapid paediatrics and child health / Helen Brough ... [et al.]. 2004.
  ISBN 978-1-4051-9330-6 (pbk. : alk. paper) 1. Pediatrics–Handbooks, manuals, etc. I. Nataraja, Ram. II. Title. III. Series: Rapid series.
  [DNLM: 1. Pediatrics–Handbooks. WS 39 B875r 2010]
  RJ48.R375 2010
  618.92–dc22
                                   2009051053
ISBN: 9781405193306

A catalogue record for this book is available from the British Library.

Set in 7.5/9.5pt Frutiger-Light by Thomson Digital, Noida, India

Printed and bound in Malaysia by Vivar Printing Sdn Bhd

1   2010

Contents

Appendices

Preface

Rapid Paediatrics and Child Health is part of a series of books for medical students that are designed to facilitate learning about core topics in a structured format. Each page is divided into our own "surgical sieve": Definition, Aetiology, Associated/Related, Epidemiology, History, Examination, Pathophysiology, Investigations, Management, Complications and Prognosis.

In the second edition we have included over 150 common conditions that cover the major topics in all paediatric medical, surgical and neonatal specialities. All of the topics have been updated with the current paediatric medical and surgical guidelines including NICE. There is also a new section called Further Reading where suggested papers for each chapter are listed in line with evidence based practice. Core knowledge, important investigative techniques and treatment modalities are all included in each chapter. The investigations suggested are for guidance and are not always necessary for a child with the condition.

This book has been designed to be easy to carry around and also to allow rapid access to information whether in the outpatient department, the ward or theatre, so you can consolidate theory with practice.

The authorship team consisting of both a paediatric and a paediatric surgical SpR means that we have brought different experiences in paediatrics to the book to create a truly unique resource. We hope you enjoy reading this book as much as we have enjoyed writing it!

List of Abbreviations

F	female	ATN	acute tubular necrosis
M	male	ATP	adenosine triphosphate
1°	primary	AUSS	abdominal ultrasound
2°	secondary	AV	atrioventricular
↑	increase(d)	AVPU	alert, verbal response, painful
↓	decrease(d)		response, unresponsive
→	to/lead(s) to	AVSD	atrioventricular septal defect
>	greater than	AXR	abdominal X-ray
<	less than	BD	twice a day
~	approximately	BCG	bacille Calmette–Guérin
×	times	BiPAP	bilevel positive airways
			pressure
ABC	airway, breathing, circulation	BM	blood monitor/monitoring
ABG	arterial blood gases	BMD	Becker muscular dystrophy
ABVD	adriamycin, bleomycin,	BMI	Body Mass Index
	vinblastine, dacarbazine	BMJ	*British Medical Journal*
ACTH	adrenocorticotrophic	BMT	bone marrow transplant/
	hormone		transplantation
AD	autosomal dominant	BP	blood pressure
ADHD	attention deficit hyperactivity	BPD	bronchopulmonary dysplasia
	disorder	bpm	beat per minute
AFP	alpha-fetoprotein	BTS	British Thoracic Society
AIDS	acquired immunodeficiency	CAD	coronary artery disease
	syndrome	cAMP	cyclic adenosine
ALL	acute lymphoblastic		monophosphatase
	leukaemia	CBT	cognitive-behavioural therapy
ALP	alkaline phosphatase	CCDC	consultant in communicable
ALT	alanine aminotransferase		disease control
ALTE	apparent life-threatening	CD	Crohn's disease
	event	CDH	congenital diaphragmatic
AML	acute myeloid leukaemia		hernia
AN	anorexia nervosa	CF	cystic fibrosis
AP	anteroposterior	CFTR	cystic fibrosis transmembrane
APTT	activated partial		regulator
	thromboplastin time	CGD	chronic granulomatous
AP50	alternative pathway		disease
	complement activation assay	CGG	cytosine-guanine-guanine
AR	aortic regurgitation	CHB	complete heart block
AR	autosomal recessive	CHD	congenital heart disease
ARDS	acute respiratory	CHF	congestive heart failure
	distress syndrome	CH100	total complement activity
ARIA	allergic rhinitis and its impact		assay
	on asthma	CLD	chronic lung disease
ARF	acute renal failure	CMV	cytomegalovirus
AFP	alpha-fetoprotein	CNS	central nervous system
ARM	anorectal malformation	COA	coarctation of the aorta
ASD	atrial septal defect	CPAP	continuous positive airways
ASOT	antistreptolysin O titre		pressure
AST	aspartate aminotransferase	CPK	creatinine phosphokinase
ATG	antithymocyte globulin	CRF	chronic renal failure

CRHD	chronic rheumatic heart disease	ERCP	endoscopic retrograde cholangiopancreatography
CRP	C-reactive protein	ESR	erythrocyte sedimentation rate
CSF	cerebrospinal fluid	ET	endotracheal
CSOM	chronic secretory otitis media	FVIII–FXI	factor VIII to factor XI
		FAB	French–American–British
CT	computed tomography	FAS	fetal alcohol syndrome
CTG	cardiotocography/graph	FBC	full blood count
CVID	common variable immune deficiency	FEV	forced expiratory volume
		FFP	fresh frozen plasma
CVP	central venous pressure	FGFR3	fibroblast growth factor receptor 3
CVS	chorionic villous sampling		
CXR	chest x-ray	FH	father's height (cm)
DD	differential diagnosis	FMR1	fragile X mental retardation 1
DDH	developmental dysplasia of the hip	FMRP	fragile X mental retardation protein
DDT	dichlorodiphenyltrichloro-ethane	FSH	follicle-stimulating hormone
		G6PD	glucose-6-phosphate dehydrogenase
DEXA	dual-energy X-ray absorptiometry	GBS	group B streptococcus
DIC	disseminated intravascular coagulation/coagulopathy	GCS	graduated compression stockings/Glasgow Coma Score
DIP	distal intraphalangeal		
DISIDA	di-isopropyl iminodiacetic acid	G-CSF	granulocyte colony stimulating factor
DKA	diabetic ketoacidosis		
DM	diabetes mellitus	GFR	glomerular filtration rate
DMD	Duchenne muscular dystrophy	GH	growth hormone
		GI	gastrointestinal
DMPK	dystrophia myotonica protein kinase	GN	glomerulonephritis
		GnRH	gonadotrophin-releasing hormone
DMSA	dimercaptosuccinic acid		
DNA	deoxyribonucleic acid	GOR	gastro-oesophageal reflux
DNAse	deoxyribonuclease	GORD	gastro-oesophageal reflux disease
DPT	diphtheria, pertussis, tetanus		
DSM-IV	*Diagnostic and Statistical Manual of Mental Disorders*, 4th edition	GP	general practitioner
		GSD	glycogen storage disease
		G&S	Group & Save
DTap	Diptheria, tetoinus, pertussis	GTCS	generalised tonic-clonic seizures
DTPA	diethylenetriamine penta-acetic acid	GU	genitourinary
		GVHD	graft versus host disease
DVT	deep vein thrombosis	HA	haemophilia A
EAS	external anal sphincter	HAV	hepatitis A virus
EBV	Epstein–Barr virus	Hb	haemoglobin
ECG	electrocardiogram/graph	HB	haemophilia B
ECMO	extracorporeal membrane oxygenation	HBV	hepatitis B virus
		HC	haemophilia C
EEG	electroencephalogram	HCG	human chorionic gonadotrophin
EHF	extensively hydrolysed formulas		
		HCV	hepatitis C virus
ELISA	enzyme-linked immunosorbent assay	HDL	high-density lipoprotein
		HFO	high-frequency oscillation
EMG	electromyogram/graph	Hib	*Haemophilus influenzae* b
ENT	ear nose throat	HIDA	hepatobiliary iminodiacetic acid
EPO	erythropoietin		

HIE	hypoxic–ischaemic encephalopathy	MCH	mean cell/corpuscular haemoglobin
His	histidine	MC&S	microscopy culture and sensitivity
HIV	human immunodeficiency virus	MCUG	micturating cystourethrogram
HLA	human lymphocyte antigen	MCV	mean cell/corpuscular volume
HR	heart rate	MDD	major depressive disorder
HS	hereditary spherocytosis	Men C	meningitis C
HSP	Henoch–Schönlein purpura	MH	mother's height (cm)
HSV	herpes simplex virus	MMR	measles, mumps, rubella
HT	hypertension	MR	mitral regurgitation
HTLV	human T-lymphotrophic virus	MRI	magnetic resonance imaging
HUS	haemolytic uraemic syndrome	MSE	mental state examination
IAS	Internal anal sphincter	MSU	mid-stream specimen of urine
IBS	irritable bowel syndrome	MVP	mitral valve prolapse
ICP	intracranial pressure	NA	noradrenaline
ICS	inhaled corticosteroids	NAI	non-accidental injury
ICSI	intracytoplasmic sperm injection	NBM	nucleus basalis magnocellularis/nil by mouth
ICU	intensive care unit	NBT	nitroblue tetrazolium
Ig	immunoglobulin	NEC	necrotising enterocolitis
IGFBP-3	insulin-like growth factor-binding protein 3	NEJM	*New England Journal of Medicine*
IHD	ischaemic heart disease	NF	neurofibromatosis
INR	international normalised ratio	NG	nasogastric
IM	intramuscular	NHL	non-Hodgkin lymphoma
IP	intraphalangeal	NICE	National Institute for Health and Clinical Excellence
IUGR	intrauterine growth restriction/retardation	NICU	neonatal intensive care unit
		NK	natural killer
IV	intravenous	NNU	neonatal unit
IVH	intraventricular haemorrhage	NO	nitric oxide
IVIg	intravenous immunoglobulin	NSAID	non-steroidal anti-inflammatory drug
IVU	intravenous urogram		
JVP	jugular venous pulse	NSPCC	National Society for the Prevention of Cruelty to Children
LABA	long-acting β_2-agonist		
LBW	low birthweight		
LCPD	Legg–Calvé–Perthes disease	OCA	oculocutaneous albinism
LDH	lactate dehydrogenase	OCD	obsessive–compulsive disorder
LFT	liver function test		
LGA	large for gestational age	OCP	oral contraceptive pill
LH	luteinising hormone	OGD	oesophagogastroduodenoscopy
LHRH	luteinising hormone-releasing hormone		
		O/N	overnight
LIF	left iliac fossa	OPV	oral polio vaccine
LN	lymph node	ORT	oral rehydration therapy
LP	lumbar puncture	OTC	over the counter
LRTI	lower respiratory tract infection	PA	pulmonary artery
		PAS	periodic acid–Schiff
LVF	left ventricular function	PCP	*Pneumocystis carinii* pneumonia
LVH	left ventricular hypertrophy	PCR	polymerase chain reaction
MAG3	mercaptoacetyltriglycine	PDA	patent ductus arteriosus
MALT	mucosa-associated lymphoid tissue	PE	pulmonary embolism
		PEN	pharmacy equivalent name

PET	positron emission tomography		SMA	superior mesenteric artery
PICU	paediatric intensive care unit		SOB	shortness of breath
PKU	phenylketonuria		SPAG	small particle aerosol generation
PNH	paroxysmal nocturnal haemoglobinuria		SSPE	subacute sclerosing panencephalitis
PO	per oral		SSRI	selective serotonin reuptake inhibitor
POS	polycystic ovary syndrome			
PPH	persistent pulmonary hypertension		STD	sexually transmitted disease
			SUDEP	sudden unexpected death in epileptic patients
PPV	positive pressure ventilation			
PROM	prolonged rupture of membranes		SUFE	slipped upper femoral epiphysis
PSC	primary sclerosing cholangitis		SVC	superior vena cava
PTH	parathyroid hormone		SVT	supraventricular tachycardia
PTSD	post-traumatic stress disorder		T_3	tri-iodothyronine
PUVA	psoralen ultraviolet A		T_4	thyroxine
QDS	four times a day		TB	tuberculosis
RAH	right atrial hypertrophy		TDS	three times a day
RBC	red blood cell/count		TFT	thyroid function test
RDS	respiratory distress syndrome		TGA	transposition of the great arteries
REAL	revised European and American lymphoma		THAM	tris(hydroxymethyl)-aminomethane
REM	rapid eye movement			
Rh	rhesus		THI	transient hypogammaglobulinaemia of infancy
rhGH	recombinant human growth hormone			
RIF	right iliac fossa		TLC	total lung capacity
RNA	ribonucleic acid		TOF	tracheo-oesophageal fistula
ROM	range of movement		TOP	termination of pregnancy
ROP	retinopathy of prematurity		TORCH	toxoplasma, other (syphilis, HIV), rubella, cytomegalovirus, hepatitis
RSV	respiratory syncytial virus			
RTA	road traffic accident			
RUSS	Renal ultrasound		TPN	total parenteral nutrition
RVH	right ventricular hypertrophy		TRH	thyrotrophin-releasing hormone
RVT	renal vein thrombosis			
SBP	systolic blood pressure		TS	transient synovitis
SC	subcutaneous		TS1&2	tuberous sclerosis 1&2
SCBU	special care baby unit		TSH	thyroid-stimulating hormone
SCID	severe combined immunodeficiency		TSI	thyroid-stimulating immunoglobulin
SCIg	sub-cutaneous immunoglobulin		TSS	toxic shock syndrome
			TTN	transient tachypnoea of the newborn
SD	standard deviation			
S/E	side effects		TTP	thrombotic thrombocytopenic purpura
SGA	small for gestational age			
SIADH	syndrome of inappropriate antidiuretic hormone		U&E	urea and electrolytes
			UC	ulcerative colitis
SIDS	sudden infant death syndrome		UDPGA	uridine diphosphoglucuronic acid
sIgAD	selective IgA deficiency		UGI	upper gastrointestinal
SIRS	systemic inflammatory response syndrome		UKALL	United Kingdom Medical Research Council protocol for childhood ALL
SLE	systemic lupus erythematosus			

URT	upper respiratory tract	VON	varicella of the newborn
URTI	upper respiratory tract infection	VSD	ventricular septal defect
		VT	ventricular tachycardia
USS	ultrasound scan	VUR	vesicoureteric reflux
UTI	urinary tract infection	VZV	varicella zoster virus
UTR	untranslated region	WAS	Wiskott-Aldrich syndrome
UV	ultraviolet	WCC	white cell count
VACTERL	vertebral, anal, cardiac, tracheal, (o)esophageal, renal, limb	WHO	World Health Organization
		WPW	Wolff–Parkinson–White (syndrome)
VE	varicella embryopathy	XLA	X-linked Bruton's agammaglobulinaemia
VF	ventricular fibrillator		

DEFINITION   Chronic inflammatory dermatosis. Classified as mild, moderate, or severe.

AETIOLOGY
Infantile acne: <3 months of life; transient and usually due to maternal androgens.
Adolescent acne:

1. ↑Sebum production: androgenic stimulation of hyper-responsive pilosebaceous units.
2. Impaired flow of sebum: obstruction of the pilosebaceous duct by hyperkeratosis.
3. *Propionobacterium acnes:* gram-positive anaerobe is implicated in the inflammation.

Associations/related: Puberty, may ↑ premenstrually, POS, excess cortisol (Cushing syndrome).

EPIDEMIOLOGY
Developed world: Affects 79–95% of the adolescent population, peaking at 14–18 years; tends to recede by early twenties.
Developing world: Acne incidence is considerably lower; likely combination of environmental and genetic factors.

HISTORY   Usually self-diagnosed, acute onset, greasy skin, may be painful.

EXAMINATION
Open comedones: Whiteheads; flesh-coloured papules.
Closed comedones: Blackheads; black colour is due to oxidation of the melanin pigment.
Other features: Pustules, nodules, cysts, scarring, and seborrhoea.
Distribution: Primarily affects the face, neck, chest and back (where sebaceous glands are most numerous).

PATHOPHYSIOLOGY   Gross distension of the pilosebaceous follicle with neutrophil infiltration. Closed comedones may contain serous fluid. Severe acne can create fistulas between inflamed glands.

INVESTIGATIONS   Not indicated unless other signs of androgen excess; prepubertal body odour, axillary/pubic hair or genital maturation; postpubertal infrequent menses, hirsutism or truncal obesity (suspect POS).
Bloods: Free testosterone, FSH, LH.
Urine: 24-hour urinary cortisol (if Cushing syndrome is suspected).

MANAGEMENT   Indication for treatment is based on classification and degree of psychosocial impact. In severe acne, therapy should be commenced early to prevent scarring. General advice should include use of non-greasy cosmetics, daily face wash. Dietary restriction is not beneficial in the treatment of acne.

Single topical preparations

1. Benzoyl peroxide: keratolytic agent, encourages skin peeling, and bactericidal (S/E: irritation and bleaching of clothes).
2. Vitamin A derivatives: retinoids reduce obstruction within the follicle.
3. Antibiotics: clindamycin or erythromycin is effective but when used as single agents may result in *P. acne* resistance.

Combination topical preparations

1. Topical retinoids and antibiotics are synergistic.
2. Topical benzoyl peroxide and antibiotics reduce the likelihood of *P. acne* resistance and are also more effective.

Systemic preparations

1. Antibiotics: tetracyclines (doxycycline, minocycline). S/E: discoloration of teeth. Macrolides (erythromycin or azithromycin) or trimethoprim-sulphamethoxazole (Septrin).
2. Vitamin A derivative: isotretinoin (Roaccutane PO): 4–6-month course only by specialist prescription for severe acne (S/E: potent teratogen, hyperlipidaemia).
3. Hormones: oestrogen-containing OCP, antiandrogens (spironolactone S/E: hyperkalaemia), cyproterone acetate in females only.

Physical treatments: Short-term efficacy from optical treatments such as lasers, light sources and photodynamic therapy.

COMPLICATIONS
Physical: Facial scarring (atrophic/keloid), hyperpigmentation, 2° infection and fistulas.
Psychosocial: Lack of self-confidence.

PROGNOSIS   Generally improves spontaneously over months/years. At 25 years, persists in 12% of women and 5% of men.

DEFINITION Inflammation of the membrane lining the nose. ARIA definition; intermittent (<4 days/week or <4 weeks) versus persistent (>4 days/week and >4 weeks). Impact on quality of life: mild, moderate or severe. 'Seasonal' (spring/summer) versus 'perennial' definition is also important in the UK.

AETIOLOGY Parental atopy. AR is more likely to occur in first-born children (hygiene hypothesis).

ASSOCIATIONS/RELATED Children with AR have an increased risk of developing asthma, sinusitis or otitis media. Allergic conjunctivitis frequently co-exists.

EPIDEMIOLOGY Seasonal AR is found in 10% and perennial AR in 10–20% of the population. Prevalence is increasing.

HISTORY Itchy nose, rhinorrhoea, sneezing, persistent nose blowing, congested nose, snoring, throat clearing, morning halitosis (post-nasal drip), chronic cough.

EXAMINATION Allergic nasal crease, allergic 'salute', allergic 'shiners' (dark circles under eyes), Dennie-Morgan (infra-orbital skin) folds, mouth breathing. On nasal inspection, pale hypertrophied inferior nasal turbinates. If polyps are seen, think of cystic fibrosis or aspirin-sensitive asthma in the older child.

PATHOPHYSIOLOGY Allergen on the nasal mucosa/eyes binds to IgE on mast cells and leads to release of inflammatory mediators (histamine/leukotriene). Mucosal cellular infiltration leads to the late phase response and chronic exposure leads to hypertrophy of the nasal turbinates and increased mucous production.

INVESTIGATIONS Skin prick tests/specific IgE for seasonal (grass/tree pollen and moulds) and perennial (house dust mite, animal dander) inhalant allergens.

MANAGEMENT Assess severity and impact on quality of life/sleep. Check compliance with medication and method of delivering intranasal steroids. Ask about asthma symptoms; treating AR will improve asthma control. Avoid irritants (e.g. cigarette smoke).

Allergen avoidance: *Pollen*: wear glasses during and shower after being outside, close windows (especially early morning and evening), don't dry clothes outside, fit pollen filter in car. *House dust mite prevention strategies*: ventilate room, bedding barrier covers, remove soft furnishings/cuddly toys, HEPA filter vacuums, acaricidal sprays.

Non-sedating antihistamines: Relieves itch, sneeze and rhinorrhoea but less effective for nasal congestion. Recommended for mild intermittent AR as a single therapy.

Decongestants: Modifies nasal obstruction. Recommended for short-term use only due to risk of rhinitis medicamentosa (rebound congestion).

Topical nasal steroids: Most effective single therapy. Relieves and prevents itch, sneeze, rhinorrhoea and congestion. Best when used regularly. S/E nasal bleed mainly if administered incorrectly. Newer formulations have minimal (<0.5%) systemic steroid absorption.

Leukotriene receptor antagonists: Second-line treatment. Synergistic effect when combined with non-sedating antihistamines but not as effective as combining antihistamines and nasal steroids.

Immunotherapy: Available in sublingual and subcutaneous preparation. Treatment shows sustained reduction in symptoms and medication scores, prevents new sensitisation to inhalant allergens and decreases the risk of developing asthma.

COMPLICATIONS Decreased quality of life: poor sleep, impairment of daily activities, problems at school (particularly during exam term).

PROGNOSIS Seasonal allergic rhinitis tends to diminish with age. If symptoms start in early childhood, the likelihood of improvement is greater than if the onset is in adulthood.

DEFINITION   Pancytopaenia (deficiency of all blood cell elements) associated with bone marrow hypoplasia.

AETIOLOGY
Idiopathic (>40%): Possibly 2° to immunological suppression of multipotent myeloid stem cells by cytotoxic T cells. Phenotypically normal but often have genetic markers of congenital marrow failure syndromes.

Acquired:

1. Viral infection (parvovirus, CMV, HIV, hepatitis, measles).
2. Drugs (chloramphenicol, alkylating agents, methotrexate).
3. Chemicals (DDT, benzene).
4. Radiation.

Inherited:

1. Fanconi anaemia, FA (autosomal recessive, error of DNA repair).
2. Dyskeratosis congenital (rare sex-linked disorder with skin and nail atrophy).
3. Shwachmann syndrome (pancytopaenia in 25%).

ASSOCIATIONS/RELATED
FA: Growth retardation, forearm bones abnormalities, heart and renal tract defects (horseshoe or pelvic kidney) and skin pigmentation.

EPIDEMIOLOGY   2–5/1,000,000/yr. Any age. M > F.

HISTORY   May present with either slow (months) or rapid (days) onset:

1. ↓ **RBC:** Tiredness, lethargy and dyspnoea
2. ↓ **Platelets:** Easy bruising, bleeding gums, epistaxis
3. ↓**WCC:** Increased frequency and severity of infections (immunodeficiency).

EXAMINATION   Signs of anaemia (pallor), petechiae, bruises, bacterial or fungal infections. No hepatomegaly, splenomegaly or lymphadenopathy.

PATHOPHYSIOLOGY
Macro: Pale or white bone marrow.
Micro: Hypocellular bone marrow composed of empty marrow spaces, fat cells, fibrous stroma and isolated foci of lymphocytes and plasma cells. Classic 'chicken wire' appearance.

INVESTIGATIONS
Blood: ↓Hb, ↓platelets, ↓neutrophils, normal MCV, low or absent reticulocytes.
Blood film: Leukaemia exclusion.
Bone marrow trephine biopsy: For diagnosis and exclusion of other causes (bone marrow infiltration: lymphoma, leukaemia, malignancies).
Chromosomal abnormalities: ↑ Random breaks in peripheral lymphocytes in Fanconi anaemia. Also prognostic guide; certain mutations associated with earlier onset of leukaemia/haematological abnormalities.
Ham test: For paroxysmal nocturnal haemoglobinuria: measures sensitivity of affected red blood cells to lysis by complement following activation in acidified serum.

MANAGEMENT
Treat the underlying cause: Medication review and underlying infection treatment.
Supportive: Blood and platelet transfusions, antibiotics (therapeutic/prophylactic).
Medical: Immunosuppression; corticosteroids, cyclosporin A, antithymocyte globulin (ATG), androgen (oxymetholone for FA), and antilymphocyte globulin (ALG). Pts who relapse or are unresponsive to an immunosuppressive regimen may benefit from a repeat or alternative course.

Surgical: CVC/Portacath placement for repeated phlebotomy/transfusions. Splenectomy with heavily transfused and allosensitised pts refractory to medical therapies and with no HSCT donor.

Haematopoietic stem cell transplantation (HSCT): Definitive treatment in severe aplastic anaemia; from an HLA-identical family member. Cure rate approaching 90%.

COMPLICATIONS

Complication of disease process: Bleeding, infections (bacterial and fungal), sepsis and ↑d risk of developing myelodysplastic syndromes or leukaemia if the duration of illness is prolonged.

Complication of HSCT: Graft rejection, graft versus host disease, infection (new or reactivated).

PROGNOSIS Poor prognostic features include: platelets $<10 \times 10^9$/l, neutrophils $<0.5 \times 10^9$/l, reticulocytes 10×10^9/l. $>50\%$ of patients with all these features lasting more than 3 weeks will die.

DEFINITION Premature erythrocyte breakdown (haemolysis) causing ↓d erythrocyte lifespan (<120 days) and anaemia (2° to bone marrow activity unable to compensate).

AETIOLOGY Intravascular or extravascular (reticuloendothelial system; by splenic macrophages). 2° to either hereditary or acquired factors.

Hereditary:
Membrane defects: Spherocytosis (abnormal spectrin: structural membrane protein which alters deformability of RBCs), elliptocytosis (elliptical RBCs), hereditary pyropoikilocytosis.
Metabolic defects: G6PD deficiency, pyruvate kinase deficiencies.
Haemoglobinopathies: Sickle cell disease, thalassaemia.

Acquired (immune):
Autoimmune: Warm or cold antibodies attach to RBCs → activation of complement → intravascular haemolysis and extravascular haemolysis in hypersplenism. *Warm antibodies:* Idiopathic or associated with SLE, lymphomas or methyldopa. *Cold antibodies:* Idiopathic/associated with infections (*Mycoplasma*, EBV) or lymphoma.
Isoimmune: Transfusion reaction, haemolytic disease of the newborn.

Acquired (non-immune):
Trauma: RBC fragmentation in abnormal microcirculation; thrombotic thrombocytopaenia purpura, haemolytic uraemic syndrome, disseminated intravascular coagulopathy, malignant hypertension, pre-eclampsia, artificial heart valves.
Paroxysmal nocturnal haemoglobinuria (PNH): Acute-onset haemoglobinuria; idiopathic or 2° to cold due to complement-mediated lysis.
Infection: Malaria.

ASSOCIATIONS/RELATED Parvovirus B19.

EPIDEMIOLOGY
Hereditary causes: Prevalent in African, Mediterranean and Middle Eastern populations.
Hereditary spherocytosis (HS): Most common inherited haemolytic anaemia in northern Europe.

HISTORY AND EXAMINATION
Depends on age: Jaundice and anaemia most common symptoms. Neonatal jaundice may require exchange transfusion. Older children may present with chronic anaemia. Hepatosplenomegaly and specific signs of underlying pathogenesis may also be present.

PATHOPHYSIOLOGY
Blood film (haemolytic anaemia): Leucoerythroblastic picture, microspherocytosis, macrocytosis, nucleated RBCs/reticulocytes, polychromasia.
Blood film (underlying cause): Spherocytes, elliptocytes, sickle cells, fragmented RBCs (DIC), malarial parasites, RBC Heinz bodies (G6PD deficiency).

INVESTIGATIONS
Bloods: ↓Hb, ↑MCV due to reticulocytes, ↑unconjugated bilirubin, ↑LDH, ↓haptoglobin, ↓red cell G6PD and pyruvate kinase assays, Hb electrophoresis (identifies variants).
Urine: ↑Urobilirubinogen 2° to excess unconjugated bilirubin, haemoglobinuria.
Direct Coombs' test: Identifies RBCs coated with antibodies using antihuman globulin. *Warm antibodies:* IgG, agglutinate RBCs at 37 °C. *Cold antibodies:* IgM, agglutinate RBCs at room temperature.
Osmotic fragility test: Detects membrane abnormalities (spherocytosis).
Ham's test: PNH.
Bone marrow biopsy (rarely required): Erythroid hyperplasia; may be hypoplastic in PNH.

MANAGEMENT
Contributing factor avoidance: Cold exposure (cold antibodies, PNH), drugs (G6PD deficiency), transfusions, folate deficiency (HS), splenectomy (postpone until after childhood).

Autoimmune (warm): Prednisolone, splenectomy, azathioprine/cyclophosphamide.

PNH: Blood transfusions (leucocyte-depleted), anticoagulants for thrombotic episodes, bone marrow transplantation is successful in a small number of patients.

COMPLICATIONS   Renal failure may develop in all cases due to accumulation of RBC breakdown products in the renal tubules. *PNH:* Can transform into aplastic anaemia or leukaemia. *HS:* Gallstones, aplastic anaemia in parvovirus infection, megaloblastic and haemolytic crises (↓folate due to hyperactive bone marrow), leg ulcers and corneal opacities.

PROGNOSIS   Depends on the cause.

DEFINITION   ↓Hb with low mean cell volume (MCV <80 fl) and depleted iron stores.

AETIOLOGY
WHO definition: Hb <11 g/dl (110 g/l) aged 1–2 years and <11.2 g/dl (112 g/l) aged 3–5 years.
General: Three stages in the pathogenesis: Fe^{2+} depletion → Fe^{2+}-deficient erythropoiesis → Fe^{2+} deficiency anaemia.
↓d Fe^{2+} stores at birth: Prematurity, multiple pregnancy, perinatal bleeding, early umbilical cord clamping, and maternal Fe^{2+} deficiency.
Nutritional (inadequate Fe^{2+} supply): Exclusive breastfeeding >6/12 (insufficient Fe^{2+} in breast milk); early cow's milk introduction (↓bioavailability of iron than breast milk and formula milk is fortified with 6 mg iron/l); excessive reliance on milk in the second year of life; ↑d infant fruit juice intake; strict vegetarian diet; behavioral (food refusal, grazing, dieting, eating disorders); Crohn's disease, coeliac disease (↓d absorption).
↑d Fe^{2+} loss: Acute haemorrhage (Meckel's diverticulum, intestinal duplication cyst, peptic ulcer); chronic haemorrhage (cow's milk protein intolerance, intestinal duplication, IBD, telangiectasia, intestinal polyp); parasites (hookworm – Ancylostoma duodenale in developing countries); menstruation.
↑d Fe^{2+} demand: Growth; prematurity; IUGR; post malnutrition.

ASSOCIATIONS/RELATED   Inner city centres (UK) and Asian communities.

EPIDEMIOLOGY   Most common nutritional deficiency disorder worldwide. *Incidence:* 5–40% depending on community. *Peak ages:* 6 months to 3 years and adolescent girls. Uncommon in non-premature infants <6/12 (fetally acquired iron reserves).

HISTORY
General: Gradual onset; failure to thrive, poor exercise tolerance, global developmental delay, headaches, and irritability.
Behavioural: Anorexia, pica (ingestion of odd materials with ↑d Fe^{2+}), irritability, impaired concentration, impaired progress at school.

EXAMINATION
General: Signs of anaemia (pallor of skin and mucous membranes, tachycardia) and systolic flow murmurs.
Rarely: Brittle nails and hair (↓epithelial cell iron), spoon-shaped nails (koilonychia), glossitis (atrophy of tongue papillae), angular stomatitis, mild hepatosplenomegaly and lymphadenopathy.

PATHOPHYSIOLOGY
Blood film: Microcytic, hypochromic (central pallor), anisocytosis (variable sizes), poikilocytosis (variable shapes).

INVESTIGATIONS
Bloods: ↓Hb, ↓serum ferritin, ↓serum Fe^{2+}, ↑TIBC, ↓haematocrit, ↓MCV.
Hb electrophoresis: Exclude β-thalassaemia trait or Sickle cell disease.
Bone marrow (only in complicated cases): Erythroid hyperplasia and ↓ bone marrow Fe^{2+} or total absence of iron.

MANAGEMENT
Preterm: Fortify breast milk with Fe^{2+}. Use Fe^{2+}-fortified milk formula.
Infants: ↑ Highly absorbable haem iron sources (meat, fish) and sources of non-haem iron (such as grains) in vegetarian families. Enhance non-haem iron absorption by eating vitamin C-rich foods at the same meal.
Oral $FeSO_4$: Maximum rise of Hb 0.25–0.4 g/dl/day.
Blood transfusion: Indicated with severe anaemia leading to CHF and cardiovascular compromise. Packed RBCs should be given slowly or partial exchange transfusion.

COMPLICATIONS   Possible impaired mental and psychomotor development. High output cardiac failure in severe cases.

PROGNOSIS   Good outcome if cause is nutritional or due to ↑d demand and prompt action is taken. If underlying GI cause, outcome dependent on underlying cause.

DEFINITION   Normocytic, normochromic, hyporegenerative anaemia in a preterm infant associated with a low serum erythropoietin (EPO) level.

AETIOLOGY

Inadequate RBC production 2° to low EPO: EPO initially produced by the fetal liver then the kidneys nearer to term. Liver EPO production stimulated with ↑d degree of anaemia and hypoxia than for the fetal kidney. With the premature neonate RBC production ↓d as liver still 1° source of EPO production.

Shortened fetal RBC lifespan: Fetal RBCs have 50–66% of the lifespan of an adult RBC. 2° to ↓d intracellular ATP, carnitine and enzyme activity combined with ↑d susceptibility to lipid peroxidation and fragmentation. At birth fetal haemoglobin represents 60–90% of haemoglobin. Adult levels of <5% by 3–6/12.

Blood loss: Intrapartum and aggravated by repeated blood sampling. A blood sampling can account for 10–15% of the total circulating volume.

Low iron stores: Combined with nutritional deficiencies of iron, vitamin E, vitamin B12 and folate may exaggerate the degree of anaemia.

Rarer pathological causes of anaemia in preterm infants

1. Haemolysis: 2° to ABO/Rh blood group incompatibility or haemoglobinopathies.
2. Bone marrow suppression: 2° to infection or renal failure.
3. Bone marrow failure: aplastic anaemia or malignancy.

ASSOCIATIONS/RELATED   Low birthweight, FHx. No association with sex/race.

EPIDEMIOLOGY   Frequency of anaemia of prematurity is inversely related to the gestational age and/or birthweight of the population. 50% of infants <32 weeks will develop symptoms secondary to this condition. Up to 80% of low-birthweight (<2.5 kg) infants require transfusions and 95% of extremely low birthweight (<1.25 kg).

HISTORY AND EXAMINATION   Symptoms and signs of anaemia in a preterm infant:

1. ↓d activity which is improved by transfusion.
2. Poor weight gain despite adequate calorie intake.
3. Tachypnoea, tachycardia, pallor and flow murmurs.
4. If severe, will result in respiratory depression; episodes of apnoea.

PATHOPHYSIOLOGY   See Aetiology.

INVESTIGATIONS

Bloods: Hb <10 g/dl, normochromic, normocytic; normal platelet count and white cell count.

Blood film: ↓Reticulocyte count (2° ↓ EPO), abnormal RBC forms (sickle cells, target cells in thalassaemia), red cell fragmentation (haemolysis).

Blood typing: ABO/Rh blood group incompatibility of neonate and mother.

MANAGEMENT

Indications for packed RBC transfusion:

1. Hb <8 g/dl.
2. Failure to thrive.
3. Cardiovascular/respiratory compromise.
4. Co-existing pathologies that may be exacerbated by anaemia.

Iron supplementation: May ↓ need for transfusion.

Recombinant EPO: Not advised (Cochrane review).

COMPLICATIONS   Transfusion-acquired infection, transfusion-associated fluid overload, electrolyte imbalances or haemolysis.

PROGNOSIS   Preterm infants are usually started on iron therapy for 2–3/12. Anaemia usually resolves spontaneously by 3–6/12, as adult haemoglobin is produced and intrinsic RBC/EPO production ↑s.

DEFINITION   Wide spectrum of congenital disorders affecting the distal anus and rectum as well as the urinary and genital tracts.

AETIOLOGY
General: Wide spectrum of defects. Exact aetiology unknown but close genetic association. All have absence of an anus in the normal position. *Mild forms*: bowel outlet via fistula in the perineal region separately from the normal sphincter complex. *Severe forms*: bowel outlet ectopically opens in the urogenital tract (males) and genital tract (females).
Classification (Wingspread): Traditional system. Relationship of the pouch to the levator muscle complex: either low, intermediate and high.
Classification (Krickenbeck): Recent international consensus. *Major group*: presence of fistula (perineal, rectourethral, prostatic, bulbar, rectovesical, vestibular) or no fistula and cloaca or anal stenosis. *Minor group*: pouch colon, rectal atresia/stenosis, rectovaginal fistula, H-fistula, others.

ASSOCIATIONS/RELATED   Associated anomalies >60%. Mulitianomaly syndromes: VACTERL, CHARGE, MURCS, OEIS. Trisomy 13, 18, 22. Hirschsprung's disease. Vertebral and sacral anomalies.

EPIDEMIOLOGY   1 in 5000 live births. M > F.

HISTORY AND EXAMINATION
General: Clinical examination by an experienced surgeon will reveal the type in >90%. The presence and position of fistula. Associated anomalies.
Specific (low lesions): Prominent midline skin bridge ('bucket-handle'), subepithelial midline raphe fistula ('chain of meconium pearls'), rectovestibular fistula, anal membrane. A flat perineum (absence of midline gluteal fold and anal dimple) may indicate absence of perineum muscle and therefore a high ARM.

PATHOPHYSIOLOGY   See Aetiology.

INVESTIGATIONS
General: Screening for associated anomalies: ECHO, CXR (NGT position/heart), RUSS, serum karotype, USS for hydrometrocolpos/spinal anomalies, sacral XR, MRI, urinalysis (?urinary tract association).
Specific: Prone cross-table lateral XR with the pelvis elevated and marker on the perineum (air column to marker <1 cm = treat as low lesion, >1 cm = colostomy), high-pressure distal colostography (distal stomal contrast to delineate distal rectum and urinary connection).

MANAGEMENT
Medical (neonatal): Resuscitation as appropriate. Associated anomalies screening, NGT, NBM, IVI, antibiotics, transfer to paediatric surgical centre. Often have 24 hours to stabilise as low obstruction. Clinically observation vital ?passage of meconium via fistula/urinary tract.
Surgical (neonatal): Ascertain provisional diagnosis of ARM level with surgical planning. *Severe*: primary diverting colostomy. *Low*: cutback anoplasty/limited PSARP. Large rectovestibular fistulas may be dilated.
Surgical (definite): Posterior sagittal anorectoplasty (PSARP) allows excellent visualisation. Colostomy closed separately. Laparoscopic-assisted approach also possible with mobilisation of the rectal pouch/ligation of fistula and delivery of the pouch to the perineum through a minimal posterior incision.
Postsurgical incontinence: Effective bowel management programme including enemas, laxatives and dietary manipulations.

COMPLICATIONS   Most common functional disorder post surgery is constipation. Possible urinary and faecal incontinence even with excellent anatomical repair 2° to poorly developed sacrum, spinal cord anomalies and deficient nerve supply.

PROGNOSIS   Generally good. Low ARM has fewer complications than high. Dependent on associated anomalies.

DEFINITION   Acute inflammation of the vermiform appendix.

AETIOLOGY   Obstruction of the appendiceal lumen, causing a cycle of progressive inflammation and bacterial overgrowth.

ASSOCIATIONS/RELATED   Poor dietary fibre intake: ↑s faecal viscosity, bowel transit time, and the formation of faecaliths.

EPIDEMIOLOGY   Most common cause of an acute abdomen in children. *Incidence*: 4/1000 children. Any age, most common >5 years of age, uncommon <2 years.

HISTORY   Large variation in clinical picture:

- Classically colicky pain starts periumbilically then localises to the right iliac fossa. Constant with peritoneal inflammation and ↑d with movement.
- Anorexia (vague abdominal pain and won't eat their favourite food).
- Vomiting (young children).
- Constipation or diarrhoea (less common).
- Low-grade pyrexia.

EXAMINATION
General: Tachycardia, pyrexia, reluctance to move.
Abdominal examination: Percussion tenderness signifies inflammation of the peritoneum. Guarding may be present in RIF (McBurney's point). Rovsing's sign (RIF pain reproduced with palpation in the LIF). There may also be pain on expansion and recession of the abdomen. Cough may exacerbate pain. Peritoneal irritation signs may be absent with a retrocaecal appendicitis.
Rectal examination: Should be performed by the most senior doctor only when diagnosis is in doubt. There is marked tenderness against anterior rectal wall, especially with a retrocaecal appendix.

PATHOPHYSIOLOGY   Obstruction of the lumen by impacted faeces or faecalith leads to mucosal inflammation. Inflammation extends into the submucosa to involve the muscular and serosal layers. Fibrinopurulent exudates from the serosal surface extend to the peritoneal surface causing localised peritonitis. The lumen subsequently becomes distended with pus and thrombosis of end-arteries leads to gangrene and perforation. Ineffective lymphatic and venous drainage allows bacterial invasion of the appendiceal wall.

INVESTIGATIONS
General: Appendicitis is a clinical diagnosis; investigations may aid diagnosis in difficult cases.
Bloods: ↑WCC (normal WCC doesn't exclude appendicitis), ↑CRP, U&Es (especially if vomiting), clotting (raised neutrophil count is the most sensitive serological investigation for appendicitis).
Urine: MC&S to exclude UTI, leucocytes may be present with an inflamed appendix against bladder wall (nitrite -ve).
Radiology: Plain AXR not indicated; if performed, may show dilated loops of bowel and a fluid level in the RIF. USS may show the inflamed appendix as a non-compressible tubular structure, presence of free fluid or appendiceal mass.

MANAGEMENT
Surgical: Once diagnosis confirmed clinically. May be performed via the traditional open approach (Lanz incision) or laparoscopically. Washout essential with complicated appendicitis.
Conservative: With a confirmed appendiceal abscess that responds to intravenous antibiotics. If this management fails then surgical intervention (+/− drain insertion) is indicated. If conservative management succeeds then the patient is offered an interval appendicectomy.

COMPLICATIONS

Perforation: <3 years old = 80–100%; >10 years old = 10–20%. Complicated appendicitis (perforated/presence of pus); wound infection/intra-abdominal abscess formation. ↓ fertility in girls after complicated appendicitis (ovarian/fallopian tube involvement), small bowel obstruction, adhesions.

PROGNOSIS   Usually excellent.

DEFINITION   Chronic inflammatory airways disease characterised by variable reversible airway obstruction, airway hyper-responsiveness and bronchial inflammation.

AETIOLOGY
Genetic factors: Positive family history of asthma or atopy.
Environmental triggers: Passive or active smoking, URTIs, exercise, cold weather, inhalant allergies (house dust mite/pollens/moulds/pets) and food allergens.

ASSOCIATIONS/RELATED   Eczema, allergic rhinitis, previous CLD of prematurity.
'Hygiene' hypothesis: Exposure to microbial products in infancy leads to switching off Th2 predisposition of T cells and increasing regulatory T cells to prevent an allergic predisposition.
DD in <2 years: Aspiration, pneumonia, tracheomalacia, CF, tracheo-oesophageal fistula (H-type), bronchiolitis.

EPIDEMIOLOGY
Prevalence: 10–15%. **Age:** 80% of asthmatic children are symptomatic by the age of 5. M: F, 2:1; equalises in adulthood. **Distribution:** Viral-associated wheeze/recurrent wheezy bronchitis ↑ in urban areas and in children of low socio-economic status families.

HISTORY
Age-related symptoms:

- **<1 year:** Persistent or recurrent nocturnal cough, wheezing with URTIs.
- **2–3 years:** Nocturnal cough, wheezing during exercise with URTIs.
- **<5 years:** Non-productive cough may be the only symptom, often worse at night and in the morning.

Assess severity: Frequency of attacks (mild: <1 attack in 2 months; moderate: >1 attack in 2 months; severe: persistent symptoms, ↓exercise tolerance), effect on school attendance, hospital attendances and admissions to PICU.

EXAMINATION
Respiratory: End-expiratory wheeze, recession, use of accessory muscles, tachypnoea, hyper-resonant percussion note, diminished air entry, hyperexpansion, Harrison sulcus (anterolateral depression of thorax at insertion of diaphragm).
Peak flow: Useful in >5 years of age; use as baseline (predicted best) and as determinant for efficacy of treatment.

BTS guidelines for assessment of acute asthma attack	
Severe asthma	**Life-threatening asthma**
Too breathless to speak or feed	Silent chest
Tachycardia:	Cyanosis
>120 bpm in 2–5 years	Poor respiratory effort
>130 bpm in <2 years	Hypotension
Tachypnoea:	Exhaustion
>30 breaths/min in 2–5 years	Confusion
>50 breaths/min in <2 years	Coma
Peak flow: <50% predicted >5 years	Peak flow: <33% predicted in >5 years

PATHOPHYSIOLOGY
Acute phase (within minutes): Contact with exacerbating factor (cigarette smoke, inhalant or food allergen or viral infection) leads to ↑ airway receptor hyper-responsiveness → narrowing of airways.
Late phase (onset after 2–4 hours, effect may last up to 3–6 months): Persistent bronchoconstriction 2° to vicious cycle of inflammation, oedema and excess mucous production.

INVESTIGATION

CXR: In acute severe cases to exclude pneumothorax or first presentation to exclude congenital anomaly.

Lung function (spirometry): Can be performed in >5 years. Obstructive airways disease: FEV1 <80%, FVC normal or reduced, FEV1/FVC <70%. Assess reversibility after 400 μg salbutamol inhalation.

MANAGEMENT

BTS guidelines 2008 for the management of acute asthma attack

- High-flow oxygen via reservoir bag.
- Salbutamol and ipratropium bromide via volumatic spacer or nebulised.
- Oral prednisolone 20 mg (2–5 years), 30–40 mg (>5 years) or IV hydrocortisone if unable to retain oral medication.
- Commence IV salbutamol (bolus then infusion) or aminophylline infusion.
- Magnesium sulphate (40 mg/kg) IV.
- If not responding (<92% O_2 saturations) or any life-threatening features present, discuss with PICU for ventilatory support.

Discharge criteria: Patients can be discharged when stable on 3–4-hourly inhaled bronchodilators. Peak flow 75% of predicted best, and O_2 saturations >94%.

Education: On adherence to medication, recognition of acute attacks, emergency protocol, maintaining normal activities.

BTS stepwise management of chronic asthma
Key principles:

1. Avoid obvious precipitants, e.g. passive smoking, allergen avoidance.
2. Ensure good inhaler technique +/− volumatic spacer.
3. Check compliance.
4. Review treatment every 3–6 months.
5. 'Rescue' prednisolone in acute deterioration.
6. If obese advise weight reduction.

When to start preventer inhaler:

1. Symptomatic/use β_2-agonist inhalers ≥3 times/week.
2. Waking one night/week.
3. Frequent exacerbations.

Children <5 years
Step 1, mild intermittent asthma: Short-acting β_2-agonist inhalers (e.g. salbutamol) as necessary.

Step 2, regular preventer control: Add low-dose inhaled steroid (200–400 μg/day budesonide equivalent) or leukotriene receptor antagonist if steroid cannot be used.

Step 3, add-on therapy: Trial of leukotriene receptor antagonist.

Step 4, persistent poor control: Refer to respiratory paediatrician.

Children 5–12 years
Step 1, mild intermittent asthma: Short-acting β_2-agonist inhalers as necessary.

Step 2, regular preventer control: Add low-dose inhaled steroid (200–400 μg/day).

Step 3, add-on therapy: Add LABA, e.g. salmeterol.

1. Good response: continue LABA.
2. Benefit from LABA but control still inadequate: ↑dose of inhaled steroids to 400 μg/day.

3. No response to LABA: stop LABA, ↑ dose of inhaled steroids to 400 μg/day, and add trial of oral theophylline (monitor plasma levels) or leukotriene receptor antagonist.

Step 4, persistent poor control: ↑ Dose of inhaled steroids to 800 μg/day.
Step 5, continuous or frequent use of oral steroids: Maintain ↑ dose of inhaled steroids. Add oral prednisolone at lowest dose to provide adequate control.
Refer to respiratory paediatrician.

COMPLICATIONS Decreased linear growth rate due to poorly controlled asthma more usual than from overprescription of inhaled steroids, chest wall deformity, recurrent infections, status asthmaticus can be fatal. One-third of deaths occur under the age of 5 years.

PROGNOSIS Asthma often remits during puberty and many children are symptom free as adults, especially those who have mild asthma and are asymptomatic between attacks, or who develop asthma at >6 years. Rates of admission and mortality in asthma have ↓ since the early 1990s.

DEFINITION Chronic inflammatory itchy skin condition. Also known as atopic dermatitis.

AETIOLOGY Parental atopy. Dysfunction in the epidermal barrier protein filaggrin (due to genetic loss of function mutations) has recently been shown to be a major predisposing factor.

ASSOCIATIONS/RELATED Eczema can be triggered by environmental factors including irritants (soaps and detergents), infections, contact with food or inhalant allergens.

EPIDEMIOLOGY Affects 15–20% of UK children; 2–3-fold increase in the last three decades.

HISTORY The majority of eczema begins in the first year of life. Intense itchy skin and chronic relapsing inflammation of the skin are cardinal features.

EXAMINATION Infantile eczema affects the face and extensor surfaces and spares the nappy area. Flexural involvement predominates in older children. In eczema herpeticum there are small uniform circular 'punched-out erosions'.

PATHOPHYSIOLOGY Acute phase is characterised by intercellular epidermal oedema (spongiosis) and leukocyte infiltration. In the chronic phase there is thickening of the epidermis, stratum corneum and dysfunction of keratinisation.

INVESTIGATIONS Infants with moderate to severe eczema with a history of immediate reaction to food warrant skin prick testing to common food allergens. Patch testing of foods in eczema produces conflicting data but in contact dermatitis it is well established.

MANAGEMENT Assess eczema severity and quality of life, including everyday activities and sleep, and psychosocial well-being. Identify and manage any trigger factors. Give advice on prompt recognition and treatment of infection (in particular eczema herpeticum) and provide a written eczema management plan.
Emollients: 'Total emollient care' includes liberal application of creams and ointments, using a soap substitute and bath oil.
Topical corticosteroids: Use a stepwise approach to topical steroids depending on the severity of eczema. Use mild steroids for the face. In children with recurrent flares, use a topical steroid for 2 consecutive days/week.
Topical calcineurin inhibitors: Can be used as second-line treatment of moderate to severe atopic eczema in children ≥2 years that is not controlled by topical corticosteroids, or where there are adverse effects to topical steroids.
Wet wraps: May be particularly effective for troublesome areas (feet/hands). Not to be used over infected skin, topical potent steroids or calcineurin inhibitors.
Dietary manipulation: In bottle-fed infants <6 months with moderate to severe eczema not controlled by optimal treatment, 6–8-week trial of an extensively hydrolysed or amino acid formula in place of cow's milk formula.
Antihistamine: If children suffer from severe itching, trial a non-sedating antihistamine.

COMPLICATIONS Skin infections leading to cellulitis. Residual pigmentation, lichenification or skin atrophy related to long-term potent steroid use. Poor quality of life for the child and parent. Psychosocial issues.

PROGNOSIS Sixty to 70% of UK children with eczema at 7 years clear their eczema as teenagers, but may go on to develop asthma or allergic rhinitis (the 'allergic march').

DEFINITION   Acyanotic congenital heart condition characterised by malformation in the atrial or atrioventricular septum.

AETIOLOGY

Secundum ASD: Patent foramen ovale (abnormal resorption of the septum primum during formation of foramen secundum).

Primum ASD/Partial AVSD: Defect in lower atrial septum, 2° to incomplete fusion of septum primum with the endocardial cushion. Immediately adjacent to the atrioventricular valves.

Sinus venosus ASD: Defect high in the atrial septum near the entry of the SVC (abnormal fusion between the embryological sinus venosus and the atrium).

Coronary sinus defect: Unroofed coronary sinus and persistent left SVC that drains into the left atrium.

Complete AVSD: Large central defect due to ASD and VSD with single large atrioventricular valve.

ASSOCIATIONS/RELATED   Wide variety of chromosomal and genetic disorders and syndromes. Trisomy 21 ~50%.

EPIDEMIOLOGY   4/100,000 live births.

HISTORY   Depends on defect size and degree of mitral regurgitation. May take decades to manifest symptoms (PHT, atrial tachyarrhythmias, mitral valve disease). Childhood diagnosis often after routine examination reveals a murmur. Large defects: recurrent respiratory infections, symptoms of congestive heart failure, dyspnoea, palpitations (older children), failure to thrive.

EXAMINATION

ASD: Left to right shunt (pink +/–breathless): Murmurs are due to ↑d flow across valves, not the ASD itself. Ejection systolic murmur (pulmonary valves). Mid-diastolic murmur (tricuspid valve). Fixed splitting of the second heart sound 2° to ↑d volume causing prolonged contraction time of the RV.

ASVD: Mixed shunt (blue and breathless): Atrial and ventricular components therefore PHT present as with a large VSD. May present with cyanosis at birth, a murmur in the first few weeks or signs of CHD at 1–2/12.

PATHOPHYSIOLOGY   See Aetiology.

INVESTIGATIONS

CXR: RAH, RVH, prominent PA and ↑d pulmonary vascular markings.

ECG: Right axis deviation, first-degree heart block, right bundle branch block, RAH and RVH.

Doppler + Echo: For diagnostic, assessment of size and congestive heart failure features.

MANAGEMENT

Supportive management: Antibiotic prophylaxis for dental surgery and other minor procedures. Medical treatment of associated CHF.

Surgical management: Closed to prevent RVH and arrhythmias. Repair of associated anomalies (e.g. PDA) under same GA. Elective repair at 2–5 years unless significant MR indicates earlier closure.

ASD/partial AVSD: Direct closure of the defect via an open median sternotomy with extracorporeal support. Use of autologous pericardium or synthetic patches made of polyester polymer (Dacron) or polytetrafluoroethylene (PTFE). Percutaneous transcatheter closure via femoral venous approach is also possible.

Complete AVSD: 3–5/12; requires treatment of pulmonary vascular resistance if present at birth.

COMPLICATIONS   Infective endocarditis, congestive heart failure, atrial fibrillation, pulmonary hypertension.

PROGNOSIS   95% remain open, 5% close spontaneously. Only large defects cause significant morbidity due to complications.

DEFINITION   Disorder characterised by attention deficit, hyperactivity and impulsiveness for $\geq$6 months which causes moderate psychological, social and/or educational impairment in $\geq$2 important settings (home, school, peers).

AETIOLOGY
Genetic factors: Twin studies 81–67% concordance; first-degree relatives 50% concordance.
Environmental factors: Intrauterine complications, maternal smoking, alcohol and drug abuse during pregnancy.

ASSOCIATIONS/RELATED   Depression, anxiety, addictive, obsessional and behavioural disorders (conduct disorder), learning difficulties including receptive and expressive language problems, tic disorders and Tourette syndrome.

EPIDEMIOLOGY   ~9% school-age children affected (DSM-IV). M:F = 4:1. Onset <7 years.

HISTORY AND EXAMINATION
Attention deficit: Inability to sustain mental effort, listen, organise or finish tasks.
Hyperactivity: Fidgeting, running, climbing or talking excessively.
Impulsiveness: Inability to wait their turn, intruding or interrupting others. Some children are predominantly hyperactive and impulsive, while others are principally inattentive.

PATHOPHYSIOLOGY   PET scan studies suggest abnormality is of ascending projections of catecholaminergic and serotonergic neurons into the frontal cortex.

INVESTIGATION   It is important to evaluate each child comprehensively and take a full developmental, educational and behavioural history. Rating scales such as the Conners Rating Scales and the Strengths and Difficulties Questionnaire (parent, teacher, child) are valuable adjuncts. Exclude medical conditions such as impaired vision and hearing or, less commonly, epilepsy (absence seizures) or hypothyroidism. ECG is warranted prior to starting central nerve stimulants if there is past medical or family history of serious cardiac disease/sudden death or abnormal findings on cardiac examination.

MANAGEMENT
Involvement of health and education: GPs, community paediatricians, educational psychologists, SENCO (special educational needs co-ordinator), social workers, CAMHS.
Child (individual) therapy: Behaviour modification programmes (home, school), CBT, training in social skills, psychotherapy to improve self-esteem.
Parent training/education programme: Parental positive reinforcement of desired behaviour and appropriate negative feedback for unacceptable behaviour.

Drug therapy
Drug treatment should always form part of a comprehensive treatment plan that includes psychological, behavioural and educational advice and interventions.

- *Methylphenidate, dexamfetamine (>6 years)*: CNS stimulant which increases arousal in areas of inactivation, thereby improving attention span and reducing impulsivity and hyperactivity. S/E: insomnia, nervousness, headache, ↓d appetite, abdominal pain, exacerbation of tics, cardiovascular effects such as tachycardia, palpitations and minor increases in BP. Weight, height and BP should be monitored every 6 months.
- *Atomoxetine (>6 years)*: Selective noradrenaline reuptake inhibitor; second-line therapy. S/E: abdominal pain, ↓ appetite, nausea and vomiting, liver damage (rare), early morning awakening, irritability, mood swings, suicidal ideation, CVS effects, dysmenorrhoea.

COMPLICATIONS   ADHD often negatively affects a person's educational achievements. This can contribute to economic, social and life adjustment problems throughout a person's life and lead to substance abuse and crime.

PROGNOSIS   Hyperactivity symptoms may improve with maturation and development of self-control. Children with appropriate educational input, support and good compliance with treatment have the best prognosis.

DEFINITION Developmental disorder affecting social interaction, social communication, rigidity of thinking and difficulties with social imagination. Autistic spectrum disorder (ASD) is an umbrella term that ranges from classic autism (severe childhood onset) to Asperger syndrome (milder social impairment with preservation of language development).

AETIOLOGY Genetic factors: 80% concordance in monozygotic twins. RF: maternal rubella infection, ↑paternal age. A link with the MMR vaccine has been proven to not exist.

ASSOCIATIONS/RELATED TS, fragile X syndrome. Epilepsy may be present in 25%.

EPIDEMIOLOGY National Autistic Society (NAS) UK prevalence: 535,000 (2006). ASD is increasing in prevalence.

HISTORY AND EXAMINATION
Motor: Stereotypical and repetitive motor mannerisms (hand flapping, body twirling), clumsy and unco-ordinated movements.
Behavioural: Repetitive activities, ritualistic behaviour, the disruption of which → violent temper tantrums, particular interests/obsessions.
Social: Indifference to others, avoiding eye contact, preferring to be alone, limited facial expressions and understanding of others' gestures, lack of understanding of social rules (e.g. turn taking), attachments to unusual objects, no danger awareness.
Speech: Delayed speech and language development, echolalia, poor comprehension and expression, abnormalities in vocal pitch or rhythm, socially inappropriate comments.
Learning disability: Varies with severity of autistic spectrum.
Other: Sensory abnormalities, difficulty with sleeping, eating, toileting, fears/phobias.

PATHOPHYSIOLOGY Normal children learn social habits without being consciously aware of them. It is these instinctive relations that are disturbed in autistic children. 'They have to learn everything via the intellect' (Hans Asperger).

INVESTIGATIONS
Diagnostic assessments:

1. Strength and Difficulties Questionnaires: parent/teacher and child.
2. School reports/observation in class.

Bloods: Chromosomes for fragile X, FBC, ferritin, thyroid function, lead.
Others: Developmental assessment, EEG (if presenting with fits/funny turns).
Multidisciplinary approach: Should be initiated as early as possible. *Behavioural interventions*: NAS EarlyBird programmes employ the SPELL (Structure, Positive (approaches and expectations), Empathy, Low arousal (calm environment), Links (child, parent and teachers)) and TEACCH (Treatment and Education of Autistic and related Communication handicapped Children) approaches. Other private interventions include Applied Behavioural Analysis and the Son-Rise programme. *Communication support*: SALT work on listening and attention skills, play, social skill and understanding; they may use picture exchange communication system (PECS) or Makaton signing in children with severe language impairment. *Educational support*: portage (preschool children) at home. School-age children may access mainstream school with support (liaison with special educational needs co-ordinator (SENCO)) or special needs school (statement of special educational needs). *Parental support*: charities (NAS, Aspergers UK, Autism UK, Contact A Family), parent partnership services (educational advice), Disability Living Allowance (DLA).

COMPLICATIONS
Physical abuse: Frustrated parents or annoyed social contacts.
Psychological/emotional: May result in aggressive or self-injurious behaviour.

PROGNOSIS Varies with degree of speech development, learning disability and severity of ASD. Adults with severe autism usually live with their parents or require care in special communities. However, many can attend higher education, be employed successfully and lead independent lives.

DEFINITION   A developmental condition in which the child experiences a brief episode of apnoea.

AETIOLOGY
Pallid (or white) breath-holding attacks: Abnormally sensitive response to carotid sinus or ocular compression with the production of temporary asystole or marked bradycardia.
Cyanotic (or blue) breath-holding attacks: Mechanism unclear; however, includes centrally mediated reduced respiratory effort and altered lung mechanics, which may inappropriately stimulate pulmonary reflexes, thus resulting in apnoea and hypoxia.

ASSOCIATIONS/RELATED   25% of children have a positive family history of breath-holding attacks.

EPIDEMIOLOGY   Occurs in 1–2% of children between the ages of 6 months and 5 years, 75% of which occur between 6 and 18 months. M = F. Breath-holding spells usually occur from 1–2×/day to 1–2×/month. 60% have cyanotic type, 20% pallid type and 20% a combination.

HISTORY

Pallid breath-holding attack

Triggered by fear or a painful stimulus such as a knock to the head or falling

↓

Child stops breathing and rapidly loses consciousness

↓

Child becomes pale and hypotonic

↓

May experience a tonic seizure as a result of cerebral underperfusion (reflex anoxic seizure)

Cyanotic breath-holding attack

Triggered by anger, frustration, upsetting event or scolding

↓

Child cries and subsequently holds breath in expiration

↓

Rapid onset of cyanosis that may progress to loss of consciousness

↓

Brief tonic-clonic jerks, opisthotonos (rigidity and arching of the back, with head thrown backwards)

↓

Bradycardia may follow

Attacks last less than a minute. There is usually full resumption of normal activity within minutes. Some children may remain lethargic and drowsy for some time after an attack.

EXAMINATION   Neurological examination to exclude focal signs suggestive of an underlying structural abnormality if unusual features in history.

PATHOPHYSIOLOGY   Involuntary reflex response to a shock, which causes overactivity of the autonomic nervous system that controls breathing and HR.

INVESTIGATIONS   Not usually required.
EEG: Shows generalised slow waves with flattening during the attack (a pattern characteristic of cerebral hypoxia). *Interictally* the EEG is normal.
ECG: If cardiac arrhythmia is suspected.

MANAGEMENT

Parental education: Reassurance and emphasis on consistency and not reinforcing the child's behaviour pattern after the attack. Child should lie flat during attack to ↑ cerebral perfusion. Atropine sulphate may be considered in refractory pallid attacks to block the vagus nerve.

COMPLICATIONS   No immediate complications except if the child collapses in an unsafe environment.

PROGNOSIS   Children usually stop having the attacks after the age of 5 or 6 years. Children who have pallid attacks have an ↑ incidence of syncope in adulthood. There is no ↑ incidence of epilepsy in either type.

DEFINITION   Respiratory condition characterised by coryza followed by a 'bronchiolitic' dry, wheezy cough, breathlessness, poor feeding, hyperinflation of the chest and expiratory wheeze in infants.

AETIOLOGY   RSV (75%); there may be multiple causative agents (rhinovirus, parainfluenza, influenza or adenovirus).

ASSOCIATIONS/RELATED

RF severe disease: Prematurity +/− chronic lung disease (CLD), congenital/acquired lung disease, congenital heart defects (CHD) and immunodeficiency. Breastfeeding and parental avoidance of smoking are protective.

EPIDEMIOLOGY   Most common LRTI in infants, especially 3–6 months. Winter epidemics: ≤3% infants are admitted to hospital.

HISTORY   Cough, breathlessness and wheeze. In more severe cases infants may become too breathless to feed, have apnoeic spells or become lethargic.

EXAMINATION
General: Mild pyrexia, tachycardia, irritability.
Respiratory distress: Tachypnoea, subcostal/intercostal recession, nasal flaring, grunting, widespread expiratory wheeze +/− fine crepitations.
Severe disease: Cyanosis, lethargy.

PATHOPHYSIOLOGY
Micro: Inflammation of the bronchioles with secretion of mucus, necrosis of ciliated epithelium, and oedema of the submucosa causing airway obstruction.

INVESTIGATIONS
Bloods: Not indicated in mild disease. May find ↑WCC, ↓Na (2° to SIADH), capillary gas (↓pO$_2$ and ↑pCO$_2$ if child is becoming exhausted).
CXR: Not indicated in mild disease; will show hyperinflation due to small airways obstruction and air trapping. Collapse (classically of the right upper lobe) and/or consolidation in secondary bacterial infection may also be seen.
Serology: RSV may be identified by immunofluorescent staining of nasopharyngeal aspirations (NPA) using specific viral antisera.

MANAGEMENT
Criteria for admission: Feeding difficulty (<50% usual amount), grunting, severe recession and/or tachypnoea, episodes of apnoea, saturations <95%, lethargy.
Infants with underlying chronic conditions, ex-premature or infants <3 months require a low threshold for admission. Consider social issues.
Supportive management: O$_2$ via nasal cannula or headbox to keep saturations >94%, 2/3 maintenance feeding via NG tube, or use IV fluids if infant is in severe respiratory distress. Physiotherapy is not indicated; rather minimal handling.
Active treatment: Bronchodilators may have only short-term benefit. Steroids are not indicated and do not prevent post-bronchiolitic wheeze. Nebulised ribavirin does not improve outcome; it is also teratogenic and may be harmful to pregnant mothers or staff.
Criteria for ventilation: Saturations <92% despite increasing oxygen therapy, signs of exhaustion, recurrent apnoeas, signs of cerebral hypoxia (drowsy/unrousable).
Prevention: Palivizumab (RSV monoclonal antibody prophylaxis) over the winter period prevents hospital admission for some infants but does not decrease length of stay or oxygen requirement. It should be considered in infants with congenital or acquired lung disease, extreme prematurity, CHD or immunodeficiency.

COMPLICATIONS Mortality 0.2%, intensive care unit admission 2.7% and need for ventilatory assistance 1.5%. Cardiac failure may occur, predominantly in infants with underlying CHD.

PROGNOSIS Difficulty breathing, wheeze and poor feeding: 6–7 days, cough: 12 days. Diarrhoea may complicate the recovery phase. Persistent cough and recurrent viral-induced wheeze recur in 20% of infants (up to 60% of infants hospitalised). Recurrent wheeze is more common in the first 5 years after RSV bronchiolitis, but there is conflicting evidence as to whether RSV bronchiolitis predisposes to asthma.

DEFINITION   Bleeds inside the extradural, subdural or subarachnoid space.

AETIOLOGY
Extradural: Direct head trauma causing arterial or venous bleeding.
Subdural: Birth trauma, forceps delivery, low-birth weight infants, high falls and non-accidental injury (NAI) caused by shaking.
Subarachnoid: Ruptured berry aneurysm or arteriovenous malformation.

ASSOCIATIONS/RELATED   May be exacerbated by coagulopathy.

EPIDEMIOLOGY
Extradural: In children 50% occur <2 years. M:F = 4:1.
Subdural: Occur mainly in young infants.
Subarachnoid: Rare in children.

HISTORY AND EXAMINATION   All intracranial haemorrhage may develop symptoms and signs of raised ICP as in all cases there is accumulation of blood within a closed cavity.
Early signs ↑ICP: Nausea, vomiting, confusion, drowsiness.
Late signs ↑ICP: Cushing response (↑BP, ↓HR), ipsilateral third nerve palsy, papilloedema, coma.
Extradural: History of trauma, force and site of impact, severe headache, boggy haematoma.
Acute subdural: Shock, seizures and coma, retinal haemorrhages.
Chronic subdural: Macrocephaly, failure to thrive, developmental delay.
Subarachnoid: Sudden-onset occipital headache, retinal haemorrhages, neck stiffness, fever, seizures and progression to coma.

PATHOPHYSIOLOGY
Extradural: Trauma affecting the middle meningeal artery over the temporal bone
Subdural: Tearing of the veins between the arachnoid and pia mater can give rise to chronic subdural. Acute subdural haemorrhage may occur in neonates by rupture of the vein of Galen.
Subarachnoid: Saccular or berry aneurysms arise because of haemodynamic stress in intracranial arteries that are susceptible (e.g. Ehlers–Danlos syndrome, Marfan syndrome).

INVESTIGATIONS
Bloods: FBC, clotting screen.
Skull X-ray: May show fracture, particularly over temporal bone region. Not usually indicated as CT is preferable mode of imaging.
CT: Best modality for detecting blood in the extradural/subdural space or CSF.
Indications for CT scan following head injury in children:

1. Witnessed loss of consciousness or amnesia (antegrade or retrograde) lasting >5 min
2. Abnormal drowsiness: paediatric GCS <15 in <1 year or <14 in >1 year in emergency department
3. ≥3 discrete episodes of vomiting
4. Clinical suspicion of non-accidental injury
5. Post-traumatic seizure but no history of epilepsy
6. Suspicion of open or depressed skull injury or tense fontanelle
7. Signs of basal skull fracture (haemotympanum, 'panda' eyes, cerebrospinal fluid leakage from ears or nose, Battle's sign)
8. Focal neurological deficit
9. Age <1 year: presence of bruise, swelling or laceration >5 cm on the head
10. Dangerous mechanism of injury

Lumbar puncture: Xanthochromia (subarachnoid).
Angiography: May show aneurysms or AV malformations in subarachnoid haemorrhage.

MANAGEMENT

Cervical spine immobilisation: If traumatic mechanism of head injury.

Supportive care: Ventilatory support and blood transfusions if shocked.

Treatment of ↑ICP: 30% head of bed elevation, mannitol, hypertonic saline.

Extradural: Surgical evacuation of haematoma and coagulation of bleeding sites.

Subdural: Surgical evacuation of haematoma.

Subarachnoid: Surgical correction of AV malformation or radiological clipping of aneurysm.

COMPLICATIONS   Hydrocephalus, uncal/central herniation 2° to ↑ICP, cerebral ischaemia, vasospasm and rebleeds in subarachnoid haemorrhages.

PROGNOSIS

Extradural: Good with early intervention. GCS prior to surgery correlates well with mortality and neurological sequelae.

Chronic subdural: Depends on the cause and associated brain injury. 3% mortality rate. At follow-up 75% have normal development.

Acute subdural and subarachnoid: >60% mortality.

DEFINITION Non-progressive disorder of movement and posture.

AETIOLOGY
Antenatal (80%): Cerebral dysgenesis/malformation, congenital infections (rubella, toxoplasmosis, CMV).
Perinatal (10%): Hypoxic ischaemic encephalopathy, birth trauma.
Postnatal (10%): Meningitis, encephalitis, extradural haemorrhage, IVH, head injury, NAI, hyperbilirubinaemia (kernicterus), prolonged hypoglycaemia.

ASSOCIATIONS/RELATED
Associated: Epilepsy, learning difficulties, visual impairment, squints, hearing loss, behavioural disorders.
Risk factors: Preterm delivery, low birthweight.

EPIDEMIOLOGY 2/1000 live births. Usually presents in infancy.

HISTORY AND EXAMINATION
General: Delayed milestones (see Global Developmental Delay chapter), poor feeding, abnormalities of tone, posture, gait, difficulties with language, impaired social skills.

Clinical types
Spastic (70%): Affected limbs show ↑ tone (clasp-knife), brisk reflexes, extensor plantar responses:

* *Hemiplegia:* unilateral, arm > leg, fisting and early hand preference < 1 year, characteristic posture of abduction of shoulder, flexion at elbow and wrist, pronation of forearm, and extension of fingers
* *Diplegia:* legs > arms, hypertonicity of hip adductors → leg 'scissoring'
* *Quadriplegia:* all 4 limbs affected – arms > legs, poor head control, paucity of movement. Abnormal primitive reflexes and fisting in the first few months.

Dyskinetic (10%): Normal progress until 6–9 months, followed by progressive dystonia of lower limbs, trunk, and mouth exaggerated by involuntary movements; athetoid (writhing) and choreographic movements (jerking).
Ataxic (10%): Hypotonia, ataxia of trunk and limbs, postural imbalance, intention tremor.
Mixed (10%).

PATHOPHYSIOLOGY
Spastic:

* *Hemiplegia:* damage to middle cerebral artery territory
* *Diplegia:* IVH, ventricular dilation or periventricular lesion
* *Quadriplegia:* widespread bilateral cerebral lesions.

Dyskinetic: Abnormality of extrapyramidal pathways (basal ganglia, thalamus).
Ataxic: Abnormal development of cerebellum.

INVESTIGATIONS Assessment of hearing and vision. EEG if seizure prone.

MANAGEMENT
Multidisciplinary approach. *Education:* mainstream school with additional support (liaison with special educational needs co-ordinator (SENCO)) or placement at a special needs school (requires statement of special educational needs). *Physiotherapy:* early to maintain full ROM, function, normal development and prevent contractures. *Occupational therapy:* splints, crutches, walking frames, wheelchairs. *SALT:* including control of drooling (oral training). *Feeding:* may be unable to suck, chew or swallow, therefore requiring gastrostomy feeds. *Orthopaedic:* surgery to correct deformity and improve function. *Neurosurgical intervention:* may be considered for reducing muscle spasticity or for disabling dystonic movements. *Medical:* baclofen or botulinum toxin injections to relieve spasticity. *Genetic counselling.*

COMPLICATIONS   Aspiration pneumonia, failure to thrive, scoliosis, dislocated hips.

PROGNOSIS
Spastic hemiplegia: Delayed but eventually normal gait.
Spastic diplegia: Characteristic gait (knees flexed, toe walking, and adducted hips).
Spastic quadriplegia: Poor prognosis related to feeding disability and immobility. Sufferers are often totally dependent and life expectancy is significantly reduced. Usually die from chest infections 2° to muscular weakness and poor chest dynamics 2° to kyphoscoliosis.
Dyskinetic: Usually unable to walk independently, quality of life can often be poor.
Ataxic: Most children walk (though often delayed) with the aid of crutches.

DEFINITION   Oxygen requirement at corrected age of term with characteristic radiological changes (also known as bronchopulmonary dysplasia).

AETIOLOGY
Multifactorial in pathology:

1. Volutrauma and barotraumas 2° to positive pressure ventilation (PPV)
2. High inspired oxygen concentration (>40%); toxic to the immature lung
3. Activation of inflammatory mediators (2° to free radicals, barotraumas and infection)
4. Inadequate nutritional supplementation.

ASSOCIATIONS/RELATED   Respiratory distress syndrome (RDS).

EPIDEMIOLOGY   Inversely related to gestation and birthweight. ↑d incidence 2° to ↑d survival of very low-birthweight infants.

HISTORY AND EXAMINATION   Most properly managed neonates are asymptomatic as they are given ventilatory support, but some CLD babies may have some chronic recession. Poor weight gain with ↑d energy intake.

PATHOPHYSIOLOGY
Theory of oxygen-mediated lung injury: Results from the generation of superoxides, hydrogen peroxide and oxygen free radicals which disrupt membrane lipids.
Histopathology: Interstitial oedema, mucosal metaplasia, interstitial fibrosis, overdistended alveoli.

INVESTIGATIONS
ABG: Compensated respiratory acidosis reflecting chronic high pCO_2.
CXR: Characteristic hyperinflation and cystic changes. Used to determine severity, and distinguishes CLD from atelectasis, pneumonia and air-leak syndrome.

MANAGEMENT
General: Factors such as PPV and oxygen therapy that cause bronchopulmonary dysplasia are necessary for survival in preterm infants; therefore management is primarily about minimisation of risk.
Ventilation: Oxygen toxicity, barotraumas and volutrauma can be minimised by strict monitoring and maintenance of pH, pCO_2 and pO_2 within small ranges dependent on age of preterm infant. There is no evidence that high-frequency ventilation is superior to conventional in prevention (Cochrane database).
Nutritional support: Early parenteral nutrition. Maximisation of the nutritional intake prevents further lung injury and aids tissue repair.
Prevention:

1. Surfactant within 2 hours with early extubation to nasal CPAP for the treatment of RDS ↓s incidence of CLD.
2. Use of steroids to prevent CLD is highly controversial as it has been shown to have an adverse affect on neurodevelopmental outcome. Steroids are generally only used in ventilator-dependent neonates who are 'stuck' on the ventilator.

Long-term: Home O_2 supported by community children's nurses; 'hospital at home' team.

COMPLICATIONS   Pulmonary hypertension → cor pulmonale, ↑ risk of respiratory infections especially RSV pneumonia (paliviazumab, monoclonal antibody prophylaxis for RSV, is currently being considered by NICE).

PROGNOSIS   Severely affected infants may require long-term home O_2 therapy.

DEFINITION   Congenital malformation, resulting in clefts that involve the lip, hard palate and the soft palate; may be unilateral or bilateral.

AETIOLOGY
CL: Results from failure of fusion of the frontonasal and maxillary processes.
CLP: Partial or total failure of fusion of the palatal shelves.

ASSOCIATIONS/RELATED   Strong genetic element. Associated with 400 syndromes especially trisomy 21. May be associated with other congenital mid-line anomalies. Suggested link with maternal smoking.

EPIDEMIOLOGY   1/1000 live births; most common congenital malformation. 20% are an isolated CL, 50% are both CL and CLP, and 30% isolated CLP.

HISTORY
At birth: Overt clefts of the hard +/− soft palate.
Postnatal:

1. *Feeding difficulties*: suckling may be compromised by the loss of an oral seal
2. *Airway difficulties*: prolapse of the tongue through the cleft into the nasal cavity, especially if associated with mandibular hypoplasia (Pierre Robin sequence).
3. *Nasal reflux of liquid or food*: in partial clefts of the soft palate
4. *Hypernasal speech or nasal emission*: may be detected later, especially in submucosal clefts.

EXAMINATION   The palate should be palpated posteriorly to exclude a posterior cleft palate and to detect an indentation of the posterior palate from a submucous cleft (postnatal baby check examination).

PATHOPHYSIOLOGY
CL: A narrow opening or gap in the skin of the upper lip, all the way to the base of the nose.
CLP: Caused by defective growth of the palatal shelves, failure of the shelves to obtain a horizontal position, lack of contact between the shelves or a postfusion rupture of the shelves. The CLP may take 2 forms: V-shape (most common in isolated) or U-shape (Pierre Robin sequence/syndromic clefts).

INVESTIGATIONS
Antenatal ultrasonography: CL diagnosed by 18–22/40 as fetal positioning is optimal after 17/40. CLP is rarely diagnosed with USS. Screening postnatally for associated anomalies.

MANAGEMENT
Multidisciplinary approach: Plastic and ENT surgeons, dentists, speech therapist, audiologists, nutritionists, specialist children's nurses and social workers.
Advice: Slower feeding, positioning the nipple along the non-cleft side and towards the back of the mouth in breastfeeding, use of cleft palate feeders, semi-upright positioning, and regular monitoring for signs of inadequate feeding or dehydration.
Surgical correction: Should occur <1 year to facilitate normal speech and language development. Various surgical techniques:

1. one-stage closure: closure of both the hard and soft palates aged 11/12
2. two-stage closure: soft palate closure aged 3/12 and hard palate aged 18/12

If there is delay in repair due to co-existing problems such as cardiac defects, repair will involve a pharyngeal flap.

COMPLICATIONS   Susceptibility to colds, hearing loss, speech defects, dental problems and otitis media.

PROGNOSIS   Good prognosis with surgical repair; for large defects, speech may still be slightly defective.

DEFINITION   Narrowing of the lumen of the aorta that produces an obstruction to flow. Defined by its relation to the ductus arteriosus (ligamentum arteriosum after regression); preductal, ductal or postductal.

AETIOLOGY   Failure of normal development of the left fourth and sixth aortic arches (5 and 6/40). Two possible theories: ductus tissue and the haemodynamic theory.

ASSOCIATIONS/RELATED   Turner syndrome, congenital rubella, VSD, PDA, hypoplastic left heart, interruption of the aortic arch (severe form of coarctation with no connection between the proximal and distal aorta).

EPIDEMIOLOGY   1/10,000, M:F $= 1.5 : 1$. Caucasians vs. Asians $= 7:1$.

HISTORY
Neonatal: Ductus arteriosus closes in the second or third week of life $\rightarrow$ sudden overflow of blood into the left ventricle which causes LVF (dyspnoea, lethargy, feeding difficulties and failure to thrive).
Infancy: Symptoms depend on the severity of stenosis and the development of collateral circulation. Preductal COA = good collateral circulation; postductal COA = variable collateral circulation.
Childhood $\rightarrow$ adulthood: Patients with good collateral circulations may be asymptomatic until childhood, adolescence or adulthood.

EXAMINATION   Nodding-type head movements accompanying each heart beat, delayed or absent femoral pulse, difference in blood pressure between upper and lower limbs (SBP >20 mmHg), loud S1 and narrow split S2, collateral flow and coarctation murmur.

PATHOPHYSIOLOGY   Collateral circulation connecting proximal and distal aspects of the aorta develops from the subclavian, scapular, internal thoracic and intercostal arteries. ↓BP and flow in the arteries distal to the constriction (lower body and legs) and ↑BP in proximal arteries (upper body and arms) = difference in BP readings. *Histology:* localised medial thickening with some infolding of the medial and superimposed neointimal tissue. Localised constriction either shelf-like structure with an eccentric opening or a membrane with a central or eccentric opening.

INVESTIGATIONS
CXR: Cardiomegaly with increased pulmonary vascular markings (LVF), a hypoplastic aortic knob with dilated poststenotic segment of the aorta.
ECG: Left ventricular hypertrophy in older children.
Doppler echocardiogram: Diagnostic and demonstrates pressure gradient.

MANAGEMENT
Medical (neonates): Infusion of prostaglandin E1 may cause the ductus arteriosus to reopen and palliate symptoms of LVF preoperatively along with fluid, sodium restriction with diuretics.
Surgical: Resection of ductal tissue with end-to-end anastomosis or subclavian artery flap repair. 5–10% incidence of re-coarctation after surgery.
Balloon angioplasty: Alternative to surgery with localised coarctation or for re-coarctation following surgery/older children. Concerns over aneurysm formation and other arterial complications. Can be combined with a stent placement.

COMPLICATIONS
Hypertension 2° to activated renin-angiotensin system: May cause aortic dissection/ rupture, subarachnoid haemorrhage from ruptured berry aneurysm and coronary artery disease.

PROGNOSIS   Untreated coarctations may survive until 35 years old although <20% survive >50 years old. Early childhood correction; 20-year survival rate is 91%. Follow-up with recurrence monitoring.

DEFINITION   A lifelong gluten-induced enteropathy of the proximal small bowel resulting in malabsorption, which remits completely on gluten withdrawal.

AETIOLOGY   Permanent sensitivity to the α-gliadin component of the cereal protein gluten. The immunological reaction in the small intestine results in mucosal damage and loss of villi.

ASSOCIATIONS/RELATED   UK prevalence in first-degree relatives is 5.6–22.5%. 95% of individuals are HLA DQ2 or DQ8 positive.

EPIDEMIOLOGY   1% positive coeliac serology (UK data). Only 1/8 cases is currently diagnosed. Recent prevalence studies describe an increase but this may be due to an increase in targeted screening.

HISTORY   Classic history of coeliac disease with symptoms of malabsorption (diarrhoea, steatorrhoea, failure to thrive or weight loss) is now considered to be quite rare. Most patients have milder symptoms of fatigue, irritability, abdominal pain, bloating, indigestion or no symptoms at all. One in four children with CD is diagnosed by targeted screening.

EXAMINATION   Many children will have no abnormal findings on examination.
Classic severe presentation: Miserable, pale, aphthous stomatitis, digital clubbing, abdominal distension, 'pot-belly' appearance, buttock wasting, delayed puberty.
Dermatitis herpetiformis: Itchy blisters on elbows, knees, face and buttocks.

PATHOPHYSIOLOGY
Macro: 'Subtotal villous atrophy' of the proximal small intestine; mucosa has a smooth flat appearance.
Micro: ↑Inflammatory infiltrates of lymphocytes and plasma cells in the lamina propria of the small bowel.

INVESTIGATIONS   Offer serological testing to any individual with autoimmune thyroid disease, dermatitis herpetiformis, irritable bowel syndrome, type 1 diabetes or first-degree relatives (parents, siblings or children) with CD.
Serology: Check IgA level as 2% of individuals with CD will be deficient.

1. Antibody directed against tissue transglutaminase (tTGA).
2. Antiendomysial antibodies if the result of the tTGA test is equivocal.

Bloods: ↓Hb, ↓MCV in iron deficiency, ↑MCV in B12/folate deficiency, ↓Ca^{2+}, ↓albumin.
Jejunal biopsy: Gold standard for diagnosis. Classic criterion on jejunal biopsy is flattened smooth mucosa with subtotal villous atrophy. 6.4–9.1% of CD cases have negative serology so biopsy should still be performed if there is clinical suspicion.
If the initial diagnosis is uncertain in children <2 years then a gluten challenge to confirm diagnosis is recommended at 6–7 years or after pubertal growth.

MANAGEMENT
Prevention: Continued breastfeeding during weaning onto wheat has been postulated as potentially protective.
Nutritional advice: Strict lifelong gluten-free diet (no wheat, barley or rye products) with dietetic input. Pure uncontaminated oats are compatible with a gluten-free diet. Vitamin, calcium and iron supplements. Advise membership of www.coeliac.org.uk. Follow up at least annually.

COMPLICATIONS   Osteoporosis and related fractures, 2° lactose intolerance due to damage of the brush border, intestinal lymphoma, bacterial overgrowth, decreased fertility and increased fetal loss/low-birth weight babies. After diagnosis of coeliac disease weight gain leading to obesity is now increasingly being recognised.

PROGNOSIS   With strict adherence to a gluten-free diet, there is a good prognosis.

DEFINITION   Aggression to people and/or animals, destruction of property, deceitfulness, theft and serious violation of rules within last 12 months (DSM-IV, ICD-10). Conduct disorder is subdivided into childhood onset (<10 years) and adolescent onset (>10 years).

AETIOLOGY
Environmental risk factors: Social disadvantage, homelessness, poverty (may exacerbate family dysfunction), overcrowding and social isolation.
Family risk factors: Parental mental illness, parental substance abuse, criminal activity, marital discord, single parenthood, large family size, child abuse and neglect, poor parental supervision, parenting style and attachment, parental rejection of the child.

ASSOCIATIONS/RELATED   ADHD, depression, learning disabilities (particularly dyslexia), substance misuse. Psychosis and ASD are less commonly associated.

EPIDEMIOLOGY   Conduct disorder is the main reason for referral to Child and Adolescent Mental Health Services (CAMHS). M : F = 3 : 1.
Childhood onset: Prevalence: 6.9% male and 2.8% female.
Adolescent onset: Prevalence: 8.1% male and 5.1% female.

HISTORY AND EXAMINATION
Childhood onset: Temper tantrums, defiance, destructiveness, hitting, biting.
Adolescent onset: Vandalism, bullying, cruelty to animals, lying, stealing, truancy, substance abuse.

PATHOPHYSIOLOGY   See Aetiology.

INVESTIGATIONS CAMHS specialist should perform formal assessment using observations and interviews with the parents, teachers and children. The Child Behaviour Check List (CBCL) is the most commonly used assessment tool.

MANAGEMENT
Child (individual)-focused therapies: Behavioural therapy, cognitive therapy, psychotherapy, social skills training, play therapy, music/art therapy.
Parent training interventions: Employs behavioural management training.

- Promote daily play and positive joint activities between parent and child.
- Encourage recognition, praise and rewards for specific desired behaviours.
- Give short specific commands about the desired behaviour, not prohibitions about undesired behaviour (e.g. 'Please eat with your mouth closed', rather than 'Don't eat with your mouth open').
- Provide consistent and calm responses to unwanted behaviour: ignoring, distracting the child or giving 'time out'.

Parent training programmes have a positive impact on childhood-onset but not adolescent-onset conduct disorder.
Family therapy interventions: A therapist meets with the whole family to explore interactions that might be contributing to the child's behavior. This intervention is more effective than individual focused therapies in decreasing behavioural problems in adolescents.
Complications: Conduct disorder has a significant impact on the child's and family's quality of life and also has a considerable cost to society. Children with conduct disorders are more likely to have poor school achievement and exclusion, unemployment, and enter into delinquency. They also have a higher risk of poor interpersonal relationships, family break-up and inflicting child abuse.

PROGNOSIS   Early conduct problems are the best predictor of future delinquency. 50% of children with conduct disorder will be diagnosed with antisocial personality disorder as adults and may also turn to substance/alcohol abuse, develop major depressive or anxiety-related disorders.

DEFINITION   Inherited disorder of adrenal steroidogenesis.

AETIOLOGY   Autosomal recessive genetic defect in the cytochrome P450 (CYP) protein enzymes involved with adrenal steroidogenesis. Resultant ↓d levels of cortisol +/− aldosterone and ↑d levels of precursor adrenocortical hormones cause symptoms (e.g. ↑d deoxycorticosterone leads to sodium retention/HT at supraphysiological levels).
Phenotypical variance: Occult (clinically asymptomatic disease), non-classic (adolescence/ adulthood mild form) and classic (severe infantile adrenal insufficiency +/− salt wasting and virilisation). 21-hydroxylase deficiency: Salt wasting/simple virilising/non-classic.
Enzyme deficiency: 21-hydroxylase (90%), 11β-hydroxylase deficiency (5%) and 17α-hydroxylase deficiency (5%).

ASSOCIATIONS/RELATED   Consanguinity, FHx.

EPIDEMIOLOGY   1/10,000 (21-hydroxylase deficiency), 1/100,000 (11β-hydroxylase and 17α-hydroxylase deficiency). Racial predilection; ↑d with Ashkenzai Jews and Yupik of Alaska.

HISTORY AND EXAMINATION
Male classic: Salt-losing crisis; occurs with severe 21-hydroxylase deficiency. Males present <1/12 old as genitalia are normal therefore diagnosis delayed. 2° to ↓d aldosterone.
Symptoms: failure to thrive, recurrent vomiting, sweating, dehydration, hyponatraemia, hyperkalaemia, hypotension and coma rapidly followed by death.
Male non-classic: Early development of 2° characteristics (pubic hair and phallic enlargement) and accelerated growth and ↑skeletal maturation.
Female classic: Ambiguous genitalia; clitoromegaly, fused labia at birth.
Female non-classic: Virilisation: acne, hirsutism, accelerated growth, ↑skeletal maturation.
17α-hydroxylase deficiency: ↑11-deoxycorticosterone (mineralocorticoid), ↓androgens causing HT and ↓Na$^+$ ↑K$^+$. Males present with ambiguous or female genitalia, females with absence of 2° characteristics at puberty.
11β-hydroxylase deficiency: May present as a salt-losing crisis in a neonate. When older, develop HT +/− ↓K$^+$ as ↑ mineralocorticoid (deoxycorticosterone) sensitivity with age.

PATHOPHYSIOLOGY
Encoding genes: CYP21A (21α-hydroxylase), CYP11B1 (11β-hydroxylase), CYP17A (17α-hydroxylase).
Adrenal histology: Hyperplasia of the adrenal cortex and disorganised architecture of cortices and medullae.

INVESTIGATIONS
Bloods: 17-hydroxyprogesterone (↑ in 21-hydroxylase deficiency and 11β-hydroxylase deficiency), testosterone, ↑basal ACTH, LH, FSH, U&E.
ACTH stimulation test: Inappropriately elevated 17-hydroxyprogesterone levels after IM ACTH.
Pelvic ultrasound: Presence of uterus/polycystic ovary syndrome/renal anomaly.
Karyotyping and molecular genetics: Mutation location and chromosomal sex.

MANAGEMENT
Acute salt-losing crisis: IV 0.9% NaCl (20 ml/kg) over first hour and repeated as necessary, dextrose and hydrocortisone, monitor for hypoglycaemia.
Medical: Glucocorticoid (hydrocortisone) and mineralocorticoid (fludrocortisone) replacement. NaCl supplementation PRN. Doses of steroids should be increased when unwell. Prednisolone +/− dexamethasone can also be used.
Surgical: Ambiguous genitalia. With female patient, possible clitoral regression followed by vaginoplasty after birth.
Counselling: Genetic with antenatal screening. Psychological counselling for parents and child.

COMPLICATIONS   ↓Female fertility. Male development of adrenal rests/tissue in the testicles. Short stature (premature epiphyseal closure 2° to steroid therapy). Steroid side effects.

PROGNOSIS   Good if diagnosed early. Undiagnosed infants may die from salt-losing crises (diagnosed as pyloric stenosis/gastroenteritis).

DEFINITION   Deficiency of thyroid hormone present at birth which if untreated leads to severe neurodevelopmental delay.

AETIOLOGY
Thyroid gland dysgenesis (85%): Agenesis (athryosis 30%), ectopic thyroid (60%) and thyroid hypoplasia (10%).
Thyroid dyshormogenesis (10%): Genetic defects in active iodine transport/hormone synthesis or secretion. Pendred syndrome (defective thyroglobulin synthesis and transport).
Maternal transmission (5%): Transplacental passage of antithyroid drugs or radio-iodine and maternal antibodies from autoimmune disease.
Central hypothyroidism: Hypothalamic defect (thyroid-releasing hormone deficiency) and pituitary defect (abnormal thyroid-stimulating hormone).
Thyroid hormone resistance: Mutation in the thyroid hormone receptor β gene.

ASSOCIATIONS/RELATED   FHx, cardiac defects, hearing impairment, constipation.

EPIDEMIOLOGY   Relatively common, incidence: 1/3500 live births. $M : F = 1 : 2$.

HISTORY
Neonates: Majority asymptomatic $2°$ to transplacental passage of moderate amounts of maternal T4 (can produce fetal level 25–50% of normal). May present with poor feeding, constipation, jaundice, thickened skin, hypothermia with poor perfusion, peripheral cyanosis, bradycardias.
Infants: First sign is often prolonged neonatal jaundice. Subsequently may develop other symptoms of hypothyroidism including lethargy, slow feeding, respiratory distress with feeds, excessive sleeping, little vocalisation and constipation.

EXAMINATION
Physical signs: Coarse dry hair, flat nasal bridge, protruding tongue $2°$ to macroglossia, hypotonia, slowly relaxing reflexes, umbilical hernia, slow pulse and cardiomegaly.
Developmental delay (untreated): Later global developmental delay, learning disabilities, delayed puberty and dentition, short stature, slow relaxation of tendon reflexes, sensorineural hearing loss.

PATHOPHYSIOLOGY   See Aetiology.

INVESTIGATIONS
Universal neonatal screening: Heel prick blood spot at 5–7/7 (Guthrie test) for TSH level ($>50 \mu U/l$ is diagnostic). Infants with TSH deficiency are not detected so clinical vigilance is still required.
Bloods: $\downarrow T_4$ (not in thyroid-binding globulin deficiency), $\downarrow$ or $\uparrow$TSH (depending on the cause), $\downarrow$Hb, unconjugated hyperbilirubinaemia.
Wrist and hand XR: Bone age < chronological age. Rough 'bone age' is calculated by analysing the number of ossification centres present.
Radio-active technetium scan: Detects functional thyroid tissue and therefore dysgenesis or ectopia.
Echocardiogram: Cardiomegaly $+/-$ pericardial effusions detection.

MANAGEMENT   Universal neonatal screening, confirmation and early treatment avoid serious sequelae.
Thyroxine replacement: PO sodium L-thyroxine (10–15 μg/kg/d).
Regular follow-up: Monitor TSH, T4 levels, development and growth, bone age (ensure adequate osseous development, delayed with undertreatment). Lifelong follow-up to monitor for adequate levels of thyroid hormone.

COMPLICATIONS   Excessive treatment with thyroxine leads to advancement of bone age and later to ↓d adult height as the epiphyses fuse prematurely; inadequate treatment leads to severe mental neurological delay.

PROGNOSIS   Prognosis is good with early detection. Some studies suggest mildly lower IQ scores, subtle neurodevelopmental delays and motor deficits in children adequately treated.

DEFINITION Antenatal transmission of a maternal infection to the fetus causing postnatal effects.

AETIOLOGY Congenital infection via transplacental transmission. Possible infective agents: TORCH (toxoplasmosis, rubella, CMV and herpes simplex) and syphilis.

CMV (most common): May occur transplacentally, intrapartum (aspiration of cervicovaginal secretions) and postnatally (during breastfeeding). ↑d neonatal sequelae with transplacental transmission. Transmission rate inversely proportional to gestational age: 1st trimester (75–90%), 2nd (35–40%) and 3rd (25–50%).

Rubella: ↑d teratogenic effect with ↓ gestational age. Occurs during the maternal viraemic phase. Fetus is most at risk within the first trimester as infection at >18/40 has a minimal risk of congenital malformations.

Syphilis: Transplacental transmission of spirochaetes, ≈100% transmission rate. Inflammatory changes after the first trimester therefore organogenesis unaffected. Most neonates are asymptomatic and only identified by prenatal screening.

ASSOCIATIONS/RELATED Lower socio-economic groups, developing countries and younger maternal age with rubella.

EPIDEMIOLOGY
CMV: 3–4/100 live births. M = F.
Rubella: Rare; ↓d incidence 2° to vaccination (possible ↑ with ↓d MMR uptake).
Syphilis: Rare.

HISTORY AND EXAMINATION
Antenatal: May cause spontaneous abortion or stillbirth in the most severe of cases.
CMV: 10% infected neonates will be symptomatic. ↓d gestational age at transmission = ↑ symptom severity.
Cytomegalic inclusion disease (CID): Most severe form of congenital CMV infection: IUGR, hepatosplenomegaly, haematological abnormalities (esp. thrombocytopenia), cutaneous manifestations including petechiae and purpura (blueberry muffin baby), CNS manifestations (microcephaly, ventriculomegaly, cerebral atrophy, chorioretinitis and sensorineural hearing loss).
Congenital rubella syndrome (classic triad): Sensorineural hearing loss; ocular abnormalities (cataracts, infantile glaucoma, chorioretinitis, retinitis pigmentosa); congenital heart disease (PDA, pulmonary artery stenosis, ASD, VSD). Also, IUGR, hypotonia, microcephaly, hepatomegaly, jaundice, hepatitis, blueberry muffin baby, later thyroid abnormalities and diabetes.
Syphilis (early onset): Mucocutaneous tissues and bone lesions (mucous patches, rhinitis and condylomatous), maculopapular desquamative rash with extensive epithelium sloughing (palms, soles, around mouth and anus), vesicular rash and bullae may develop (highly contagious), hepatomegaly.
Syphilis (late onset): Neurosyphilis, involvement of the teeth, bones, eyes, and CN VIII.

PATHOPHYSIOLOGY
CMV: Herpesviridae family of large DNA viruses.
Rubella: Togaviridae family RNA virus.
Syphilis: *Treponema pallidum* (Spirochaetaceae family).

INVESTIGATIONS
Antenatal: Amniotic fluid culture (18/40).
Virology: Direct viral/spirochaetes isolation from saliva, tears or urine, CSF.
Bloods: Serum IgM and IgG (↓ sensitivity and specificity). Automated reagin test (ART). Treponema-specific tests.
Imaging: CT (cerebral calcification), AUSS (hepatosplenomegaly), ECHO, CXR (pneumonitis or pulmonary oedema).

MANAGEMENT

Multidisciplinary: Paediatricians, surgeons, neurologists, ophthalmologist, ENT, audiology; regular follow-up to identify and treat disease sequelae as they occur.

Medical treatment: 1° supportive and symptomatic control. Ganciclovir ↓s sensorineural hearing loss in affected CMV neonates treated for 6/52 (frequent side effect 2° to mutagenic, teratogenic and carcinogenic effects). Rubella contact isolation. Congenital syphilis treated with aqueous penicillin G.

Surgical: Cardiac defects, ophthalmic intervention, gastrostomy insertion (enteral supplementation).

COMPLICATIONS   See History and Examination.

PROGNOSIS Intracerebral calcifications typically demonstrate a periventricular distribution and are a poor prognostic sign in congenital CMV infection. First year congenital rubella mortality: 10–20% 2° to multiorgan pathology (life-long morbidity). Good prognosis with early diagnosis and treatment of syphilis.

DEFINITION   A delay or difficulty in defaecation, present for >2/52 and sufficient to cause significant distress.

AETIOLOGY
Functional: 90–95% of cases; idiopathic as nil underlying medical condition 2° to vicious cycle of pain on defaecation and retention.
Slow transit constipation (STC): Causes intractable symptoms and normally refractory to medical management.
Nutritional: Cow's milk protein allergy, inadequate fluid intake, malnutrition, high refined carbohydrate and protein diet or a low-fibre diet.
Organic (rare): Gastrointestinal anomalies; Hirschsprung's disease, anorectal stenotic lesions, anal fissures. Spinal/neuromuscular disease. Hypothyroidism.

ASSOCIATIONS/RELATED   Cerebral palsy, delayed passage of meconium, failure to thrive, positive FHx, encopresis.

EPIDEMIOLOGY   Extremely common; 3–5% of outpatient consultations and 35% of gastroenterology consultations. Peak incidence 2–4 years of age. M = F (prepuberty), F>M (postpuberty).

HISTORY
General: Detailed history including diet and social setting, onset of constipation. Delayed passage of meconium >24 hours at birth is characteristic of Hirschsprung's disease. Infants have a wide normal range of stool frequency, depending on type of milk (breastfeeding/formula) and amount of solids.

EXAMINATION
General: Abdominal distension and palpable stools. Presence of sacral dimples/pits.
Digital rectal examination: Anus position on perineum, presence of fissures/fistulae/stool/mass, anal wink and sensation, size of anal canal/rectum.

PATHOPHYSIOLOGY
Functional constipation: Association of pain with defaecation and withholds stools in an attempt to avoid discomfort. ↑d retention = ↓d sensory feedback, rectal wall is stretched and loses contractile strength (normal urge to defaecate gradually disappears), ↑d water absorption from faecal matter causing larger and harder stool. Chronic rectal distension; ↓d rectal sensitivity and loss of the urge to defaecate which can lead to encopresis.

INVESTIGATIONS
Radiology: AXR is not helpful in the initial assessment.
Anorectal manometry: Delineating child's defaecation dynamics, evidence of megarectum, exclusion of ultra-short segment Hirschsprung's disease.
Radionuclear transit scintography: Identifies slow colonic transit. May also be done with plain AXR after ingestion of different shaped markers.

MANAGEMENT
General: Evacuation of the colon, elimination of pain and establishment of regular defaecation routines.
Medical: Dietary changes (↑d fibre, adequate fluids), exercise, laxatives/faecal softeners, enema programme, lignocaine gel (anal fissures).
Surgical intervention: Endorectal pull-through for confirmed Hirschsprung's disease. Antegrade continence enema (ACE) either proximally (pACE/Mallone procedure) or distally (dACE). Allows the administration of enemas directly into the caecum or the distal colon. Some centres recommend rectosigmoid resections for refractory constipation.
Other: Interferential therapy (transcutaneous electrical stimulation) is a possible future therapy.

COMPLICATIONS   Faecal overload, overflow incontinence, encopresis, 2° emotional and behavioural difficulties.

PROGNOSIS   50% recover within 1 year and 65–70% recover within 2 years; the remainder require regular laxative therapy +/− have encopresis.

DEFINITION   Immune-mediated hypersensitivity reaction to cow's milk protein.

AETIOLOGY   Cow's milk proteins are casein (80%) and whey (20%)($\alpha + \beta$ lactoglobulin).

ASSOCIATIONS/RELATED   Parental atopy. Atopic eczema. 25% CMPA have other food allergies.

EPIDEMIOLOGY   Incidence 2–2.5% at 1 year (2002).

HISTORY AND EXAMINATION   Symptoms appear within the first weeks of introducing cow's milk. CMPA usually affects more than one organ system.

Immediate IgE mediated (occurs within 2 hours)

1. **Skin:** Flush, itch, urticaria, angio-oedema
2. **Respiratory:** Wheeze/cough 2° to bronchospasm, stridor 2° to laryngeal oedema
3. **CVS:** Tachycardia, hypotension
4. **GI:** Vomiting, diarrhoea, abdominal pain

Mixed IgE and non-IgE mediated (2–12 hours)

1. **Skin:** Atopic eczema
2. **GI:** Eosinophilic eosophagitis (reflux, food aversion, dysphagia), proctocolitis (bloody stools in an otherwise thriving breastfed infant)

Delayed non-IgE mediated (12–24 hours)

GI: Food protein-induced enterocolitis (FPIES) presents with vomiting and possibly diarrhoea, shock and metabolic acidosis. Failure to thrive, constipation (classically straining followed by passage of normal stool).

PATHOPHYSIOLOGY AND INVESTIGATIONS   See Food allergy chapter.

MANAGEMENT

Prevention: Exclusive breastfeeding for ≥ 4 months reduces allergic disease (eczema), especially in atopic families. In children from atopic families who are unable to receive breast milk, hypoallergenic formulas have been shown to reduce allergic disease in the first few years of life.

Avoidance: All mammalian dairy products (under dietetic review as cow's milk is an important source of calcium).

Cow's milk alternatives

- Breast milk is still the best milk for children with CMPA. Strict maternal avoidance of dairy may be required (dietetic input).
- Hypoallergenic formulas:
  (a) Extensively hydrolysed casein or whey formulas (EHF)
  (b) Amino acid-based formula: if symptoms do not improve on EHF or if infant is failing to thrive.
- Soya milk formula: 3–14% of IgE-mediated and up to 40% of non-IgE mediated children with CMPA are also allergic to soya milk. Due to the phyto-oestrogen content, soya should not be used <6 months.
- Rice, oat and pea milk (calcium fortified) are alternative milks for children who are CMPA and allergic to soya who cannot tolerate hypoallergenic formulas. Rice milk is not recommended in children <4.5 years due to arsenic content.

Reintroduction of cow's milk: Child should be seen every 6–12 months to assess possible reintroduction of cow's milk in hospital (oral challenge).

COMPLICATIONS   Anaphylaxis is a real and severe complication of cow's milk protein allergy and can be fatal. Mortality is increased if the child has poorly controlled asthma.

PROGNOSIS In IgE-mediated CMPA, one-third will resolve by 2 years, half by 3 years and two-thirds by 4 years. In non-IgE mediated CMPA, two-thirds will be tolerant by 2 years and >90% by 3 years. CMPA children have ↑ risk of developing eczema, allergic rhinitis and asthma.

DEFINITION   Common condition characterised by progressive spread of inflammation down the respiratory tract starting at the larynx, followed by trachea and bronchi 2° to a viral infection.

AETIOLOGY   Parainfluenza virus is the most common cause but other viruses can produce a similar picture, such as RSV, influenza, rhinoviruses.

ASSOCIATIONS/RELATED
DD of acute stridor:

1. *Acute epiglottitis*: child is toxic, no cough, drooling symptoms develop over shorter period of time (hours)
2. *Foreign body*: acute onset, clear history
3. *Anaphylaxis*: known allergy, urticaria, wheals
4. *Tracheitis*: toxic child, croupy cough, no drooling
5. *Infectious mononucleosis*: marked tonsillar swelling
6. *Diphtheria*: rare but important, always check immunisation status.

May be more severe with underlying conditions: laryngomalacia, subglottic stenosis.

EPIDEMIOLOGY   Commonly affects children from 6 months to 5 years old. Occurs in the winter months and children may have repeated episodes.

HISTORY
Coryza: Symptoms preceded by 1–3 days of coryza +/– fever.
Laryngitis: Barking, croupy cough and hoarse voice.
Tracheitis: Onset of stridor (seal-like yelp) 1–2 days after cough.
Bronchitis: ↑ Respiratory effort as infection spreads down bronchial tree.

EXAMINATION   Examine the child in a calm environment with minimal disturbance. Do not examine the child's throat as this may precipitate acute airway obstruction.

Classification of severity of croup to determine management

Sign	0	1	2	3
Stridor	None	When agitated	At rest	Severe, inspiratory/expiratory
Recession	None	Mild, subcostal	Moderate/ tracheal tug	Severe with marked use of accessory muscles
Colour	Normal	Normal	Dusky	Central cyanosis
Level of consciousness	Normal	Restless when disturbed	Anxious and agitated	Lethargic and drowsy

Mild ≤3 signs, moderate 4–5 signs, severe >5 signs.

PATHOPHYSIOLOGY   Mucosal inflammation and ↑ secretions affect the larynx, trachea and bronchi. Narrowing of the subglottic area causes stridor and is potentially dangerous in young children because of their narrow trachea.

INVESTIGATIONS   Blood tests are seldom taken as croup is a clinical diagnosis and the aim is to cause the least distress to the child.

MANAGEMENT
Mild croup: During the day may be managed at home with careful observation Advise plenty of fluids. Humidity is popular with parents but is of unproven value. Paracetamol PRN may be used for symptomatic relief and to ↓ temperature.

Moderate croup: Oral steroids (dexamethasone) or nebulised budesonide have been shown to shorten duration and severity of disease. Observe for 2–4 hours post administration of steroids to watch for deterioration.

Severe croup: Nebulised adrenaline with O_2 may be used as a temporary measure as it is effective in reducing upper airway oedema but watch for rebound obstruction. Treat with steroids as in moderate croup. May require intubation and admission to PICU.

COMPLICATIONS   Upper airway obstruction may be fatal.

PROGNOSIS   Duration usually 2–3 days, occasionally 2–3 weeks. 2–5% of children hospitalised for croup require intubation.

DEFINITION   Failure of normal descent of the testicle to a scrotal position.

Undescended testes (UDT): Testes are found at any point within the normal path of descent with a patent processus vaginalis.

Ectopic: Descended through the inguinal canal but positioned abnormally outside the scrotum, e.g. perineum, femoral, suprapubic regions.

Acquired: Failure of the growth of the spermatic cord in proportion to the scrotal growth. Scarring caused by inguinal hernia repair.

AETIOLOGY

Normal testicular descent

First stage (transabdominal): The fetal gubernaculum enlarges under the control of INSL3 +/− MIS/AMH and testosterone. This anchors the testicle near the inguinal region during growth of the fetal abdominal cavity.

Second stage (inguinoscrotal): Involves the migration of the gubernaculum to the scrotum with elongation of the PV within it, under androgen control.

The testicles remain retroperitoneal until 28/40.

ASSOCIATIONS/RELATED   Prematurity, low birthweight, hypospadias, patent processus vaginalis (always present with UDT), if bilateral may be due to hypopituitarism.

EPIDEMIOLOGY   3% of full-term male infants. 30% of premature infants.

HISTORY   Usually asymptomatic, picked up during child health surveillance, although may present with the associated inguinal hernia.

EXAMINATION   Examine child relaxed in a warm room. The most common location of the cryptorchid testis is in the inguinal canal (72%), followed by prescrotal (20%) and abdominal (8%) locations.

DIFFERENTIAL DIAGNOSIS   Retractile testis with a positive cremesteric response, rarely congenital absence, atrophic testis caused by a neonatal torsion.

PATHOPHYSIOLOGY   See Aetiology.

INVESTIGATIONS   Diagnosis is clinical. Divided into palpable and impalpable. Palpable do not require further preoperative investigation. USS may aid location in impalpable, although some centres will perform an examination under anaesthetic +/− laparoscopy. Bilateral impalpable testicles require hormonal investigation (β-HCG stimulation) and chromosomal mapping.

MANAGEMENT   Orchidopexy performed traditionally at 1 year of age but now recommended at 6/12 in some centres. PPV ligation at same operation. Orchidectomy may be performed with abnormal testicle with contralateral orchidopexy.

COMPLICATIONS   Failure of correct intrascrotal position can lead to infertility, spermatogenesis defects, increased malignancy risk (60% seminomas) and also late detection of malignancy.

PROGNOSIS   Good with appropriate surgical intervention.

DEFINITION   AR condition characterised by recurrent lung infections, malabsorption and failure to thrive.

AETIOLOGY

Common genotype (70–80%): Phenylalanine deletion at position 508 (ΔF508) results in a defective gene on chromosome 7 q. There are $\geq$900 known mutations of this gene. Defective gene codes for abnormal transport protein (CFTR) in the cell membrane.

ASSOCIATIONS/RELATED   Obstructive azoospermia (may occur without other CF symptoms).

EPIDEMIOLOGY   1/2500 live births; 1/25 carrier rate in Caucasians.

HISTORY

Neonatal: 15% present with meconium ileus (bowel obstruction by thick meconium).
Infancy: Recurrent chest infections, steatorrhoea, failure to thrive, developmental delay.
Older children: Asthma, allergic bronchopulmonary aspergillosis (episodic wheeze, low-grade fever, brown sputum), recurrent sinusitis.

EXAMINATION

Signs of malnutrition: $\downarrow$ Muscle mass, protuberant abdomen.
Respiratory: Hyperinflation (air trapping), coarse crepitations, expiratory rhonchi.
Others: Jaundice, early digital clubbing, nasal polyps, rectal prolapse.

INVESTIGATIONS

Sweat test (gold standard). Sweat Cl$^-$ of $>$50 mmol/L and Na^{2+} of $>$60 mmol/L by pilocarpine iontophoresis, weight of sweat $>$100 mg on 2 occasions.
Lung function: Obstructive picture with air trapping and hyperinflation ($\downarrow$FEV1, $\uparrow$TLC).
Guthrie's test: $\uparrow$ Serum immunoreactive trypsin (all UK newborns are now screened).
Antenatal tests: First trimester CVS (95% sensitivity). Second trimester $\downarrow$ intestinal ALP in amniotic fluid (90% sensitivity).

PATHOPHYSIOLOGY

Genetic: Defective CFTR acts as cAMP chloride channel blocker. $\downarrow$Cl$^-$ transport accompanied by $\downarrow$Na$^+$ and H$_2$O transport across epithelial cells results in dehydrated viscous secretions causing luminal obstruction, destruction and scarring of exocrine glands.
Respiratory: Lung is normal at birth but as it matures, mucous gland hyperplasia occurs and thick viscid mucus is formed in the small airways. Patients are predisposed to chronic infection with *Staphylococcus aureus*, *Haemophilus influenzae* and *Pseudomonas* which leads to areas of fibrosis, consolidation and bronchiectasis.
Pancreatic: Exocrine enzyme insufficiency causes malabsorption and steatorrhoea.

MANAGEMENT

Multidisciplinary approach
Respiratory:

1. Flucloxacillin prophylaxis for *Staphylococcus aureus*
2. 80% of CF patients are chronically infected by adolescence with Pseudomonas. This is treated with nebulised antibiotics (colomycin $+/-$ gentamicin/tobramycin) and intermittent courses of IV antibiotics to decrease size of colony (every 3 months)
3. Allergic bronchopulmonary aspergillosis: steroids $+/-$ itraconazole
4. $\uparrow$Airway responsiveness presents with asthma-like symptoms: bronchodilators $+/-$ inhaled steroids if responsive
5. Nebulised recombinant human DNAse acts as a mucolytic.

Nutritional: $\uparrow$ Calorie, $\uparrow$ protein diet for $\uparrow$ energy requirements and malabsorption often with overnight supplementation. Some CF patients have a gastrostomy inserted to facilitate ↑ calorie intake. Enteric-coated pancreatic enzyme (e.g. Creon) and fat-soluble vitamin supplementation. Ursodeoxycholic acid to prevent gallstones.

Immunisations: Usual schedule + pneumococcal, influenza.

Physiotherapy: >2 × daily to be continued even when well; swimming is ideal exercise.

Heart-lung transplant: If lung function deteriorates to <30% predicted best.

Gene therapy: Viral vectors/liposomes to deliver normal copies of the CF gene to make the CFTR protein. Still at research stage.

COMPLICATIONS

Respiratory: Bronchiectasis, cor pulmonale, pneumothorax, haemoptysis.

GI: Cirrhosis, portal hypertension, distal intestinal obstruction syndrome; viscid mucofaeculent material obstructs the bowel.

Endocrine: DM, ↓ fertility. 99% of males are infertile due to obstruction and abnormal development of vas deferens. Females are often subfertile but there have been many successful pregnancies.

Psychological/behavioural problems: Due to compromised lifestyle and morbidity.

PROGNOSIS   Most sufferers now survive into adult life (median survival 40 years). Children with Pseudomonas colonization have a 2–3-fold increased mortality over 8 years.

DEFINITION Onset of puberty spontaneously at a time that is more than two standard deviations later than the mean time of breast development in girls (13.4 years) or ↑ in testicular volume in boys (14.0 years).

AETIOLOGY

Puberty: Process involving the acquisition of 2° sexual characteristics with an associated growth spurt and attainment of reproductive function.

Normal gonadotrophins (LH, FSH) (pubertal delay):

1. *Constitutional delay*: due to late activation of the hypothalamic-pituitary-gonadal axis, delay is synchronous for height and bone age.
2. *Chronic illness*: inflammatory bowel disease, cystic fibrosis, renal disease, severe asthma, CNS disorders (Langerhans cell histiocytosis, congenital defects)
3. Anorexia nervosa, starvation, excess physical training (ballet, athletes)
4. Deprivation.

Hypergonadotrophic hypogonadism/unresponsive gonad (pubertal failure):

1. *Congenital*: Turner syndrome (45X karyotype), Klinefelter syndrome (47XXY)
2. Steroid hormone enzyme deficiency
3. *Acquired gonadal damage*: chemotherapy, radiotherapy, trauma, torsion, autoimmune.

Hypogonadotrophic hypogonadism/failure of hypothalamic or pituitary function (pubertal failure):

1. *Hypothalamo-pituitary disease*: panhypopituitarism, intracranial tumours
2. Kallmann syndrome (LHRH deficiency, anosmia) and Prader-Willi syndrome
3. Hypothyroidism (acquired)
4. Idiopathic.

ASSOCIATIONS/RELATED FHx (constitutional delay).

EPIDEMIOLOGY Physiological or constitutional delay: 1/200 sex: M > F

HISTORY Elicit FHx, symptoms of chronic disease (failure to thrive, lethargy) and SHx.

EXAMINATION

General: Full examination to detect any indication of underlying disease, neurological signs (fundi, visual fields), dysmorphic features.

Testicular size: Orchidometer: 4 ml at 10–14 years, 12 ml at 12–17 years.

Tanner stages of puberty

Male genital stages:
1. Preadolescent
2. Lengthening of penis
3. ↑ Length and circumference
4. Glans penis, scrotal darkening
5. Adult genitalia

Female breast stages
1. Prepubertal
2. Breast bud
3. Juvenile smooth contour
4. Areola/nipple project above breast
5. Same shape nipple and breast

Pubic hair changes in males and females
1. Preadolescent, no sexual hair
2. Long downy hair along labia/base of penis
3. Dark, coarser, curlier hair
4. Filling out towards adult distribution
5. Adult in quantity and type, medial thigh spread

PATHOPHYSIOLOGY   See Aetiology.

INVESTIGATIONS
Bloods: TFTs, LH/FSH/androgen/oestrogen levels.
Karyotype: Chromosomal abnormalities.
Radiology: Determination of bone age, USS pelvis to assess uterine size and endometrial thickness.

MANAGEMENT
General: 1° treatment of the underlying cause. Induction of hormone treatment should be the patient's and family's choice.
Females: Oestrogen replacement therapy (treatment of choice). Administration PO or transdermally. After 12–18/12 of unopposed oestrogen therapy or after vaginal bleeding occurs, progesterone should be added.
Males: Hormonal replacement with intramuscular testosterone.

COMPLICATIONS   Complications of individual conditions and psychosocial complications including poor self-esteem, ↓d academic performance and socialising with peers.

PROGNOSIS   Dependent on underlying pathology.

DEFINITION

ICD-10 cardinal features: Depressed mood, anhedonia, low energy and fatigue leading to significant impairment of personal and social function.

Other features:

1. ↓ Concentration and attention
2. ↓ Self-esteem and self-confidence
3. Guilt and unworthiness
4. Bleak view of the future
5. Ideas or acts of self-harm or suicide
6. Disturbed sleep
7. Diminished appetite.

Mild depressive episode: 2 cardinal + 2 other features for >2 weeks; mild intensity.
Moderate episode: 2 cardinal + 3–4 other features for >2 weeks; moderate intensity.
Severe episode: 3 cardinal + >4 other features for >2 weeks; severe intensity.
Somatic symptoms (appetite, sleep): Present in severe episode but may not be in mild–moderate episode.

AETIOLOGY

Genetic: Positive family history.
Environmental: Parental mental health problems, unemployment and poverty. Substance abuse, neglect, family break-up, single-parent families, life 'events', 'looked after' children, poor support network, lack of friends, isolation, abuse.
Systemic disease: Anaemia, postviral syndrome (e.g. EBV), hypothyroidism, chronic illness.

ASSOCIATIONS/RELATED Learning disability, anxiety and behavioural disorders (50–80%), conduct disorder (25%), OCD (15%), eating disorders (5%) and obesity.

EPIDEMIOLOGY Twelve-month prevalence increases with age: 1% of children and 3% of adolescents. M : F equal during childhood, but F > M during and after adolescence.

HISTORY AND EXAMINATION Manifestation of depression in children is affected by developmental stage and ability to identify and communicate internal emotions. Children and adolescents will often use other means of expression such as:

1. Somatisation (frequent non-specific physical complaints) (children > adolescents)
2. Poor academic performance, truancy/school refusal
3. Being bored, lack of interest in anything
4. Disorganised or reckless behaviour
5. Separation anxiety, loss of interest in friends, social withdrawal
6. Outbursts of shouting, complaining, unexplained irritability or crying
7. Alcohol or substance abuse
8. Hitting, biting and scratching

PATHOPHYSIOLOGY Reduction in serotonergic and NA nerve transmission within the brain is thought to contribute to depression. There is a reduction in activity within the prefrontal cortex, which may have a part in 5-HT and NA neuron regulation.

INVESTIGATIONS

Bloods: FBC, LFTs, TFTs, U&E if clinical suspicion of systemic disease.

MANAGEMENT Child and family should be involved and supported.
Psychological therapies: Individual and group CBT, interpersonal psychotherapy (IPT), family therapy, relaxation.
Medical: SSRIs (only fluoxetine is licensed in children) require careful monitoring for the appearance of suicidal behaviour, self-harm and hostility.

COMPLICATIONS Poor school performance, unemployment, criminality, difficulty maintaining relationships.

Self-harm: A desperate attempt to draw attention to a perceived irresolvable situation. High rate of recurrence. Majority are *not* clinically depressed.

Suicide: 3% risk over following 10 years; most common in adolescent boys, ↑ risk if combined with alcohol/substance abuse.

PROGNOSIS Ten percent recover spontaneously within 3 months. A further 40% recover within the first year. At 12 months 50% remain clinically depressed. By 24 months this figure is around 20–30%. Approximately 30% recur within 5 years.

DEFINITION   Abnormal growth of the hip resulting in dislocation or instability.

AETIOLOGY   Multifactorial; racial association, intrauterine positioning, gender and ligamentous laxity.

ASSOCIATIONS/RELATED   FHx (first-degree relative; 20%), first born (smaller uterus), oligohydramnios, breech delivery, caesarean section, neuromuscular disorders, metatarsus adductus, torticollis.

EPIDEMIOLOGY   1–2/1000; M : F = 1 : 4. Caucasians > Asians.

HISTORY   Elicit family history and any risk factors.

EXAMINATION   DDH examined for routinely in newborn checks. With a relaxed child, the hip and knee are flexed to 90°, examiner's thumbs placed on the medial proximal thigh, and long fingers placed over the greater trochanter.
Ortolani manoeuvre: Contralateral hip is held still while the thigh of the hip being tested is abducted and gently pulled anteriorly. With a +ve Ortolani test, the femoral head glides over the ridge of pathological hypertrophic acetabular cartilage into the acetabulum. A palpable clunk occurs with the reduction. Therefore manoeuvre relocates a dislocated hip.
Barlow manoeuvre: The hip is adducted while pushing the thigh posteriorly. With a +ve Barlow test, the femoral head is dislocated posteriorly from the acetabulum. Dislocation is confirmed by performing the Ortolani manoeuvre to relocate the hip. Therefore manoeuvre dislocates an unstable hip.
Other physical signs: ↓ abduction on the affected side, standing or walking with external rotation, and asymmetry; leg positions, leg length, gluteal thigh or labral skin folds.

PATHOPHYSIOLOGY   Normal acetabular growth requires normal epiphyseal growth of the triradiate cartilage and the three ossification centres (os acetabulum, ilium and ischium). This is dependent on the presence of the femoral head and normal interstitial appositional growth within the acetabulum. Absence of the femoral head therefore leads to abnormal acetabular growth.

INVESTIGATIONS
USS hip: Reveals relationship between femoral head and acetabulum, existence of any acetabular dysplasia. High false +ve rate in infants <6 weeks.
X-ray hip: >4 months (2 views: adduction and abduction).

MANAGEMENT
Supportive: Pavlik harness abduction splints until age 5–6 months. USS monitoring.
Surgical correction: Late diagnosis (>6 months): preoperative traction (2–3 weeks) then closed reduction (arthrography guided). Surgical release of the hip adductor longus and iliopsoas muscles may be required. >18 months: open reduction with femoral +/− pelvic osteotomy may be required to correct severe deformities.

COMPLICATIONS
Iatrogenic: Skin irritation from reduction devices, 1–5% incidence of avascular necrosis of the femoral head with Pavlik harness splinting.
Long-term: Osteoarthritis of the hip.

PROGNOSIS   Pavlik harness has good results <6/12. ↑d age at diagnosis = worse outcome. Untreated, can be severely disabling.

DEFINITION Chronic metabolic disorder characterised by hyperglycaemia 2° to an absolute or relative deficiency of insulin secretion.

AETIOLOGY Insulin production in the pancreas by the β-cell of the islets of Langerhans is disrupted by their absence or destruction. There is a strong genetic influence (50% concordance in monozygotic twins).

Autoimmune: 85% of patients have circulating islet cell antibodies; majority directed against glutamic acid decarboxylase (GAD) within pancreatic β-cells.

Environmental: Viral infections initiate or modify the autoimmune process (mumps, rubella, coxsackie B4, ↑d with cow's milk protein exposure in infancy, ↑d with late vitamin D supplementation.

Non-type 1 paediatric diabetes: Neonatal diabetes (transient/permanent), maturity-onset diabetes of youth (MODY), obesity-associated paediatric type 2.

ASSOCIATIONS/RELATED Human leukocyte antigen DR-3 and DR-4, thyroid autoimmune disorders (Graves disease, Hashimoto thyroiditis), viral infections in pregnancy, ↑d maternal, blood group incompatibility, cow's milk proteins.

EPIDEMIOLOGY ↑ing paediatric incidence: 15/10,000/yr. Peaks at ages 4–6 years and 10–14 years (most common). Racial and geographical variation. M > F.

HISTORY AND EXAMINATION
General: Polyuria (nocturnal enuresis/persistently wet nappies/nappy rash), polydipsia, weight loss, recurrent infections, necrobiosis lipoidica (well-demarcated, red atrophic area, usually on lower leg), blurred vision, fatigue.

Diabetic ketoacidosis (DKA): Abdominal pain, vomiting, dehydration, drowsiness progressing to coma, Kussmaul breathing (rapid deep breathing) 2° to acidosis, acetone smelling breath.

Hypoglycaemia (2° to insulin treatment): Sweating, tremor, palpitations, irritability. Late (progressive) symptoms seizures, coma.

PATHOPHYSIOLOGY
HbA1c: Stable product of non-enzymatic irreversible glycosylation of the β-chain of Hb by plasma glucose.

INVESTIGATIONS
Urinalysis: Ketonuria, glycosuria.
Bloods: Random plasma glucose >11.0 mmol/l or fasting >7.0 mmol/l. HbA1c >7.5%. Islet cell antibodies.
DKA: Low blood bicarbonate, ↓pH, heavy ketonuria.
Hypoglycaemia: Plasma glucose <2.5 mmol/l.

MANAGEMENT
Initial: Home-based or inpatient management according to clinical need, family circumstances and wishes. Home-based diabetes care team with 24-hour telephone advice is as effective as inpatient care.

Parental/patient education: Nature of diabetes, recognition of hypoglycaemia, insulin regime and technique, ↑d insulin requirements in illness, diet and maintenance of active lifestyle.

Total insulin requirement: DNA recombinant human insulin 0.5–1 unit/kg/d in prepubertal children. Insulin resistance in adolescents may require 2 units/kg/d.

Insulin regimes: Short-acting combined with intermediate-acting insulin (BD) given in combined solution by pen. May use TDS or QDS regimes in older children with short-acting insulin before main meals and intermediate insulin ON.

Insulin pump therapy: ↑ing numbers of children are using continuous subcutaneous insulin infusion using long-acting insulin glargine and bolus doses at meal times.

Conservative: Blood glucose monitoring (aim for 4–6 mmol/l), dietary changes (high fibre, ↓refined carbohydrate but ↑complex carbohydrate consumption), psychological support. Medic-Alert bracelet/necklace. HbA1c level <7.5%. Coeliac/thyroid disease monitoring, retinopathy, microalbuminuria and BP screening.

Surgical/future: Stem cell therapy and pancreatic transplant (severe cases).

Diabetic ketoacidosis:

Appropriate fluid resuscitation with IV normal saline

↓

Insulin sliding scale: short-acting soluble insulin via syringe driver (0.25 units/kg/h)

↓

Hourly U&Es + K⁺ replacement on passing urine (plasma K⁺ falls as K⁺ enters cells with treatment)

↓

Switch to IV dextrose when glucose levels fall to 12 mmol/l

Hypoglycaemia: Mild (food, e.g. apple/sandwich), moderate (PO glucose drink), severe (intrabuccal Hypostop/IV dextrose).

COMPLICATIONS

Acute: Hypoglycaemia, hyperglycaemia and DKA.

Chronic: Microvascular (retinopathy, neuropathy, nephropathy, cataracts) and macrovascular (ischaemic heart disease, hypertension, CVA) disease.

PROGNOSIS Depends on quality of glycaemic control. ↑d morbidity and mortality with DKA.

DEFINITION   Third extra non-sex (autosomal) chromosome 21. Normally homologous pairs.

AETIOLOGY
Non-dysjunction at meiosis (95%): Extra maternal chromosome: karyotype 47XX + 21 or 47XY + 21. Increased incidence of trisomy 21 2° to non-dysjunction with increasing maternal age, especially >35 years and is independent of paternal age.
Robertsonian translocation (4%): Chromosome 21 usually translocated onto chromosome 14.
Mosaicism (1%): Some cells normal, some trisomy 21 due to non-dysjunction during mitosis after fertilisation; usually less severely affected.

ASSOCIATIONS/RELATED
Congenital heart disease (40%): AVSD, VSD, ASD, Fallot tetralogy, PDA.
Gastrointestinal: Anal, oesophageal and duodenal atresia (one-third of infants with duodenal atresia are syndromic), Hirschsprung's disease.
Chronic secretory otitis media: Gives rise to conductive hearing loss.
Others: Recurrent respiratory infections, cataracts, squints, hypothyroidism.

EPIDEMIOLOGY   1/700 live births. Most common genetic cause of learning difficulties. Second affected child is 1/200 if >35 and double the age-specific rate if <35.

HISTORY AND EXAMINATION   Most cases of Down syndrome are now diagnosed antenatally (see Investigations).
General: Neonatal hypotonia, short stature.
Developmental: Mild–moderate learning disability (IQ 25–70, with social skills exceeding other intellectual functions).
Craniofacial: Microcephaly, brachycephaly (shortness of skull), round face, epicanthic folds, upward sloping palpebral fissures, protruding tongue, flat nasal bridge, small ears, excess skin at back of neck, atlantoaxial instability.
Eyes: Strabismus, nystagmus, Brushfield spots in iris, cataracts.
Limbs: Fifth finger clinodactyly, single palmar crease, wide gap between first and second toes, hyperflexible joints in infants.
CVS: Murmurs dependent on congenital heart disease, arrhythmias, signs of heart failure.
GI: Constipation.

PATHOPHYSIOLOGY   See Aetiology.

INVESTIGATIONS
Antenatal screening: Maternal age combined with the 'triple test' at 19/40 on maternal serum: AFP ($\downarrow$), unconjugated oestriol ($\downarrow$) and β-hCG ($\uparrow$).
Confirmation of diagnosis: Prenatal examination of fetal cells from amniocentesis or chorionic villus sampling, postnatal chromosomal analysis.
Screening for complications: Echocardiography, TFTs, hearing and vision tests.

MANAGEMENT
Multidisciplinary approach: Parental education and support, genetic counselling, IQ testing with appropriate educational input.
Medical: Antibiotics in recurrent respiratory infections, thyroid hormone for hypothyroidism.
Surgical: Congenital heart defects, oesophageal/duodenal atresia.

COMPLICATIONS   Decreased fertility. 15 × decreased risk of leukaemia; transient myeloproliferative disorder and AML (mutations in the haematopoietic transcription factor gene, *GATA1*). ↑d incidence of Alzheimer's disease by 40 years (amyloid protein coding gene located on chromosome 21).

PROGNOSIS
Antenatal: 75% of trisomy 21 spontaneously abort.
Childhood: 15–20% of Down syndrome children die <5 years, usually due to severe congenital heart disease.
Adulthood: 50% survive longer than 50 years but undergo premature ageing.

DEFINITION X-linked recessive degenerative muscle disorders, characterised by progressive muscle weakness and wasting of variable distribution and severity.
DMD: Rapidly progressive form.
BMD: Slowly progressive form.

AETIOLOGY
DMD: Gene mutations on Xp21 result in the absence of dystrophin (<5% of normal). Two-thirds are inherited, one-third are *de novo* mutations. Dystrophin protein forms part of a membrane-spanning protein complex of the muscle sarcolemma. This connects the cytoskeleton to the basal lamina.
BMD: Exon deletions exist in the dystrophin gene Xp21 in 70% of cases. Dystrophin levels are 30–80% of normal. Abnormal translation of the dystrophin gene produces abnormal but partially functional dystrophin.

ASSOCIATIONS/RELATED Family history.

EPIDEMIOLOGY
DMD: 1/3000 live male births.
BMD: 3–6/100,000 live male births.

HISTORY
DMD: Child appears healthy at birth. Onset of symptoms from 1–6 years with a waddling gait, toe-walking, difficulty running, climbing stairs or getting up from a seated or lying position. By 10 years braces are required for walking, by 12 years most children are wheelchair bound. In 20% there is associated learning disability.
BMD: Symptoms appear around 10 years and are a milder version of those in DMD.

EXAMINATION
Distribution of muscle weakness: Symmetrical pelvic and shoulder girdle weakness
Calf muscle pseudohypertrophy: Excess adipose replacement of muscle fibres.
Gower's sign: Child pushes hands down against thighs to overcome proximal muscle and pelvic girdle weakness to stand up from seated position on floor.

PATHOPHYSIOLOGY Variation in muscle fibre size, segmental necrosis of fibre groups. Initially, fibre regeneration occurs, but this fails and → loss of muscle and replacement by adipose cells and connective tissue.

INVESTIGATIONS
Bloods: ↑CK present from birth.
Genetic testing.
EMG: Establishes myopathic nature; excludes neurogenic causes of muscle weakness.
Muscle biopsy: Immunostaining for dystrophin.
Lung function: ↓ vital capacity (VC) 2° to ↓ muscle strength leads to hypoventilation and atelectasis.

MANAGEMENT
Multidisciplinary approach
Medical:

1. Oral glucocorticoids improve muscle strength over 6 months to 2 years. Observational studies suggest improved function over 5 years
2. Early aggressive management of cardiomyopathy
3. Respiratory care and assisted respiration may be required at a later stage
4. Immunisations: usual + pneumococcal and influenza
5. Prophylactic antibiotics for children with low VC.

Orthopaedic: Contracture correction and scoliosis repair to maintain mobility and preserve lung function. Scapular fixation.

Occupational/physiotherapy: Moderate physical exercise, mobility aids, night splints, braces and spinal supports.

Education: Mainstream with support or special schools for children with physical disabilities and/or learning disability.

Genetic counselling of female family members: CVS is 95% accurate.

Psychological: Support and counselling for parent and child. Respite care.

COMPLICATIONS   Loss of mobility, limb contractures, scoliosis, osteoporosis, respiratory insufficiency and infection, dilated cardiomyopathy at >15 years. Side effects of long-term oral steroids.

PROGNOSIS

DMD: Respiratory and cardiac failure is the main cause of death. Few live beyond their late twenties.

BMD: Disease develops later and less rapidly. Most patients walk beyond 16 years of age and may maintain this into adulthood.

DEFINITION   Inflammation of the brain parenchyma.

AETIOLOGY
Viruses: Enteroviruses, HSV1, HSV2, VZV, arboviruses, adenoviruses, HIV, mumps (rare now due to immunisation), rubella and rabies.
Post-measles: Subacute sclerosing panencephalitis (SSPE).

ASSOCIATIONS/RELATED   Foreign travel, measles, immunosuppression, active maternal HSV2 infection.

EPIDEMIOLOGY
Prevalence: 1/100,000.
Peak age: 3–8 months. Most common in <4 years.

HISTORY
General: Lethargy, poor feeding, irritability, hypotonia, behavioural change, vomiting.
Neurological: Headache, drowsiness, confusion, photophobia, neck pain, seizures (focal fits suggestive of HSV encephalitis).

ASSOCIATIONS/RELATED   Pharyngitis, conjunctivitis, myositis.

EXAMINATION
General: Fever, ↓GCS, positive Kernig sign; pain on extension of the knee with hips and knees flexed whilst in a supine position.
Neurological: Cranial nerve and motor abnormalities, ataxia (varicella-associated encephalitis)

PATHOPHYSIOLOGY
Infectious: Viruses enter the bloodstream during systemic febrile illness and affect several organs. There is further viral replication and subsequent invasion into the brain parenchyma with cell destruction, localised inflammation, swelling and inflammation of the meninges. HSV probably reaches the brain directly via neuronal axons.
Postinfectious: Immune-mediated reaction to viral antigens that → perivascular inflammation and demyelination

INVESTIGATIONS
Bloods: FBC, blood culture, glucose, U&Es, serum and urine osmolality (SIADH).
LP for CSF: WCC normal/↑ lymphocytes, protein mildly ↑/normal, glucose ↓/normal.
CSF microscopy: Gram stain, culture and sensitivity.
CSF PCR: HSV.
CSF serology: HSV antibody can be detected in the CSF in later stages.
Radiology: CT/MRI brain may show oedema or focal lesions (particularly in the temporal lobes) with HSV encephalitis.
EEG: Shows diffuse slow wave activity usually without focal changes.
Intracranial pressure monitoring: May be required in severe cases.

MANAGEMENT
Empirical antibiotic therapy: Third-generation cephalosporin is indicated until bacterial meningitis is excluded.
Supportive: Fluid resuscitation and correction of electrolyte imbalance (SIADH), anticonvulsants for seizures, analgesia for headache.
Antivirals: All children with suspected encephalitis should initially be treated with aciclovir to cover the possibility of HSV encephalitis. Confirmed HSV encephalitis requires a 3-week course of IV aciclovir.
Follow-up: Regular neurological and audiological assessment.
Prevention: MMR vaccine.

COMPLICATIONS   HSV encephalitis may cause hemiparesis, deafness, epilepsy, visual impairment, bilateral motor impairment, learning and language difficulties. Neurological deficits also occur following arbovirus and 2° viral infection in HIV patients.

PROGNOSIS   Many cases of encephalitis make a full recovery but this is dependent on age, aetiology and severity. There is a 70% mortality rate with untreated HSV encephalitis, and survivors often have severe neurological defects.

DEFINITION Uncommon life-threatening emergency 2° to inflammation of the epiglottis and supraglottic structures causing upper respiratory obstruction.

AETIOLOGY Traditionally caused by an infection with the bacterium *Haemophilus influenzae* B (Hib). Since immunisation, *Staph. aureus* or group A streptococci most common organism. Traumatic epiglottitis from direct trauma or thermal injury can occur +/− *Staph. aureus* infection.

ASSOCIATIONS/RELATED ↑d risk in the non-immunised child.

Acute stridor differential diagnosis: Acute laryngotracheobronchitis (croup); child is less toxic, and develops over greater period of time (days), foreign body, measles, EBV and diphtheria.

EPIDEMIOLOGY Rare condition (UK) since introduction of the Hib vaccine. Most common between 2 and 4 years. M > F.

HISTORY

Sudden onset: Very unwell child, pyrexia, drooling 2° to inability to swallow due to pain in pharynx. Not usually hoarse and rarely has a cough (to differentiate from croup).

EXAMINATION

General: Unwell, toxic looking, pyrexial (>38.5 °C), ↑HR.

Specific signs:

1. Difficulty breathing and stridor (harsh inspiratory noise)
2. Unable to talk and swallow due to intensely painful throat
3. Drooling, with characteristic sitting posture (sitting upright with the throat thrust forward).

Don't examine the child's throat as this may precipitate acute airway obstruction.

PATHOPHYSIOLOGY Epiglottis looks cherry-red and swollen due to inflammation 2° to acute bacterial infection. Supraglottic tissues surrounding the epiglottis, including the aryepiglottic folds, arytenoid soft tissue and occasionally the uvula may also be affected. The tightly bound epithelium on the vocal cords halts oedematous spread at this level.

INVESTIGATIONS

Take bloods only after intubation to prevent acute airway obstruction.

Bloods: ↑WCC with neutrophilia and ↑d CRP.

Blood cultures: ? causative bacteria.

ABG: To determine severity of respiratory compromise.

MANAGEMENT

Fast action is imperative to avoid acute airway obstruction.

1. Admit and transfer to intensive care unit accompanied by ENT surgeon equipped to perform emergency tracheostomy if necessary.
2. Call for senior anaesthetist to make diagnosis by laryngoscopy.
3. If appearance on laryngoscopy is typical of epiglottitis, electively intubate before obstruction occurs.
4. Third-generation cephalosporin, e.g. cefotaxime IV as Hib strains resistant to ampicillin and chloramphenicol are prevalent; continue for 5 days. Or antibiotic therapy to target likely pathogens in the context of the clinical setting.
5. Hydrocortisone is often given, but is of unproven value.

Prophylaxis: With rifampicin is offered to close household contacts.

COMPLICATIONS Acute airway obstruction leading to hypoxia and 2° ischaemic injuries.

PROGNOSIS With prompt diagnosis and management, most children recover within 3–5 days. Expect to extubate after 24–48 hours. Mortality can be 10% with an unprotected airway.

DEFINITION   Two or more seizures unprovoked by any immediately identifiable cause.

CLASSIFICATION   The International League Against Epilepsy (ILAE) classifies epilepsy seizures by localisation (in which part of the brain the epileptic activity starts) and aetiology:

1. *Generalised*: large part of cortex is involved, consciousness is impaired
2. *Localised (focal, local, partial)*: begins in a focal area of the cerebral cortex
3. *Symptomatic epilepsy*: cause is known
4. *Cryptogenic epilepsy*: presumed to be symptomatic but the aetiology is not known
5. *Idiopathic epilepsy*: no apparent cause.

At present, a task force is revising this classification.

AETIOLOGY
Idiopathic: Many have positive family history.
Symptomatic: Head trauma, encephalitis, meningitis, CNS tumours, hypoxic–ischaemic injury, intrauterine infections, cerebral dysgenesis and specific aetiologies (e.g. TS).

ASSOCIATIONS/RELATED   Non-epileptiform attack disorder (also known as pseudo-seizures).
DD: 'Fits, faints and funny turns' such as postural hypotension or cardiac arrhythmias.

EPIDEMIOLOGY   1% of children suffer from epilepsy.

HISTORY
Generalised seizures
Absence seizures: Onset 4–12 years. Short episodes (<20 s) during which the child stares or blinks, with no apparent awareness of the surroundings. Can occur >100×/d. No aura or postictal phase. May present as 'day-dreaming' in class or ↓ in school performance. Usually undergo spontaneous remission during adolescence.
Myoclonic seizures: Sudden brief muscle contractions; often cluster within a few minutes. If they evolve into rhythmic jerking movements, they are classified as a clonic seizure.
Atonic seizures: Consist of brief loss of postural tone, often resulting in falls and injuries. This seizure type occurs in people with significant neurological abnormalities.
Clonic seizures: Rhythmic, jerking movements.
Tonic seizures: Sudden-onset tonic extension or flexion of the head, trunk and/or extremities for several seconds.
Generalised tonic-clonic seizure (GTCS): Tonic extension lasting for a few seconds followed by clonic rhythmic movements and a prolonged postictal phase. Often associated with tongue biting, urinary or faecal incontinence.
Status epilepticus: A generalised convulsion lasting ≥30 minutes or repeated convulsions occurring over 30 minutes without recovery of consciousness between each convulsion.

Partial-onset seizures
Simple partial seizures: Seizure with preservation of consciousness; includes sensory, motor, autonomic and psychic experiences. Tonic or clonic movements are initially localised but may move to different parts of the body if the seizure is propagated.
Complex partial seizures: Similar to simple partial seizure but consciousness is impaired and the episode is followed by postictal phase.
Partial seizures with 2° generalisation: Focal seizure is followed by GTCS.

Epilepsy syndromes
Infantile spasms: Affect infants aged 4–8 months. Clusters of myoclonic spasms; classic 'salaam' attack where child jerks forward with arms flexed and hands extended. Usually have chronic epilepsy and developmental delay.

Lennox–Gastaut syndrome: Affects children aged 1–3 years. Characterised by multiple seizure types (tonic-axial, atonic and absence seizures), developmental regression and learning disability. Often chronic epilepsy resistant to therapy.

Benign childhood epilepsy with centrotemporal spike: Affects children aged 4–10 years. Clonic seizures affecting face and upper limbs usually during sleep; may progress to GTCS. Also known as benign Rolandic epilepsy. Usually undergo spontaneous remission during adolescence.

Juvenile myoclonic epilepsy: Affects adolescents; idiopathic generalised epileptic syndrome characterised by myoclonic jerks, GTCS and sometimes absence seizures, usually on awakening. Usually require lifelong treatment but not associated with intellectual impairment.

EXAMINATION   General and neurological examination to rule out specific aetiologies (TS) and focal neurological signs.

PATHOPHYSIOLOGY   Imbalance between excitatory and inhibitory neurotransmission resulting in high-frequency burst activity seen as spike and wave on EEG. Seizure propagates if sufficient surrounding neurons are recruited.

INVESTIGATIONS

EEG: Epileptiform spike and wave activity correlates with different forms of epilepsy (hypsarrhythmia in infantile spasms).

MRI: To rule out underlying pathology, e.g. glial tumour.

Lumbar puncture. If infective cause suspected.

ECG/ECHO/lying/standing BP: To exclude other causes of fit, faints and funny turns.

MANAGEMENT

Education: Explain nature of epilepsy to parent and child. Aim is to give child the most confidence and independence possible. Avoid precipitating factors such as alcohol, sleep deprivation, drugs. Supervision when in swimming pools or baths. Information on driving and insurance. Advice on sudden unexpected death in epilepsy (SUDEP). Side effects of AED (e.g. teratogenicity of sodium valproate).

Follow-up: All children with epilepsy should have structured review at least yearly.

Acute treatment of seizure (see Appendix 11): Long-term antiepileptic medication (AED) is used in the following situations.

Generalised epilepsy. *Absence seizures*: sodium valproate, lamotrigine, ethosuximide, topiramate. Exacerbated by carbamazepine. *Myoclonic*: sodium valproate, lamotrigine, topiramate, levetiracetam (adjunct). *Tonic-clonic*: sodium valproate (first-line), topiramate, lamotrigine, levetiracetam (adjunct).

Partial epilepsy: Carbamazepine (first-line), topiramate, lamotrigine, gabapentin.

Epilepsy syndromes. *Infantile spasms*: ACTH, prednisolone, vigabatrin. *Lennox–Gastaut syndrome*: lamotrigine, topiramate, vigabatrin. *Benign childhood epilepsy with centrotemporal spike*: carbamazepine (problematic or daytime seizures only). *Juvenile myoclonic epilepsy*: sodium valproate.

Ketogenic diet: May be considered in children with drug-resistant epilepsy.

COMPLICATIONS   Developmental delay, poor school performance, SUDEP (500 deaths/year).

PROGNOSIS   Remission depends predominantly on the type of epilepsy. Patients with epilepsy have a mortality rate 2–3 × that of the general population.

DEFINITION   Congenital anterior wall defects resulting in herniation of abdominal viscera.

AETIOLOGY

Embryology: Abdominal wall formation is 2° to infolding of the cranial, caudal and two lateral embryonic folds. Migration of the rapidly growing intestine occurs through the umbilical ring during 6/40. At 10–12/40 the abdominal wall is formed and the intestine undergoes 270° counter-clockwise rotation before returning to the abdominal cavity.

Exomphalos: The bowel does not return to the abdomen, remaining in the umbilical cord. Unknown exact aetiology but probably 2° to failure of abdominal wall folding. From Greek meaning 'outside the navel', also called omphalocoele.

Gastroschisis: Likely to be 2° to an ischaemic injury to the developing anterior abdominal wall. Right paraumbilical area is at risk as it is dependent on right umbilical vein and right omphalomesenteric artery for its blood supply until they involute. Disruptions in this involution process may lead to ischaemia. Translation: 'stomach cleft'.

ASSOCIATIONS/RELATED

General: Factors affecting placental insufficiency; maternal illness and infection, drug dependency, smoking.

Exomphalos: Common associated anomalies resulting from chromosomal abnormalities (most commonly trisomy 18 and 13). ↑d maternal age. *Pentalogy of Cantrell*: cranial fold deficits; epigastric exomphalos, anterior diaphragmatic hernias, sternal clefts, pericardial and cardiac defects.

Gastroschisis: Rare associated anomalies, intestinal atresia 25%, cryptorchism. ↓d maternal age.

EPIDEMIOLOGY

Exomphalos: 3/10,000.

Gastroschisis: 4–5/10,000.

HISTORY AND EXAMINATION

Antenatal: USS detection common. *In utero* transfer to paediatric surgical centre with antenatal parental counselling.

Exomphalos: Herniation of the bowel, liver +/− other organs into the intact umbilical cord. Herniated viscera are covered by a membrane.

Gastroschisis: Intact umbilical cord and evisceration of the bowel through a defect generally to the right of the cord. No membrane covering. Appearance of red matted bowel loops.

PATHOPHYSIOLOGY   See Aetiology.

INVESTIGATIONS

Ultrasound: Screening for associated anomalies.

Amniocentesis: Antenatal diagnosis of karyotyping and chromosomal abnormalities.

MANAGEMENT

General: Postnatal resuscitation, NGT with frequent aspirations, IV access with dextrose infusion. Possible intubation with ventilation +/− surfactant therapy. Broad-spectrum prophylactic antibiotics. Minimisation of insensible losses (cling-film therapy).

Surgical (initial): Prompt assessment to ensure that the bowel is not compromised by twisting of its mesenteric vascular pedicle. If compromise present, needs urgent surgical intervention.

Surgical (definitive): Majority of lesions repaired by 1° closure. Larger lesions may require a prefabricated spring-loaded Silastic silo which may be applied on the neonatal unit or theatre as appropriate. Gentle staged reduction is then achieved over the next 1–2/52. With complete closure and reduction then intra-abdominal pressure should be monitored with intragastric pressure monitoring (<20 mmHg).

COMPLICATIONS Adhesions, short gut syndrome, syndrome-specific complications, antenatal volvulus.

PROGNOSIS The prognosis is good with antenatal diagnosis, adequate supportive and surgical management in a specialized centre. In exomphalos ↓d prognosis with co-existing abnormalities.

DEFINITION   Voluntary or involuntary passing of faeces in inappropriate places after the age at which faecal continence is considered normal (>4 years).

AETIOLOGY
Retentive encopresis: Most common; 2° to functional constipation (constipation not associated with abnormality/medication use). Constipation → progressive rectal distension and stretching of the internal/external anal sphincters (IAS/EAS) → chronic rectal distension and loss of normal defaecation sensation.
Non-retentive faecal soiling: Occurs without constipation.
Emotional: May have an impact although not primarily a behavioural problem. Low self-esteem, parent–child conflict results from the disorder rather than being causative.

ASSOCIATIONS/RELATED   Surgical interventions for Hirschsprung's disease and anorectal malformations, neuropathy, behavioural problems, low birthweight and enuresis.

EPIDEMIOLOGY   1–3/100 (age dependent; $4 = 3/100$, $>10 = 1–2/100$), M:F = 4:1.

HISTORY   Detailed history from child and carer important: stooling/sensation/constipation. Children on average are symptomatic for 5 years prior to presentation. Nocturnal encopresis uncommon.

EXAMINATION
Abdominal: Distension or palpable stool.
Digital rectal examination: Anal fissures or tears. Stool around perianal region. Anal sphincter may appear lax 2° to massive rectal distension and relaxation of the IAS. Normal anal wink and sensation. Rectum normally filled with soft stool.

PATHOPHYSIOLOGY   See Aetiology.

INVESTIGATIONS
Anorectal manometry: Delineating child's defaecation dynamics, evidence of megarectum, exclusion of ultra-short segment Hirschsprung's disease.
Radionuclear transit scintography: Identifies slow colonic transit. May also be done with plain AXR after ingestion of different shaped markers.

MANAGEMENT
Medical: Constipation management with diet control. Colonic evacuation (disimpaction) may be required before the establishment of routine laxative therapy. Laxative (e.g. Sennakot) at night encourages a motion in the morning after breakfast (gastrocolic reflex). Movicol is a commonly used medication. An enema programme may also be initiated.
Behavioural strategies: May be used in combination with medical therapy. Regularly scheduled toileting, maintenance of a symptom diary and an age-appropriate incentive scheme.
Parental and child education: Techniques to reinforce good behaviour, including encouragement during periods of relapse. Exploration of the child's self-perception and its relationship with soiling; behavioural programmes can help the child to recognise their own body signals.
Biofeedback training: Children with chronic encopresis have paradoxical constriction of their EAS (anismus) during attempted defaecation; biofeedback training allows EAS relaxation during active straining.
Surgical intervention: Antegrade continence enema (ACE) either proximally (pACE or Mallone procedure) or distally (dACE). Allows the administration of enemas directly into the caecum or the distal colon to treat constipation causing retentive encopresis.

COMPLICATIONS   Low self-esteem with associated social acceptance problems.

PROGNOSIS   Depends on the underlying cause. Unusual for encopresis to persist beyond middle teenage years.

DEFINITION   Failure to thrive (also known as faltering growth) is a description applied to children whose current weight or rate of weight gain is significantly below that of other children of similar age and sex.

Continual assessment: Crossing two major growth percentiles for weight.

AETIOLOGY
Functional (most common cause):

1. *Nutritional neglect:* poor understanding of feeding techniques, exclusion diets.
2. *Emotional neglect:* stimulus deprivation.
3. *Abuse:* physical, sexual, fabricated and induced illness (also known as Munchausen's syndrome by proxy).
4. *Psychiatric:* AN, depression.

Organic:

1. *Feeding difficulties:* mechanical (cleft palate disorders), neurological (CP).
2. *Poor retention of food:* GORD, eosinophilic oesophagitis.
3. *Poor absorption of food:* coeliac disease, inflammatory bowel disease, CF.
4. *Poor metabolism of food:* metabolic (hypothyroidism, GH deficiency), inborn errors of metabolism (glycogen storage disorders, galactosaemia).
5. ↑ *Metabolism:* CHD, CF.
6. *Chronic disease:* anaemia, recurrent UTIs, CRF, HIV.
7. *Chromosomal abnormalities:* Down syndrome, Turner syndrome.

ASSOCIATIONS/RELATED   Poor socio-economic circumstances, parents with psychiatric illness.

EPIDEMIOLOGY   Between 6 weeks to 1 year prevalence is mild in 5% and severe in 1%.

HISTORY
General: Antenatal history, perinatal/postnatal complications, birth weight.
Feeding history: Record of food consumption, e.g. frequency of breastfeeding or meals/day + snacks, reflux symptoms, frequency of stools, mucus, blood in stools.
Social history: Assess parenting skills and any possibility of neglect or abuse.

EXAMINATION
General: Observe child's demeanour, level of activity, interaction with parent and and sibling.
Measure: Height, weight, head circumference (restriction is a late sign) and plot serially on a standard growth chart. Look at Red Book.
Signs of malnutrition: Wasting, muscle loss (buttocks, particularly in coeliac disease).
Developmental assessment: Milestones, school performance, pubertal development

PATHOPHYSIOLOGY   See Aetiology.
INVESTIGATIONS
Bloods: Hb, TFTs, U&E, CRP, ESR, coeliac screen (if indicated).
Specific tests: May be indicated if an organic cause is suspected, e.g. sweat test in CF, karyotype, USS renal tract.

MANAGEMENT   Frequent follow-up.
Nutritional cause: Can be treated with a balanced diet of proteins, carbohydrates, vitamins, minerals and parental education. Involve paediatric dietitian.
Functional cause: A multidisciplinary approach is required, with involvement of social workers, GP, teachers and psychologists.
Organic cause: Treat the underlying disorder.
Hospitalisation May be required for assessment and observation of feeding and behavioural patterns.

COMPLICATIONS   Developmental delay, stunting of growth, complications of underlying condition, psychological implications.

PROGNOSIS   Depends on the duration before effective treatment begins. The longer the delay before diagnosis, the less likely that normal growth and development will be achieved.

DEFINITION   Seizure associated with fever occurring in a child between 6 months and 5 years. Febrile seizures usually arise from infection/inflammation outside the CNS in an otherwise neurologically normal child. Seizures arising from fever due to meningitis or encephalitis are *not* included in the definition of febrile convulsion.

Simple febrile seizure: Isolated, brief, generalised clonic/tonic-clonic seizure.

Complex febrile seizure: >15 minutes, focal features, repeat seizure within the same illness or incomplete recovery from seizure <1 hour.

Febrile status epilepticus: Duration >30 min (up to 5% present as status epilepticus).

AETIOLOGY

Genetic: >50% concordance rate in monozygotic twins, family history of febrile seizures.

ASSOCIATIONS/RELATED

DD: CNS infection, epilepsy.

EPIDEMIOLOGY   3–4% in Western Europe and USA, up to 9% in Japan.

Peak age: 18 months.

HISTORY   Determine the cause of the fever: viral URTI, otitis media, pneumonia, UTI or gastroenteritis. Febrile seizures may occur after immunisation (not a contraindication to future immunisation with the same vaccine).

EXAMINATION   Assess cause of fever: respiratory distress, ENT examination.

Exclude signs of CNS infection:

- **Meningitis:** Strongly consider in febrile child <12 months old.
- **Encephalitis:** Change in behaviour, persistent drowsiness or irritability.

PATHOPHYSIOLOGY   The mechanisms causing febrile seizures are not known.

INVESTIGATIONS   MSU, CXR, LP (if suspicion of meningitis/encephalitis), contraindicated if focal neurology or signs of ↑ICP.

Bloods: Glucose, U&Es, WCC, CRP, blood cultures as appropriate.

MANAGEMENT

Termination of seizure: Majority require no medical intervention. Rectal diazepam/buccal midazolam if seizure persists longer than 3–4 min.

Status epilepticus requires full protocol (see Appendix 11).

Reassurance and education:

1. *Antipyretics*: controlling fever does not prevent recurrence but does make the child more comfortable if they are distressed. Explain that aim of controlling fever is to ease symptoms and prevent dehydration. Tepid sponging and fanning are not recommended. Advise parents how to assess for dehydration and signs of more serious disease (non-blanching rash/signs of meningism).
2. Prevent accidental injury from fall during seizure but do not restrain.
3. Inform of excellent prognosis with very minimal risk of epilepsy.

Criteria for admission:

1. First febrile convulsion
2. Diagnostic uncertainty about the underlying cause of the seizure
3. Complex febrile seizure
4. <18 months of age
5. Pretreatment with antibiotics (masked meningitis)
6. 'Unwell child'
7. Social circumstances.

Seizure prophylaxis (Children at risk of/with history of prolonged/multiple seizures):

1. Rectal diazepam at onset of febrile illness
2. Regular antiepileptics are rarely indicated.

COMPLICATIONS   Mesial-temporal sclerosis is associated with prolonged febrile status epilepticus (>90 min).

PROGNOSIS

Recurrence: One-third of children will experience a recurrence. Risk factors for recurrence include <18 months, family history of febrile seizures or epilepsy, complex febrile seizure and day care nursery attendance (increased frequency of febrile episodes).

Developmental sequelae: No subsequent deficit in cognitive ability/school performance.

Epilepsy: 1–2% will develop epilepsy; ↑ risk if family history of epilepsy, neurodevelopmental abnormality or complex febrile seizure.

Mortality: Low even in febrile status epilepticus.

DEFINITION Immune-mediated hypersensitivity reaction to food proteins.

AETIOLOGY Parental atopy. Atopic eczema.

ASSOCIATIONS/RELATED Eczema, asthma, allergic rhinitis – the 'allergic march'.

EPIDEMIOLOGY 6–8% of children. 90% of food-allergic reactions in children are caused by six major foods: cow's milk (prevalence 2–2.5%), egg (prevalence 1.6–3.2%), peanut (prevalence 1.4–1.8%), fish (1.3%), soybean and wheat (0.25%). Other important allergenic foods include crustaceans, tree-nuts, celery, mustard, sesame seeds, sulphites (EU labelling regulations).

HISTORY AND EXAMINATION
Immediate IgE mediated (occurs within 2 hours):

1. *Skin*: Flush, itch, urticaria and angio-oedema
2. *Respiratory*: Wheeze/cough 2° to bronchospasm, stridor 2° to laryngeal oedema
3. *CVS*: Tachycardia, hypotension
4. *GI*: Vomiting, diarrhoea, abdominal pain.

Mixed IgE and non-IgE mediated: (2–12 hours):

1. *Skin*: Atopic eczema (cow's milk, egg, soya or wheat)
2. *GI*: Eosinophilic eosophagitis; reflux, food aversion, dysphagia (cow's milk, egg, soya or wheat).

Delayed non-IgE mediated (occurs 12–24 hours after):

1. *GI*: Food protein-induced enterocolitis (FPIES)/enteropathy/enterocolitis, commonly cow or soya milk but also solids (fish, wheat). Failure to thrive.

PATHOPHYSIOLOGY
IgE mediated: Exposure to food protein in a presensitised individual leads to IgE cross-linking on mast cells. This triggers degranulation releasing inflammatory mediators such as histamine and leukotrienes.
Non-IgE mediated: Food protein is taken up by antigen-presenting cells and presented to T cells. Th2 cells interact with B cells and produce allergic cytokines and interleukins leading to inflammation.

INVESTIGATIONS
IgE mediated: Skin prick tests and specific IgE 95% positive predictive values have been validated for cow's milk, egg and peanut. Gold standard for diagnosis remains a double-blind placebo-controlled food challenge. Open challenges are often performed in clinical practice.
Non-IgE mediated: There are no good diagnostics tests for non-IgE mediated reactions apart from diagnostic trial of exclusion followed by reintroduction under dietetic review.
Bloods: Signs of gut inflammation/malabsorption ($\uparrow$plts, $\downarrow$albumin, $\downarrow$Hb, $\downarrow$iron).

MANAGEMENT
Avoidance: Once allergy has been confirmed, dietitian input is important to ensure adequate alternative sources of nutrients and advice on eating out, hidden sources and 'may contain' labelling.
Emergency plan: Families must be provided with a written emergency plan. Parent/patient should be taught how to assess severity of allergic reaction, whether and how to administer self-injectable adrenaline device. Advise Medic-Alert bracelets.

Indications for self-injectable adrenaline device
Absolute: Previous cardiorespiratory symptoms, exercise-induced anaphylaxis, idiopathic anaphylaxis and persistent asthma with food allergy.

Relative: Any reaction to a small amount of food (contact/airborne), peanut or tree-nut allergy, remoteness from medical facilities, food allergy in a teenager.

COMPLICATIONS   Anaphylaxis is a real and severe complication of food allergy and can be fatal. Peanuts have been shown to be responsible for the majority of fatal food-induced anaphylaxis in the UK and USA.

PROGNOSIS   Children are likely to grow out of cow's milk, egg, wheat and soya allergy. Peanut (80%), tree-nut (>90%), fish and shellfish allergy usually persists into adulthood.

DEFINITION   Disruption in the integrity and continuity of bone associated with soft tissue injury.

AETIOLOGY

Trauma: Force applied to bone exceeds its strength. Direct force (penetrative, crushing) or indirect (tension, compression or rotation injuries).

Greenstick: Incomplete fracture with angulation on the opposite side due to stronger fibrous periosteum in children.

Pathological: Minor force causes fracture 2° to underlying bone weakness (malignancy, congenital).

Salter-Harris classification: Epiphyseal injuries: involve growth plate, types I–V depending on involvement of the physis, metaphysis and epiphysis.

ASSOCIATIONS/RELATED   Contact sports, trampoline use, RTAs and other traumas, rickets, osteogenesis imperfecta, non-accidental injury (NAI).

EPIDEMIOLOGY   Common. M>F. Incidence ↑d with age. Majority 2° to sports and leisure activities, minority 2° to assaults, RTAs, pathological causes.

HISTORY   Mechanism of injury; whether this is consistent with the child's developmental stage and injury sustained. Additionally, where, time elapsed, force, possibility of glass contamination, associated head injury, medications, previous injury or fractures and SHx. Low threshold for suspecting NAI.

EXAMINATION

Closed fracture: Pallor and swelling over fracture site, obvious deformity.

Open fracture: Bleeding and bruising over fracture, associated soft tissue injury.

Neurovascular status: Assess for distal numbness, tingling, paralysis or loss of pulse.

Musculoskeletal examination: Examine joint above and below for crepitus, effusion and pain.

Tuning fork test: Exacerbates pain over small stress fractures.

PATHOPHYSIOLOGY   Healing involves inflammation, followed by granulation tissue formation. Chondroblasts and osteoblasts form in the granulation tissue, leading to callus formation. Finally lamellar bone replaces mesh-like callus and is remodelled by osteoclasts.

INVESTIGATIONS

X-ray: Rule of 2s: 2 views (frontal/lateral), 2 joints. Repeat 7–14/7 later in fracture clinic if fracture not immediately apparent.

MRI: May be required to assess ligamentous/soft tissue injury.

Bone scan: Occasionally required to exclude stress fractures.

MANAGEMENT

Initial: Resuscitation, analgesia, stabilisation with splints.

Closed reduction: Manipulation under anaesthetic (MUA).

Open reduction and internal fixation: Adequate exposure before fracture is reduced using wires, plates, screws or nails.

External fixation: Avoids soft tissues that are adjacent to the fracture.

Immobilisation: With plaster casts, braces or splints attached from joint above to joint below to allow healing. Traction by application of tension aligns ends of fracture.

Physiotherapy: Prevents contractures and loss of function.

COMPLICATIONS

Short term: Neurovascular damage, malunion, non-union, delayed union of the fracture, infection (cellulitis/osteomyelitis), thromboembolic events (DVT, PE), avascular necrosis (scaphoid, femur), psychological impact of disabling condition.

Medium term: Compartment syndrome.

Long term: Fractures involving the growth plate may arrest growth. Fractures involving joint surfaces may lead to arthritis.

PROGNOSIS Typically upper limb fractures require 3–4 weeks and lower limb 6–8 weeks to heal (depends on site of fracture and health of child).

DEFINITION   Abdominal pain of sufficient severity to interfere with daily activities without demonstrable evidence of a pathological condition.

AETIOLOGY   Intermittent or continuous. Rome III criteria classification. Chronic pain >1–2/ 12. Often misdiagnosed. Unknown exact aetiology; proposed mechanisms include:

1. *Enteric nervous system (ENS)*: abnormal bowel reactivity to physiological stimuli (meal, luminal distension, hormonal changes), noxious stressful stimuli (inflammatory processes) or psychological stressful stimuli (parental separation, anxiety).
2. *Visceral hyperalgesia*: ↓d pain threshold to changes in intraluminal pressure 2° to sensitisation of afferent nerves by infections, allergies or 1° inflammatory diseases.
3. *Biopsychosocial model*: child's response to biological factors, governed by an interaction between the child's temperament and the family/school environments.

ASSOCIATIONS/RELATED   Possible psychological disturbances.

EPIDEMIOLOGY   4–25% of school-aged children.

HISTORY AND EXAMINATION   FAP needs to be distinguished from anatomical, infectious, inflammatory or metabolic causes of abdominal pain. May present with symptoms typical of functional dyspepsia, irritable bowel syndrome (IBS), abdominal migraine or functional abdominal pain syndrome.

1. *Irritable bowel syndrome (IBS)*: pain is often worse before and relieved by defaecation, stools contain excess mucus, children experience bloating, sensation of incomplete defaecation and constipation.
2. *Functional dyspepsia*: epigastric pain, postprandial vomiting, early satiety and GOR.
3. *Abdominal migraine*: paroxysmal pain with anorexia, N&V +/− pallor. Maternal migraine history.
4. *Functional abdominal pain syndrome (FAPS)*: FAP without the characteristics of dyspepsia, IBS or abdominal migraine.

PATHOPHYSIOLOGY
Organic disease biopsy microscopy: Marked basal layer hyperplasia, vascular ectasia and numerous intraepithelial eosinophils/lymphocytes (oesophagus), lymphoid aggregates (gastric antrum/fundus), crypt hyperplasia, moderate/marked villous atrophy, or ↑d intraepithelial lymphocytes (duodenum).

INVESTIGATIONS   If symptoms and signs indicate an organic cause: involuntary weight loss, deceleration of linear growth, gastrointestinal blood loss, significant vomiting, chronic severe diarrhoea, persistent RUQ/RIF pain, unexplained pyrexia, FHx IBD.
Endoscopy with negative biopsies (see above) may exclude organic disease. USS for RIF/RUQ pain (gallstones/ovarian cyst/appendiceal pathology).

MANAGEMENT
Supportive: FAP diagnosis should be made as a positive diagnosis (not exclusion), therefore limiting unnecessary investigations. Careful explanation, headache analogy (functional disorder rarely associated with serious disease), establishment of reasonable goals, reassurance of absence of organic disease.
Psychological: Cognitive-behavioural therapy and biofeedback; some supporting evidence (Cochrane database). General positive effect on children with true FAP.
Medical: Time-limited use of medications; H2-antagonists/proton pump inhibitors, peppermint oil enteric-coated capsules can aid symptom control. Poor evidence base (Cochrane database).
Dietary modifications: No evidence that fibre supplements, lactose-free diets or lactobacillus supplementation are effective (Cochrane database).

COMPLICATIONS Psychological impact and changed family dynamics. School absences may interfere with education.

PROGNOSIS Usually self-limiting (>50% spontaneously resolve) although may continue into adulthood as IBS.

Ringworm

DEFINITION Dermatophytosis (fungal infection) of keratin layer of skin, nails or hair. Called *ringworm* due to annular skin lesions produced.

AETIOLOGY Dermatophyte fungi infect the skin, nails or hair, reproduce by spore formation, and induce inflammation by delayed hypersensitivity or metabolic effects. Three genera of fungi responsible:

1. *Microsporum* (infect skin and hair)
2. *Trichophyton* (infect skin, nails and hair)
3. *Epidermophyton* (infect skin and nails).

Infections include: tinea capitis (scalp), tinea pedis (feet = athlete's foot), tinea unguium (nails), tinea corporis (trunk and limbs), tinea cruris (groin). (*Tinea* = Latin for worm.)

ASSOCIATIONS/RELATED Humid, sweaty conditions, e.g. occlusive footwear, moist bodyfolds, hyperhidrosis. Topical steroid use. Tinea capitis is often acquired from cats and dogs.

EPIDEMIOLOGY Tinea capitis is more common in children of Afro-Caribbean descent in whom scalp and hair are more susceptible to fungal infection.

HISTORY Generally itchy, red patches. In tinea capitis, hairs break just above the scalp, producing a *black dot* appearance.

EXAMINATION Ringworm occurs as asymmetrical, scaly, erythematous annular patches with an advancing raised border, central clearing and occasional vesicles/pustules at edge. In tinea capitis patchy alopecia occurs. In tinea pedis typical annular lesions are rarely seen; usually skin in toe clefts is white and fissured.

PATHOPHYSIOLOGY Dermatophytes infect keratin as branching hyphae. Silver stains and neutral polysaccharide stains (PAS) react with cell walls and reveal dermatophytes.

INVESTIGATIONS
Wood's light: Some fungi fluoresce greenish/yellow under Wood's light (filtered UV light).
Microscopy: Skin scrapings placed on a slide with 10% aqueous potassium hydroxide to examine for hyphae. Gives almost immediate diagnosis.
Culture: Skin scrapings, nail clippings or hair may be cultured in a medium for 3 weeks to identify the fungus.

MANAGEMENT
Topical antifungals: Imidazoles (Canesten) for tinea pedis and localised skin lesions.
Systemic antifungals: Griseofulvin for scalp infections. Terbinafine for nail infections.

COMPLICATIONS Kerion formation – severe inflammatory, pustular scalp ringworm patch.

PROGNOSIS Resolves with appropriate treatment.

Pityriasis versicolor

DEFINITION Chronic, asymptomatic, fungal infection characterised by pigmentary changes on the trunk.

AETIOLOGY Overgrowth of commensal yeast *Pityrosporum orbiculare (Malassezia furfur)*.

ASSOCIATIONS/RELATED Humid tropical conditions.

EPIDEMIOLOGY Common yeast infection in adolescence.

HISTORY Asymptomatic rash on trunk and upper arms.

EXAMINATION   Caucasians: reddish brown scaly macules. Dark-skinned patients: macular areas of hypopigmentation.

PATHOPHYSIOLOGY   Microscopic: 'grapes and bananas' appearance of spores and short hyphae.

INVESTIGATIONS   Skin scrapings for microscopy and culture, fluorescence by Wood's light.

MANAGEMENT   Selenium sulphide shampoo/topical imidazoles/oral itraconazole.

COMPLICATIONS   Inappropriate topical steroids spread the rash.

PROGNOSIS   Pigmentation takes months to recover. Recurrences are common.

DEFINITION   Inflammation of the gastrointestinal tract 2° to an acute infection by an enteropathogen.

AETIOLOGY
General: ↑ bacterial-induced gastroenteritis in the developing countries, ↑d viral in developed.
Viruses: Rotavirus (most common), adenovirus, calicivirus, coronavirus and astrovirus.
Bacteria:

1. *Neurotoxin producing*: *Staphylococcus aureus* and *Bacillus cereus*; cause severe vomiting shortly after ingestion, rarely cause diarrhoea.
2. *Enterotoxin producing*: *Escherichia coli* and *Vibrio cholerae* act directly on secretory mechanisms primarily by ↑d activation of cAMP and produce typical copious watery (rice water) diarrhoea. No mucosal invasion occurs.
3. *Cytotoxin producing*: *Shigella dysenteriae, Vibrio parahaemolyticus, Clostridium difficile* and enterohaemorrhagic *E. coli* result in enterocyte destruction, leading to bloody stools with inflammatory cells.
4. *Mucosal invasion*: *Shigella, Campylobacter* organisms and enteroinvasive *E. coli* cause mucosal destruction and inflammatory diarrhoea. *Salmonella* and *Yersinia* species invade the enterocytes but do not induce cell death so dysentery does not usually occur. However, bacterial translocation occurs via the lamina propria, causing enteric fever such as typhoid.

ASSOCIATIONS/RELATED   Poverty, malnutrition, lack of infrastructure, bottle feeding, antibiotic use and immunocompromise.

EPIDEMIOLOGY
Worldwide: 3–5 billion cases/year.
UK: Average child experiences two episodes of diarrhoea/year.

HISTORY
General: Pyrexia, anorexia, vomiting, abdominal pain and diarrhoea.
Specific: Features of diarrhoea (frequency/duration/character) and time-lapse between ingestion of food and symptoms may suggest infective organism (see Aetiology).

EXAMINATION   Assess degree of dehydration:

1. *Mild (<4%)*: no clinical signs
2. *Moderate (>5%)*: dry mucous membranes, ↓d skin turgor, cool peripheries, ↓CRT
3. *Severe (10%)*: skin laxity, sunken eyes and fontanelle, impaired peripheral circulation, acidotic breathing, restlessness, lethargy and oliguria
4. *Extreme (10–15%)*: anuric, shock or coma.

Stool examination: Mucus, blood (streaks/large amounts).

PATHOPHYSIOLOGY   Dehydration is the result of impaired absorption of water, electrolytes and sugars following mucosal damage or increase in secretory mechanisms.

INVESTIGATIONS
General: Weight and temperature monitoring.
Bloods: FBC, U&Es, LFTs.
Stool: MC&S.

MANAGEMENT
General: Mild–moderate dehydration may be managed at home with ORT.
Oral rehydration therapy (ORT): ESPGHAN recommendation for treatment of mild–moderate dehydration, also recommend rapid rehydration over 3–4 hours.
Mild dehydration: Short-term substitution of normal feeds with maintenance type of oral glucose-electrolyte solution 'Dioralyte', until ↓d symptoms.

Moderate dehydration: 6-h trial of oral rehydration (PO/NG) with 100 ml/kg. If no improvement >6 h, intravenous rehydration.
Severe dehydration: IV rehydration. Treat shocked patients with plasma expanders. Fluid deficit replacement as well as maintenance fluid requirement with allowances for future losses. Potassium supplementation should commence once the patient is passing urine.

COMPLICATIONS   Dehydration, post-gastroenteritis syndrome, acute renal failure in severe dehydration.

PROGNOSIS
Developing countries: 5 million children <5 years die/year (improvement with WHO-administered ORT programmes).
Developed countries: 1% mortality.

DEFINITION Abnormal retrograde flow of gastric contents from the stomach into the oesophagus.

AETIOLOGY
Gastroesophageal reflux (GOR): Normal in infants (60–70% have physiological reflux), predisposing factors include supine position, short and straight intra-abdominal length of the oesophagus (affecting angle of His), immature lower oesophageal sphincter (LES) function with multiple transient relaxations and a primarily milk diet.
Gastroesophageal reflux disease (GORD): When reflux frequency and duration produce symptoms. Common mechanisms: delay in neurological maturation (e.g. preterm infants), neurological impairment (cerebral palsy, hypoxic ischaemic encephalopathy, trisomy 21), excessive frequent spontaneous reductions in sphincter pressure (crying, coughing or defaecating).

ASSOCIATIONS/RELATED Cow's milk protein intolerance, oesophageal atresia, hiatus hernia.

EPIDEMIOLOGY 1/3000 infants. GORD is often overdiagnosed 2° to difficulty in differentiation between physiological and pathological reflux.

HISTORY AND EXAMINATION Wide range of clinical presentations, ranging from mild irritation to severe disease depending on degree of reflux. Respiratory symptoms may be the 1° complaint.
General: Feeding avoidance (associating feeding with discomfort) or constant eating/drinking (milk is alkali), irritability (discomfort of acid indigestion), failure to thrive, tooth enamel decay, may present with ALTEs.
Gastrointestinal: Difficulty/pain on swallowing, frequent spitting up or vomiting hours after feed, haematemesis, gastric/abdominal/retrosternal pain.
Respiratory: Apnoea, intermittent stridor, recurrent chest infections.

PATHOPHYSIOLOGY See Aetiology. The angle of His = acute angle between the gastric cardia and distal oesophagus.

INVESTIGATIONS
24-hour pH monitoring of the oesophagus: Calculated reflux index (time at which the lower oesophagus is pH < 4).
Impedance testing: More sensitive technique for testing small changes in pH levels by measuring resistance to electrical currents within oesophagus. Detects non-acid reflux.
Contrast studies: Upper GI tract to exclude anatomical abnormalities, reflux can be demonstrated.
Endoscopy: Confirms oesophagitis, biopsies of the lower oesophagus, fundus and the duodenum.

MANAGEMENT
Conservative: Time and reassurance unless child is exhibiting failure to thrive. Thickened feeds, ↓ volume, ↑ frequency of feeds, position infant upright for 30 minutes after feeding.
Pharmacological: H2-antagonists with prokinetic (ranitidine and domperidone) used with symptomatic infants or confirmed GORD with 24-h pH study/contrast/OGD.
Surgical: Only with children who have failed conservative/medical management. Fundoplication performed is either complete (Nissen 360°) or partial (Toupet 180° or Belsey/Thal 270°). May involve the placement of a gastrostomy and the laparoscopic approach can be used.

COMPLICATIONS
General: Failure to thrive, Sandifer syndrome (dystonic movements of the head and neck).
Gastrointestinal: Oesophagitis, peptic stricture, Barrett oesophagus.
Respiratory: Pulmonary aspiration due to neurological immaturity, leading to pneumonia and apnoea in preterm infants.

PROGNOSIS 60% will resolve by 6/12 of age 2° to the maturation of the lower oesophageal sphincter.

DEFINITION   Genetic disorders of skeletal development and growth, which can be divided into the chondrodysplasias (e.g. achondroplasia) and the osteodysplasias (e.g. osteogenesis imperfecta).

AETIOLOGY
Chondrodysplasia: Mutations in genes for cartilage matrix proteins, transmembrane receptors, transcription factors and ion transporters.
Achondroplasia: Autosomal dominant condition involving mutation in the FGFR3 gene on chromosome 4 (50% *de novo* mutations).
Osteodysplasia: Mutations in genes → abnormal development of bone.
Osteogenesis imperfecta (brittle bone disease): Autosomal dominant mutations that code for type I procollagen.

ASSOCIATIONS/RELATED   Achondroplasia is associated with higher paternal age.

EPIDEMIOLOGY
Achondroplasia: Incidence 0.5–1.5/10,000/year.
Osteogenesis imperfecta: Incidence 1/20,000/year.

HISTORY AND EXAMINATION
Achondroplasia: Average trunk length with shortened limbs, megalocephaly, short stature, and angular deformities of the extremities. Cervicomedullary compression may present with ataxia, pain, apnoea or incontinence.
Osteogenesis imperfecta:

- *Type I (mild):* recurrent childhood fractures, blue sclera, early deafness
- *Type II (most severe):* may be stillborn or die in infancy from respiratory insufficiency. Extreme fragility, low birthweight, small thorax.
- *Type III:* in utero fractures, macrocephaly, triangular facies, scoliosis, and vertebral compression.
- *Type IV:* moderate short stature and bowing of legs; sustain fractures but are often mobile in the community.

PATHOPHYSIOLOGY
Achondroplasia: ↑ function of the FGFR3 gene → reduced endochondrial ossification.
Osteogenesis imperfecta: In normal bone formation, type I collagen contains three chains composed of uninterrupted repeats of glycine-X-Y. In osteogenesis imperfecta, the matrix of bone is composed of abnormal type I collagen caused by substitution of glycine by other residues.

INVESTIGATIONS
Achondroplasia
Radiology: Large skull cap bones, small cranial base and facial bones.
MRI cervical spine: For cervical stenosis.
Osteogenesis imperfecta
DEXA scan: Bone mass density is ~75% of normal.
Lumbar spine X-rays: For compression fractures.
Collagen synthesis analysis.

MANAGEMENT
Achondroplasia: GH/insulin-like growth factor, neurological follow-up, surgical decompression of cervical stenosis, leg-lengthening procedures.
Osteogenesis imperfecta: Prompt fracture splinting or casting and correction of deformity to restore function, physiotherapy in younger children, mobility aids (braces, wheelchairs).

COMPLICATIONS

Achondroplasia: Craniocervical stenosis may lead to spinal cord compression, quadriparesis and respiratory arrest.

Osteogenesis imperfecta: Recurrent pneumonia, brainstem compression, hydrocephalus, and syringohydromyelia.

PROGNOSIS

Achondroplasia: Individuals have normal lifespan and intelligence.

Osteogenesis imperfecta:

- *Type I* and *IV* are associated with a normal lifespan
- *Type III* are susceptible to respiratory problems and have a ↓ lifespan
- *Type II* usually die in infancy.

DEFINITION   A significant delay (>2 SD) in >2 areas of development (motor, speech/language, cognition, social/personal, and activities of daily living) in child <5 years of age.

AETIOLOGY   In many cases no cause is found. A review of 261 GDD children <5 years identified a cause in 38%:

1. Intrapartum asphyxia (22%)
2. Cerebral dysgenesis (16%)
3. Chromosome abnormalities (13%): Down, fragile X syndrome
4. Genetic syndromes (11%): tuberous sclerosis, Angelman/Prader-Willi syndrome
5. Psychosocial deprivation (11%)
6. Term periventricular leucomalacia (9%)
7. Fetal alcohol syndrome (6%).

Other causes: Metabolic (congenital hypothyroidism, phenylketonuria), traumatic brain injury, lead poisoning, congenital infections (rubella, CMV), child abuse.

EPIDEMIOLOGY   Prevalence 1–3%. Most children have impairment in all five domains.

ASSOCIATIONS/RELATED
Co-morbidity: Autistic spectrum disorder, ADHD, depression, self-harm (especially fragile X), epilepsy. Physical co-morbidities associated with chromosomal/genetic conditions; cardiovascular, malignancies, metabolic.

HISTORY   Consanguinity, antenatal and birth history, maternal alcohol/substance abuse in pregnancy, family history of development delay/chromosomal abnormality, social history. Assess whether child has developmental delay, arrest or regression.

EXAMINATION   Growth parameters (head circumference), physical/neurological examination, developmental assessment (schedule of growing skills, Bailey or Griffith scales).

Assessment of dysmorphic/characteristic syndromic features
Down syndrome: See relevant chapter.
Fragile X: Large ears, narrow facies, strabismus, macro-orchidism, gaze aversion.
Tuberous sclerosis: Ash leaf macules (depigmentation), adenoma sebaceum (facial angiofibromas), shagreen patch over the sacrum/back.
Angelman syndrome: Strabismus, hypopigmented skin and eyes, prominent mandible, wide mouth, wide-spaced teeth.
Prader-Willi syndrome: Obesity, almond-shaped eyes, narrow forehead, down-turned mouth, small hands and feet.

PATHOPHYSIOLOGY   Depends on the cause. May be heritable or may be due to brain insult before, during or after birth.

INVESTIGATIONS   Benefits of identification of cause include identifying treatable conditions, genetic counseling, prognostic information and referral to support groups.
Diagnostic:

1. Chromosomal analysis and fragile X screening
2. Thyroid function testing (hypothyroid now rare since neonatal screening)
3. *Neuroimaging*: especially in children with microcephaly (congenital infection, metabolic disorders) or macrocephaly (fragile X, hydrocephaly)
4. *Metabolic testing*: especially if developmental regression; plasma and urinary amino and organic acids, acid/base, plasma VLCFA, lyzosomal enzyme analysis, ammonia
5. *EEG*: seizure activity or developmental regression (epileptic encephalopathy, Rett syndrome).

Co-morbidities: Echocardiogram, spinal X-ray.

MANAGEMENT
Multidisciplinary team approach: Co-ordinated by a community paediatrician.
Educational input: Mainstream school with additional support (liaison with special educational needs co-ordinator (SENCO)) or placement at a special needs school (requires statement of special educational needs).

Assessment of vision and hearing:
Therapist input: SALT, physiotherapy, occupational therapy.
Orthopaedic referral: Scoliosis or muscle spasticity/contractures.
Treatment of co-morbidity: Physical and mental health problems.
Genetic counselling: Screening in future pregnancies.

COMPLICATIONS Depends on the aetiology. Psychological/emotional: may result in aggressive or self-injurious behaviour.

PROGNOSIS Varies with the degree of learning impairment. Early input of resources can encourage child to attain milestones with the appropriate support and learning environment. Most children with GDD are dependent on parents/carers for support in activities of daily living.

DEFINITION   Bilateral inflammation of the renal glomeruli with proliferation of cellular elements 2° to an immunological mechanism.

AETIOLOGY

Post-infectious: 2° to group A β-haemolytic streptococcus; glomerular inflammation 2° to streptococcal proteins derivatives. Serotype 12 (post-URTI) and serotype 49 (post-skin infection). Other causative organisms: diplococcal, staphylococcal, mycobacterial, CMV, coxsackie virus, EBV.

Haemolytic uraemic syndrome: Haemolytic anaemia, thrombocytopenia and endothelial damage to glomerular capillaries 2° to infection by *E.coli* 0157, *Shigella* or *Salmonella*.

Henoch–Schönlein purpura (HSP): Hypersensitivity vasculitis and inflammatory response within the glomerular capillaries.

Berger disease: Diffuse mesangial deposition of IgA and IgG.

Systemic lupus erythematosus (SLE) nephritis: The immune system produces antinuclear antibodies. Antibodies and complement complexes accumulate in the kidneys resulting in an inflammatory response.

ASSOCIATIONS/RELATED   Preceding sore throat/impetigo (post-infectious GN), URTI (HSP) or GI infection (HUS). Hepatitis and diabetes.

EPIDEMIOLOGY   Typically 2–12 years old, although may be any age. $M:F=2:1$. Incidence depends on underlying cause but generally rare. SLE is uncommon in children.

HISTORY AND EXAMINATION

General: Characterised by the sudden onset of haematuria, proteinuria and red cell casts. Often associated with hypertension, oedema (face, ankles and ascites) and impaired renal function. Flank pain may be present 2° to renal capsule swelling.

HSP: Characteristic petechial/purpuric rash on buttock and extensor surfaces, arthralgia commonly at the ankles, symptoms of nephritis, abdominal pain.

PATHOPHYSIOLOGY

Histopathology: Swelling of the glomerular tufts and infiltration with polymorphonucleocytes.

Immunofluorescence: Immunoglobulins and complement deposition.

INVESTIGATIONS

Urine: Microscopy; RBC +/− casts and culture, 24-hour collection; protein and creatinine clearance.

Bloods: ↓Hb, ↑WCC, ↓Plt (HUS), ↑urea, ↑ESR/CRP, metabolic acidosis, GFR.

Specific: ↑ Antistreptolysin titre, (↑d in 1–3/52 and peaks at 3–5/52), RBC fragmentation, stool culture (HUS), IgA antibodies, antinuclear antibodies (SLE).

Imaging: Renal USS.

Surgical: Renal biopsy may be necessary.

MANAGEMENT

General: Correction of any electrolyte abnormalities/acid–base imbalances. Fluid restriction if severe oedema present.

Medical: PO antibiotics for post-infective causes (penicillin for streptococcus), antihypertensive therapy, treatment of pulmonary oedema, possible use of steroids +/− cytotoxic/immunosuppressive agents (HSP, vasculitis).

COMPLICATIONS

Hypertension: Encephalopathy, convulsions, end-organ damage, cerebral haemorrhage.

Renal failure: Uraemia, metabolic acidosis, electrolyte abnormalities, fluid overload.

PROGNOSIS

General: 10% may develop chronic glomerulonephritis. Mortality depends on cause.

Post-infection: Good for >95%; acute phase lasts 1–2/52, hypertension for 3–4/52 and microscopic haematuria for <12/12 but rapidly progressive to CRF in 1%.
HUS: Life-threatening condition: mortality 5–30%; some may relapse.
IgA nephropathy: 10–30% progress to CRF.
HSP: Usually resolves spontaneously without treatment. 1–2% develop CRF.

DEFINITION Bacterial infection caused by *Streptococcus agalactiae* (gram-positive β-haemolytic streptococcus) potentially causing neonatal sepsis.

AETIOLOGY GBS is a common infection in the adult population. May be subclinical infection therefore many patients are carriers; it colonizes the gastrointestinal tract, vagina, bladder or throat. Most common cause of neonatal sepsis, either by vertical (*in utero*) or intrapartum (maternal vaginal tract) transmission. Early > late infections.

Early: Occurs between $24^\circ \rightarrow 1/52$ of age. Vertical transmission. Commonly presents with sepsis, pneumonia, $+/-$ meningitis.

Late: Occurs between $1/52 \rightarrow 3/12$ of age. Vertical transmission (delayed infection after early colonisation) or horizontal infection (hospital or community). Meningitis is the most common presentation (85%).

ASSOCIATIONS/RELATED Prematurity, prolonged rupture of membranes (>18 hours), maternal pyrexia, maternal GBS bacteriuria during pregnancy, chorio-amnionitis, previous delivery of a GBS neonate (regardless of current maternal colonisation status).

EPIDEMIOLOGY 1–3/1000 live births. Maternal colonisation rates: 20–30%. Vertical transmission rate: 50%. 1–2% of colonised neonates have invasive disease.

HISTORY AND EXAMINATION
Sepsis:

- Pyrexia, temperature instability or hypothermia
- Shock, irritability, seizures, lethargy, drowsiness, neutropenia or hypo/hyperglycaemia
- Vomiting, abdominal distension, jaundice or poor feeding
- Apnoea and bradycardia, respiratory distress.

Meningitis:

- As for sepsis with tense or bulging fontanelle and head retraction (opisthotonos).

Pneumonia:

- Respiratory distress: tachypnoea, laboured breathing with chest wall recession and nasal flaring, expiratory grunting, tachycardia and cyanosis.

PATHOPHYSIOLOGY *S. agalactiae* is an invasive encapsulated organism producing a polysaccharide toxin. Immunity mediated by antibodies against the capsular polysaccharide and is serotype specific (multiple different serotypes have been identified).

INVESTIGATIONS
Radiology: CXR.
Bloods: FBC and WCC, glucose, inflammatory markers (CRP), U&Es and LFTs.
Microbiology: Blood cultures, urine and CSF (lumbar puncture).

MANAGEMENT
Preventive:

- Identification of at-risk infants/colonised mothers (vaginal introitus and anorectum cultures)
- Intrapartum IV penicillin G (clindamycin if allergic) should be used.

Treatment:

- Admission to the neonatal unit with IV access, IVI fluids, bloods and blood cultures
- Broad-spectrum intravenous antibiotics, started after blood cultures obtained but before results available
- IV penicillin and gentamicin (which act synergistically against GBS), or ampicillin and gentamicin.

Future:

- Vaccination possibility.

COMPLICATIONS   Hearing and vision loss and neurodevelopmental impairment.

PROGNOSIS   Morbidity is 5% in infected neonates for infection although neonatal meningitis has a mortality of 20–50%.

DEFINITION   Infestation of the head with lice.

AETIOLOGY
Pediculus humanus capitis: Six-legged, flat, wingless, blood-sucking louse up to 3 mm long with legs adapted to cling onto hair shafts.
Mechanism of spread: Head-to-head contact, sharing of hats, combs, hairbands, towels. Eggs (nits) can live for up to 1 month away from the body.

ASSOCIATIONS/RELATED   Young age, close crowded living conditions, warm weather.

EPIDEMIOLOGY
Incidence: Under-reported due to social stigma, namely the preconceived notion that lice are related to poor personal hygiene. F > M due to social acceptance of close physical contact – sharing hats, combs, hairbands.
Peak age: 3–11 years 2° to close contact in Class-rooms and day-care facilities.
Race: Caucasians > Afro-Caribbeans.

HISTORY   Parents often seek assessment after becoming aware of an outbreak at school. Pruritus is the major complaint.

EXAMINATION
Neck: Urticarial papules and/or excoriations, post-occipital +/− cervical lymphadenopathy.
Scalp: Live lice on scalp and empty egg cases (nits) on hairs. The eggs are cemented firmly to the scalp hairs and appear as small white oval capsules when empty; they remain attached to the hair as it grows.

PATHOPHYSIOLOGY   The louse bite introduce enzymes, an Anti-clotting agent and a local anaesthetic into the scalp. This produces a typical allergic reaction. With repeated exposure to the bites, sensitisation occurs with an inflammatory papular dermatitis.

INVESTIGATIONS   Wood's light examination reveals yellow and/or green fluorescence of the lice and their nits.

MANAGEMENT   There is no need for children with head lice to stay away from school.
Non-drug management

1. *Wet-combing*: after shampooing and applying conditioner, the wet comb is used to mechanically remove adult lice and nymphs. Wet combing should be performed twice weekly until no full-grown lice have been seen for three consecutive sessions.
2. *Dimeticone 4%*: a silicon polymer that covers lice and disrupts their ability to manage their water balance. Consequently, treated insects fail to excrete surplus water and die.

Drug management

1. *Pediculicides*: malathion 0.5% or phenothrin 0.5% aqueous liquid are recommended (available over the counter). Apply liquid overnight and following day remove lice and nits with a fine-toothed comb. This is not very effective against developing nits so a second treatment is required after 7 days.
2. If there is resistance then first ensure compliance, then use the alternative first-line treatment and subsequently consider carbaryl 1% aqueous liquid.

Drug resistance: Pediculicide resistance is increasingly common, and rotational treatment strategies are recommended by health authorities.
Environmental eradication: Pillow-cases, linens, towels, toys and hats should be washed in hot water and dried.
Treatment of contacts: Treatment of family members, friends and/or other close contacts is very important in helping to prevent further spread of lice and reinfestation.

COMPLICATIONS

2° bacterial infection: Impetigo requires treatment and may mask underlying lice infestation.

Psychosocial impact: 2° to stigma associated with lice infestation.

PROGNOSIS   Good with appropriate treatment, environmental eradication and treatment of contacts.

DEFINITION   Normal hearing at any frequency is ≤20 dB.

Conductive hearing impairment: Sound vibrations are not conducted via the ear canal, tympanic membrane or the ossicles. Maximum 20–60 dB hearing loss.

Sensorineural hearing impairment: Dysfunction of the cochlear (sensory) components or the auditory nerve. May have profound >90 dB hearing loss.

AETIOLOGY
Conductive:

1. *Ear canal*: Wax, foreign body.
2. *Tympanic membrane*: Most cases 2° to chronic secretory otitis media (CSOM). Also perforation due to trauma, pressure change in aircraft or acute otitis media.
3. *Ossicles*: Absent/defective ossicles due to congenital malformation.
4. *Eustachian tube dysfunction*: Cleft palate, Down syndrome.

Sensorineural:

1. *Genetic (50%)*: AR/AD or part of a syndrome, e.g. Waardenburg syndrome
2. *Intrauterine (10%)*: congenital infections (rubella, CMV, herpes)
3. *Perinatal (10%)*: HIE
4. *Postnatal (30%)*: measles, mumps, meningitis, encephalitis, head injury, neurodegenerative disorders, aminoglycosides, loop diuretics, hyperbilirubinaemia.

ASSOCIATIONS/RELATED   Recurrent otitis media, URTIs, atopy

EPIDEMIOLOGY
Severe: 1/1000 children require special schooling (sensorineural or mixed).
Moderate: 2/1000 children require hearing aids and educational support.
Mild: 1/100 school age children affected (usually 2° to glue ear and transient).

HISTORY   Usually suspected by mother when the baby consistently fails to respond to noise. May report delayed language development, behavioural or educational difficulties. Elicit family history, consanguinity, intrauterine, perinatal or postnatal complications, recurrent otitis media, atopy or URTIs.

EXAMINATION   Look for dysmorphic features. Examine ENT for signs of wax, CROM or perforated ear drum. Weber and Rinne tests (tuning fork) can be used to differentiate between conductive and sensorineural hearing loss.

PATHOPHYSIOLOGY   See Aetiology.

INVESTIGATIONS
NHS Newborn Hearing Screening Programme (NHSP): Uses automated otoacoustic emission test and/or auditory brainstem-evoked responses.
Distraction test (>4 months): Infant is held on parent's lap and distracted by a toy in front. The examiner stands behind parent and creates noises of different intensities and pitches (voice, keys, rattle) to test each ear separately. Normal head-turning responses are elicited towards the side of the sound stimulus.
McCormick's toy discrimination test (>2 years): Phonetically similar-sounding toys (duck/cup, tree/key) are named and the child is asked to identify them.
Tympanogram: Tests the condition of the middle ear, mobility of the tympanic membrane and conduction bones by creating variations of air pressure in the ear canal.
Audiometry testing (>5 years): Child sits in a sound proof booth wearing a set of head/earphones connected to an audiometer. The audiometer produces tones at specific frequencies and set volume levels to each ear independently. An audiogram is plotted which describes the child's hearing ability at different frequencies.

MANAGEMENT
Conductive:

1. *CSOM (see chapter on otitis media)*: If there is persistent hearing loss, 'grommets' (tiny plastic tubes) inserted into the tympanic membrane allow fluid to drain out
2. Myringoplasty for persistent tympanic membrane perforation
3. Reconstruction for congenital ossicular chain abnormalities.

Sensorineural:

1. Early diagnosis is key. Hearing aids or cochlear implants if insufficient amplification. Auditory training by peripatetic teacher, who can later advise on school placement. Lip-reading and sign language are additional means of communication
2. Parental counselling on safety hazards.
3. Genetic counselling.

COMPLICATIONS   Delayed speech and language, falling behind at school, behavioural problems.

PROGNOSIS
Conductive: Most causes are treatable or resolve spontaneously.
Sensorineural: Good if detected early to implement necessary support and prevent educational and behavioural problems.

DEFINITION

Heart failure: Results when the heart can no longer meet the metabolic demands of the body.

Congestive heart failure (CHF): Refers to ↑ venous congestion in the pulmonary (left heart failure) or systemic (right heart failure) veins. This occurs when the compensatory mechanisms used to improve cardiac output are no longer adequate, and heart failure becomes uncompensated.

AETIOLOGY

Overcirculation: Normal forward blood flow is disrupted and the heart becomes an inefficient pump.

1. *Congenital heart disease (CHD)*: hypoplastic left heart (HLH), severe aortic stenosis, interrupted aortic arch, coarctation of the aorta (COA), patent ductus arteriosus (PDA), total anomalous pulmonary venous drainage (TAPVD), large VSD, transposition of the great arteries (TGA), truncus arteriosus.
2. Postoperative repair of CHD.
3. Arteriovenous malformation, e.g. hepatic.
4. Severe anaemia, e.g. hydrops fetalis.

Pump failure: Heart muscle is damaged and no longer contracts normally.

1. Viral myocarditis/cardiomyopathy
2. Metabolic cardiomyopathy (e.g. Pompe disease)
3. Arrhythmias: SVT, VT or congenital heart block (CHB)
4. Ischaemia (post Kawasaki disease)
5. Duchenne muscular dystrophy
6. Medications e.g. chemotherapy

ASSOCIATIONS/RELATED CHD is more common in Down, Turner, Marfan and Noonan syndromes.

EPIDEMIOLOGY Rare in children; more common in infants with CHD.

HISTORY

Infants: Breathlessness, wheeze (cardiac asthma), grunting, feeding difficulties, sweating, failure to thrive, recurrent chest infections.

Older children: Fatigue, exercise intolerance, dizziness or syncope.

EXAMINATION

General: Tachycardia (not in CHB); absence of a heart murmur does not exclude heart disease (TGA, HLH, COA).

Left CHF: Tachypnoea, respiratory distress (recession), gallop rhythm, displaced apex

Right CHF: Hepatosplenomegaly +/− oedema or ascites. Jugular venous distension is not a reliable indicator in infants and young children.

Uncompensated CHF: Hypotension, cool peripheries, prolonged capillary refill time, thready pulse, ↓ urine output, signs of renal and hepatic failure in severe cases.

PATHOPHYSIOLOGY

Cardiac output = stroke volume × HR.

BP = cardiac output × systemic vascular resistance (SVR). In progressive heart failure, cardiac output drops and is initially compensated for by ↑HR, then ↑SVR (cool peripheries). Once these are no longer sufficient, ↓BP is preterminal.

INVESTIGATIONS

Bloods: Acid/base balance, electrolytes and osmolality (likely SIADH), liver and renal function.

CXR: Cardiomegaly, ↑ pulmonary vascular markings and fluid collection in the horizontal fissure/pleural effusions may be detected.

ECG: Rate, rhythm, atrial/ventricular hypertrophy or hypoplasia. Evidence of myocarditis/ cardiac ischaemia or ventricular strain.

ECHO: Diagnostic for CHD.

Cardiac catheterisation: Measures intracardiac pressures and shunts.

MANAGEMENT

This is an emergency requiring admission to a specialist unit.

Newborn/infant: Duct-dependent CHD is the most likely cause for heart failure so IV prostaglandins should be commenced immediately.

Goals of medical therapy: Reducing the preload (loop and thiazide diuretics), enhancing cardiac contractility (inotropes), reducing the afterload (ACE inhibitors), improving oxygen delivery, and enhancing nutrition.

Surgical: Cardiac transplantation.

COMPLICATIONS   Arrhythmias, SVT, VT, CHB, cardiogenic shock.

PROGNOSIS   Poor in children in the absence of correctable CHD.

DEFINITION   Congenital defect in the formation of the diaphragm that leads to the protrusion of abdominal contents into the thoracic cavity.

AETIOLOGY
General: More commonly unilateral although may be bilateral. Lt > Rt. Bowel or intra-abdominal viscera may herniated. Common for liver (Rt) and also spleen (Lt) to be herniated. There may be associated abnormal hepatic vasculature. Associated with abnormalities of the pulmonary tree, vasculature and surfactant deficiency (hypoplastic lungs).
Posterolateral Bochdalek hernia: 90% of cases, commonly left-sided, posterolateral defect.
Morgagni hernia: 3% of cases, commonly right-sided (90%), anteromedial defect.
Congenital hiatus hernia: Rare, stomach herniates through the oesophageal hiatus.

ASSOCIATIONS/RELATED   Previous affected sibling, cardiac anomalies (25%), renal anomalies, persistent pulmonary hypertension, malrotation of the small bowel (40%).

EPIDEMIOLOGY   1/2000–4000 live births. M : F = 1.5 : 1.

HISTORY AND EXAMINATION   Infants may have a history of polyhydramnios. Most commonly present with a history of cyanosis and respiratory distress in the immediate neonatal period. If there is a left-sided posterolateral hernia, there may be poor air entry on the left and a shift of cardiac sounds into the right chest. Smaller defects may present later in infancy with a diagnosis of a 'wheezy child' or recurrent chest infection.

PATHOPHYSIOLOGY   Diaphragmatic development is from four structures embryologically: dorsal oesophageal mesentery, pleuroperitoneal membranes, body wall and septum transversum. Defect occurs from failure of these to fuse.

INVESTIGATIONS
Karyotype: Chromosomal studies.
Radiology: CXR (with prior placing of an orogastric tube to aid gastric positioning), cardiac ECHO (? right-sided aortic arch) and renal USS.

MANAGEMENT
Medical: NGT to decompress the bowel. If respiratory support is indicated, should be via ETT and mechanical ventilation with avoidance of high peak inspiratory pressures. Bag and mask ventilation should be avoided. UAC/UVC placement with ABG monitoring. Surfactant administration after intubation. May require stabilisation with HFOV, NO therapy or extracorporeal membrane oxygenation (ECMO) or the use of inotropes.
Surgical: Post-stabilisation of the neonate. The approach can be via an open subcostal incision approach (+/− thoracotomy incision), the laparoscopic transabdominal approach or the thorascopic approach. The approach depends on surgeon's choice and the position of the hernia (right CDH are unsuitable for laparoscopic approach due to the liver). Surgical technique involves careful reduction of the herniated contents, definition of the posterior rim and repair with non-absorbable sutures +/− a synthetic patch (depending on the size of the defect). A chest drain may be left *in situ*.

COMPLICATIONS   Pulmonary hypoplasia, intestinal malrotation (40%), gastric and mid gut volvulus, gastric or other gastrointestinal perforations, gastric volvulus and bilateral renal hypertrophy.

PROGNOSIS   Reported mortality is 25–60%. Mortality closely associated with the degree of pulmonary hypoplasia.

DEFINITION   Abnormal protrusion of an intra-abdominal structure through the inguinal canal into the inguinal region or scrotum.

AETIOLOGY   The testicle develops retroperitoneally and begins descent to the scrotum at 28/40. This is under control of both hormones and the gubernaculum. Peritoneal evagination creates the processus vaginalis and allows testicular descent thorough the ventral abdominal wall to the scrotum. This normally obliterates by term but if it remains open (patent processus vaginalis), will allow the passage of bowel (inguinal hernia) or fluid (hydrocoele) through the inguinal canal. In females, the gubernaculum becomes the ovarian ligament and round ligament; with a patent processus vaginalis, it extends into the labium majus and is known as the canal of Nuck. Hernia content most commonly ileum (male), ovary (female).

ASSOCIATIONS/RELATED   Preterm infants, low birthweight, FHx (10%), undescended testicles, gastroschisis, exomphalos, hypospadias, Ehlers–Danlos syndrome, cystic fibrosis, connective tissue disorders and other conditions that ↑ intra-abdominal pressure.

EPIDEMIOLOGY   3–5% full-term infants and 30% premature infants. M>F 5:1. Right-sided (60%), left-sided (25%), bilateral (15%). 7% develop metachronous hernia post-repair (contralateral exploration is not recommended).

HISTORY AND EXAMINATION
Infant: History of intermittent inguinal/inguinoscrotal swelling. First presentation may be with incarceration. Unable to palpate the cord superiorly (possible with hydrocoeles). Reducible unless incarcerated (tender/red/firm). Non-transluminable.
Child: Supine and standing positions, expansile cough impulse and as above.
Incarceration: Unsettled, pain, tender non-reducible inguinal scrotal mass, erythema, oedema, vomiting and abdominal distension (late signs).
Differential diagnosis of inguinal hernia: Hydrocoeles, retractile testes, undescended testes, femoral hernias and lymphadenopathy.

PATHOPHYSIOLOGY   See Aetiology.

INVESTIGATIONS   USS used rarely to enable diagnosis in difficult cases.

MANAGEMENT
General: Herniotomy is performed. Hernia sac is located in the inguinal canal, separated from the vas deferens and testicular vessels, transected and ligated. Traditional repair using an inguinal open approach. Some centres use the laparoscopic approach with the placement of an intraperitoneal purse string for closure. Concerns over ↑d recurrence with laparoscopic technique.
Neonate: Reducible; elective repair at the next available theatre session with overnight post-operative cardiorespiratory monitoring.
Infant/Child: Elective repair as a day-case.
Incarceration: Manual reduction of the hernia contents under sedation (IV morphine) with repair after 48 hours to allow oedema to settle. Rarely operative reduction and repair if manual reduction fails.

COMPLICATIONS
Inguinal hernia: Incarceration (50% within first year of life).
Inguinal herniotomy: Recurrence (1–2%), damage to the vas deferens and testicular vessels (testicular atropy), ascending ipsilateral testicle 2° to scarring.

PROGNOSIS   Excellent with surgical repair.

DEFINITION Congenital disorder of the enteric nervous system, 2° to aganglionosis of the myenteric (Auerbach) and submucosal (Meissner) plexuses, resulting in a functional obstruction.

AETIOLOGY
General: Affects the anus and variable distance of bowel proximally. Classified according to the length of bowel affected (short segment, long segment, total colonic, total intestinal or ultra-short segment).
Embryology: Failure of neural crest-derived ganglion cells to migrate from proximal to distal bowel during development leading to the rectum $+/-$ colon without parasympathetic nerve innervation. Affected bowel has only sympathetic nerve innervations $\rightarrow$ hypertonicity and lack of appropriate relaxation in response to proximal distension $\rightarrow$ narrow/contracted segment of bowel and stool stasis proximally.

ASSOCIATIONS/RELATED Trisomy 21, Waardenburg syndrome, MEN2, FHx (long segment disease). Exclude other causes of neonatal abdominal distension (atresia, meconium ileus or plug syndrome).

EPIDEMIOLOGY 1/5000 live births; accounts for 20% of all neonatal obstruction. M : F = 4 : 1. 90% of patients present in the neonatal period and 95% before the first year.

HISTORY
Neonatal presentation:

1. Failure to pass meconium in first 24–48 hours
2. Acute intestinal obstruction; abdominal distension, poor feeding, bilious vomiting
3. Severe life-threatening enterocolitis.

Infantile presentation:

1. Chronic obdurate constipation with abdominal distension without soiling
2. Intermittent abdominal pain and fever during episodes of retained faeces
3. Failure to thrive.

EXAMINATION Depends on the age of presentation. Typically abdominal distension with dilated loops of bowel. PR examination reveals a sudden explosive 'gush' of stool as the digital examination bypasses the aganglionic segment. Septic signs if associated enterocolitis.

PATHOPHYSIOLOGY Absence of ganglion cells in the Auerbach and Meissner plexuses, ↑d amounts of acetylcholinesterase stained nerve endings, and hypertrophied nerve trunks in the lamina propria and muscularis propria.

INVESTIGATIONS
Bloods: ↑WCC/CRP with enterocolitis. Blood cultures and venous gas (acidosis).
Radiology: AXR – dilated bowel (important to exclude atresia as a differential diagnosis in the neonatal period). Gastrograffin enema – may demonstrate the transition zone.
Suction rectal biopsy: Three biopsies taken at 2, 3 and 4 cm from the anal margin above the dentate line. Full-thickness biopsy under a GA may be required if insufficient sample with SRB.
Anorectal manometry: Older children with chronic constipation.

MANAGEMENT
Initial: Neonates should be managed with broad spectrum IV antibiotics, NGT decompression, and rectal washouts (typically 15 ml/kg TDS). If this fails (rare) then may require a colostomy to decompress the colon.

Surgical: Pull-through procedure performed (>3/12 of age); Swenson, Duhamel, Soave (endorectal). Can be performed with laparoscopic assistance; biopsies for identification of the transition zone and mobilisation of the sigmoid colon and rectum.

COMPLICATIONS   Hirschsprung enterocolitis, encopresis, constipation, incontinence.

PROGNOSIS   Prognosis is poor with non-adequately treated enterocolitis (80% mortality). Postoperatively good outcome although majority will still have intestinal motility problems.

DEFINITION   Virus that infects and disables the host's CD4 T cells.

AETIOLOGY
Vertical transmission (>75%): *In utero*, perinatally or via breastfeeding.
Sexual transmission: Abuse in children, intercourse in adolescents.
IV drug abuse: Rare in children.

ASSOCIATIONS/RELATED
DD: Immunodeficiency (DiGeorge syndrome, chronic granulomatous disease). Co-infections: tuberculosis, hepatitis B/C and sexually transmitted diseases.

EPIDEMIOLOGY   2,000,000 children worldwide were suspected to be infected in 2007. 1,800,000 of those children live in sub-Saharan Africa. Higher rates of prevalence within children from ethnic minority groups.

HISTORY AND EXAMINATION
General: Failure to thrive, developmental delay, chronic diarrhoea, lymphadenopathy, bilateral non-tender parotitis, hepatosplenomegaly.
Infections:

1. Recurrent bacterial infections and viral infections
2. Opportunistic infections (PCP is an AIDS-defining disease)
3. *Oral candidiasis*: white/yellow plaques and loss of tongue papillae
4. *Herpes simplex*: herpes labialis, gingivostomatitis, oesophagitis or chronic skin vesicles
5. *VZV*: recurrent/persistent/severe infection
6. *Human papillomavirus*: flat warts covering large areas of the body
7. *Fungal infections*: tinea capitis resistant to treatment.

Neoplasm: B-cell lymphoproliferative disease.

PATHOPHYSIOLOGY   Virus enters CD4 lymphocytes by binding with CD4 and a chemokine receptor, using its glycoprotein receptor (gp120). Viral reverse transcriptase converts RNA to DNA, which is incorporated into the host genome.

INVESTIGATIONS
Neonatal bloods: HIV serology and DNA for PCR are taken at birth before antiretroviral prophylaxis is commenced. Repeat bloods are taken at 6 weeks and 3 months and serology is repeated until the child is >18 months when maternal antibodies will have disappeared.
Confirmatory tests: HIV RNA PCR, CD4 count, baseline resistance screen.
Endoscopy: If oesophageal candidiasis is suspected.
Screen for other diseases: TB (Mantoux), hepatitis B/C, syphilis and toxoplasmosis.

MANAGEMENT
Prevention: Without preventive measures 25–40% of children will acquire vertical transmission of HIV.

1. All pregnant women are offered antenatal screening for HIV and hepatitis B/C.
2. Mothers with HIV should not breastfeed their child (UK guidelines). Risk decreases from 25–40% to ~15% when breastfeeding is avoided.
3. Reduce maternal viral load with antiretroviral drugs antenatally, perinatally and post-natally; reduces transmission rate to 5%.
4. Elective caesarean section to avoid contact with the birth canal; reduces transmission rate to 1% (less with low maternal viral load).
5. Empirical treatment with antiretroviral medication (usually zidovudine) post-natally.

Prophylaxis: Co-trimoxazole against PCP, routine immunisation schedule but no live vaccines (except MMR).

Screen for opportunistic infection regularly.

Regular monitoring and follow-up: Viral load/CD4 count. Start highly active antiretroviral therapy (HAART) if these indicators of disease progression start to deteriorate:

1. Nucleoside analogue reverse transcriptase inhibitors (zidovudine)
2. Non-nucleoside reverse transcriptase inhibitors (nevirapine)
3. Protease inhibitors (indinavir).

COMPLICATIONS   Drug side effects, e.g. myelosuppression with zidovudine. Poor compliance rapidly leads to drug resistance. Opportunistic infections with progression of disease.

PROGNOSIS   Children with untreated HIV infection progress rapidly and approximately 25% develop AIDS in the first year of life. Mortality is >50% by 2 years of age in poorly resourced areas.

DEFINITION   Excess CSF from abnormal flow, absorption or production.

AETIOLOGY
Obstructive hydrocephalus: Disruption in the flow of CSF within the ventricular system.

1. *Aqueductal stenosis or atresia*: most common site of intraventricular obstruction in infants with congenital hydrocephalus.
2. *Obstruction of the 4th ventricle*: Dandy–Walker syndrome (cystic dilatation of the 4th ventricle with cerebellar hypoplasia).
3. *Obstruction due to intracranial mass lesion*: tumours of the posterior fossa (medulloblastoma, astrocytoma, ependymoma), haematomas, vein of Galen aneurysm.

Communicating hydrocephalus: Disruption in the flow of CSF in the surface pathways.

1. *Arnold–Chiari malformations*: herniation of cerebellar tonsils through the foramen magnum, frequently associated with neural tube defects:
   a) *Myelomeningocoele*: outpouching of the spinal cord through the posterior bony vertebral column.
   b) *Cranial meningocoele*: meningeal sac protrudes through a skull defect.
2. *Encephalocoele*: protrusion of cerebral tissue through midline cranial defect located in frontal or occipital regions.
3. *Meningeal adhesions*: 2° to inflammation (meningitis) or haemorrhage (intraventricular or subarachnoid).

↑ **Production of CSF:**

1. *Choroid plexus papilloma*: rare cause of hydrocephalus.

ASSOCIATIONS/RELATED   Family history, NF.

EPIDEMIOLOGY
Congenital hydrocephalus: 3–5/1000 live births.

HISTORY

Infants
Slow progression: Infants may thrive and develop normally apart from poor head control.
Rapid progression: Irritability, lethargy, failure to gain weight and achieve developmental milestones, vomiting.

Older children
Posterior fossa tumours: Cerebellar signs: ataxic gait, dyspraxia, slurred speech.
'Arrested' hydrocephalus: Rare condition in which there is stable ventriculomegaly in the presence of a child with stable neurology.

EXAMINATION
Signs of hydrocephalus include:

1. Progressive ↑ in occipitofrontal head circumference or >97th centile
2. Wide open bulging anterior fontanelle
3. Widening of the coronal, sagittal and lambdoidal sutures
4. Eyes deviate downwards ('setting sun' sign)
5. Papilloedema (uncommon in congenital hydrocephalus).

PATHOPHYSIOLOGY   Accumulation of CSF in a confined space leads to ↑ intraventricular pressure and ↑ICP. In infants there is initial compensation from open fontanelles.

INVESTIGATIONS
CT/USS: May show dilation of ventricles and any tumours or cysts present.

MRI: Shows greater anatomical detail, and with contrast illustrates flow through the aqueduct.

MANAGEMENT

Surgical: Insertion of a shunt with a one-way valve from the ventricle to the peritoneum (or the right atrium).

Supportive: Requires long-term multidisciplinary follow-up to provide support for neurological sequelae.

COMPLICATIONS

Shunt complications: Obstruction, infection, especially *Staphylococcus epidermidis*. Overdrainage can lead to subdural haemorrhage.

Long-term sequelae: Global developmental delay, impaired memory and vision, precocious puberty.

PROGNOSIS   Some forms of hydrocephalus are temporary, such as meningeal adhesion 2° to infection or haemorrhage; some forms give rise to limited ventricular enlargement and then cease: compensated hydrocephalus. However, in most cases the ventricles will continue to enlarge and compress brain matter, resulting in a very poor prognosis.

DEFINITION   Overactivity of the thyroid gland, which → an increase in levels of circulating T_3 and T_4.

AETIOLOGY
Graves disease: An autoimmune disorder in which antibodies stimulate the thyroid-stimulating hormone (TSH) receptor.
Transient neonatal hyperthyroidism: 2° to maternal Graves disease; circulating TSH receptor-stimulating antibodies cross the placenta and stimulate the fetal thyroid.
Permanent neonatal hyperthyroidism: Germline mutation in the TSH receptor results in its constitutive activation. Autosomal dominant or *de novo* mutation.

ASSOCIATIONS/RELATED   Other autoimmune disorders. Toxic multinodular goitre and toxic thyroid adenoma present in adults rather than children.

EPIDEMIOLOGY
Graves disease: Peak in teenage years, very rare in early childhood. M : F = 1 : 5.
Transient neonatal hyperthyroidism: Incidence 1/50,000 live births; 1–2% of neonates of mothers with Graves disease will be affected.
Permanent neonatal hyperthyroidism: Rare.

HISTORY   Anxiety, restlessness, weight loss, rapid growth in height, advanced bone maturity, learning difficulties/behavioural problems, psychosis.

EXAMINATION
Graves disease: The clinical features in children are similar to those of adults although the eye signs are less common.
General: Sweating, diarrhoea, weight loss, tremor, tachycardia with a wide pulse pressure, warm vasodilated peripheries, goitre.
Eye signs: Exophthalmos, ophthalmoplegia, lid retraction, lid lag.
Transient neonatal hyperthyroidism: Irritability, weight loss, diarrhoea, exophthalmos.

PATHOPHYSIOLOGY
Graves disease: Thyroid stimulating antibodies act on the TSH receptor as an autoimmune phenomenon due to interactions between T and B lymphocytes. Eye symptoms are caused by mucopolysaccharides and lymphocytes infiltrating the orbital, skin and subcutaneous tissues.

INVESTIGATIONS
Antenatal monitoring: CTG trace may indicate tachycardia in the fetus of an affected mother.
Graves disease: $\uparrow T_4$ +/− $\uparrow T_3$, TSH levels are highly suppressed (<0.1 µU/l).
Transient neonatal hyperthyroidism: $\downarrow$TSH, $\uparrow T_4$, and $\uparrow T_3$

MANAGEMENT
Medical treatment:

1. Carbimazole or propylthiouracil are the first-line treatment options
2. β-blockers are given for symptomatic relief of tremor, anxiety and tachycardia, and to protect the patient from cardiac arrhythmias.

Treatment usually lasts for 2 years. 40–75% of patients relapse when medical treatment is stopped; these patients need a second course of medical therapy, radio-iodine treatment or surgery.

Radio-iodine treatment: Highly successful although it may cause hypothyroidism.
Surgical: Subtotal thyroidectomy is indicated if there is failure of medical management and in permanent neonatal hyperthyroidism as first-line treatment.

COMPLICATIONS

Cardiac arrhythmias: Important and life-threatening complication.

Complications of treatment: Some patients will become hypothyroid with treatment and will therefore require T_4 replacement therapy for life.

PROGNOSIS   In all cases prompt treatment is of paramount importance to prevent complications. Following successful treatment, there is good prognosis with a normal life expectancy.

DEFINITION   Abnormally low plasma glucose levels sufficient to cause a potential long-term neurological injury (<2.5 mmo/l in a symptomatic neonate).

AETIOLOGY
General: May be transient (<1/52) or persistent. Neonates have limited hepatic glycogen stores and impaired ketone production so any condition that ↑s metabolic demand will quickly ↓ glycogen and ultimately glucose. Infants are most at risk between 6 and 12 hours post-partum unless underlying condition. Majority is caused by either transient or prolonged hyperinsulinism.

Transient: Prematurity, IUGR, perinatal asphyxia, Beckwith–Wiedemann syndrome, hypothermia, sepsis, maternal diabetes (β-cell hyperplasia), erythroblastosis fetalis (↑d insulin and pancreatic β-cells), β-agonist tocolytics (e.g. terbutaline).

Prolonged: Congenital hyperinsulinism (most common cause), inborn errors of metabolism (alterations in hepatic enzyme function impairing glucogenolysis and gluconeogenesis). Nesidioblastosis/islet cell adenoma.

ASSOCIATIONS/RELATED   Neonatal seizures, hyperthyroidism.

EPIDEMIOLOGY   Common (10%) of neonates if first feed is delayed by >6 hours. Hyperinsulinism has racial variation (1 in 2500–50,000).

HISTORY AND EXAMINATION
General: Irritability, tremulousness, brisk Moro reflex, poor feeding, apnoea, respiratory distress, lethargy, drowsiness, low core temperature and seizures.

Specific: Macrosomia (hyperinsulinism), jaundice (in galactosaemia or sepsis), hepatomegaly (glycogen storage diseases).

PATHOPHYSIOLOGY   See Aetiology.

INVESTIGATIONS
Routine bloods: ↓Glucose, ↑ketones (in ketotic hypoglycaemia).

Specific bloods: Insulin (hyperinsulinism), c-peptide, cortisol (hypoadrenalism), GH (hypopituitarism), lactate/pyruvate (types I – V glycogen storage diseases), ketone bodies, ammonia.

Urine analysis: Ketones, reducing sugars, organic acids.

MANAGEMENT
Mildly symptomatic infants: If no contraindications, hypoglycaemia is managed with ↑d enteral feeds. Monitor at-risk infants until blood sugar stabilisation.

Severely symptomatic infants, refractory hypoglycaemia or contraindications to feeding:

1. *IV dextrose*: a bolus of 2–5 ml/kg of 10% dextrose followed by an infusion to prevent rebound hypoglycaemia; 5–8 mg/kg/min in an infant (matches normal hepatic production).
2. If ↑s to the glucose intake are required, the volume of the fluid should be ↑d rather than strength of the fluid wherever possible.
3. Dextrose >12.5% must be infused through a central venous device such as an umbilical vein catheter.
4. If the baby is requiring >10 mg/kg/min IV dextrose infusion then consider:
   - Glucagon IM/IV (↑s glycogenolysis and gluconeogenesis)
   - Diazoxide +/– octreotide with suspected hyperinsulinism (inhibits pancreatic insulin production)
   - Hydrocortisone if adrenal insufficiency is suspected.

Surgery: May be required for nesidioblastosis/islet cell adenoma. Laparoscopic or open pancreatectomy may be necessary for persistent hyperinsulinaemic hypoglycaemia of infancy.

COMPLICATIONS   Untreated, ↓d head size / IQ / specific regional brain abnormalities revealed by MRI. Epilepsy and cerebral palsy.

PROGNOSIS   50% of patients who survive hyperinsulinaemic hypoglycaemia of infancy have long-term neurological complications.

DEFINITION   Abnormality of anterior urethral and penile development resulting in an ectopically located urethral opening on the ventrum of the penis proximal to the tip of the glans penis.

AETIOLOGY
General: Ectopic meatus can be located from a glandular level to the perineum. Distal hypospadias is more common than proximal; subcoronal position most common. Several factors including genetic, endocrine and environmental have been suggested.
Genetic: Polygenic inheritance; $8\times$ increased incidence with monozygotic twins, 8% of fathers and 14% of brothers are affected.
Endocrine: Defects in androgen synthesis or androgen sensitivity are associated with hypospadias. Especially associated with 5α-reductase mutation. IVF pregnancies are $5\times$ affected 2° to progesterone administration.
Environmental: Androgen disruption by environmental agents such as oestrogen use in pesticides has been implicated.

ASSOCIATIONS/RELATED   Cryptorchidism, patent processus vaginalis (inguinal hernia/hydrocoele). Majority have a hooded prepuce +/− chordee (abnormal curvature of the shaft).

EPIDEMIOLOGY   1/200 live births (↑ing incidence).

HISTORY AND EXAMINATION   Majority detected postnatally as associated hooded prepuce. Micturition unobstructed but stream will be directed inferiorly. Glandular hypospadias with a normal prepuce may present later. Appearance depends on the level of the urethral meatus. Meatal position (distal to proximal): glandular, coronal, subcoronal, distal shaft, mid-shaft, proximal shaft, penoscrotal, perineal. Can be associated with bifid scrotum in severe proximal hypospadias.

PATHOPHYSIOLOGY   Urethral development occurs at 8–20/40. Classic theory and Baskin modification (2000).

INVESTIGATIONS   RUSS. Further investigation with proximal severe hypospadias and karyotyping. Severe hypospadias with bilateral cryptorchidism should be carefully examined (exclusion of ambiguous genitalia).

MANAGEMENT
Initial: No circumcision as foreskin sometimes used in the reconstructive surgery. Parental counselling.
Surgical: 9/12 to 1 year old and before toilet training. Reconstruction of the urethra to allow straight voiding of urine, a satisfactory cosmetic appearance and normal ejaculation process. Mild glandular hypospadias may be managed conservatively if there is no compromise to flow. Repair as either a single procedure for distal hypospadias or as a staged procedure for more proximal defects. The tubularised incised plate (TIP) or Snodgrass procedure is the technique most commonly used for repair of distal hypospadias although >300 techniques are described in the literature. Normally surgical repair is over a stent that remains *in situ* with the dressing for 1/52.

COMPLICATIONS
Surgical: Neo-urethral stenosis, fistula formation, urethrocoele, wound infection and dehiscence as major complications.
Non-treatment: Psychological as well as functional issues. Associated with infertility (abnormal ejaculation).

PROGNOSIS   Generally very good. Complications depend on technique as well as experience of paediatric urologist. Many will require further operations or procedures under general anaesthetic. Distal hypospadias is associated with less morbidity than proximal.

DEFINITION   Clinical manifestation of brain injury ≤48 h after hypoxic event; whether antenatal, intrapartum or postnatal.

AETIOLOGY
Obstructed labour: Malpresentation, cephalopelvic disproportion, multiple births (particularly second twin due to prolapsed cord or malpresentation), postmature neonates.
Hypotension: Maternal haemorrhage (placental abruption, placenta praevia).
Hypertension: Fulminant pregnancy-induced hypertension.
Infants at risk: Preterm infants, infants with CHD.

ASSOCIATIONS/RELATED   Other systems affected by inadequate oxygenation and perfusion: persistent pulmonary hypertension of the newborn, meconium aspiration syndrome, acute renal failure, necrotising enterocolitis, hypoglycaemia, disseminated intravascular coagulation, myocardial ischaemia.

EPIDEMIOLOGY   Moderate–severe HIE in 2–4/1000 live births.

HISTORY   Determine maternal/infant risk factors and details of neonatal resuscitation; low cord gas pH, low APGAR scores at 10 minutes, ventilator/cardiovascular resuscitation required.

EXAMINATION
Classification of HIE:

- *Stage 1*: hyperalert (eyes wide open, ↓ blinking, excessive response to stimulation), impaired feeding 2° to weak suck but normal tone
- *Stage 2*: lethargic, mild hypotonia, reduced spontaneous movement, seizures
- *Stage 3*: no spontaneous movements, withdrawal or decerebrate posturing only to pain, variable abnormal tone (hypotonia/hypertonia), suppression of primitive (Moro, tonic neck, sucking) and brainstem (corneal, gag) reflexes. Prolonged seizures refractory to treatment.

PATHOPHYSIOLOGY   Occurs following perinatal events that reduce oxygen and glucose delivery to the brain. These factors are often inter-related. The exact pathology is unclear but involves excitatory neurotransmitters (glutamate, glycine), cell death by apoptosis, and an inflammatory reaction.

INVESTIGATIONS
CTG: Poor correlation between specific patterns and neurological outcome.
Fetal cord pH: Poor association of low pH and long-term neurological outcome.
CFAM/EEG: Progressively more abnormal with worsening HIE.
USS brain: Useful to detect IVH and gross ischaemia.
MRI brain: Detects focal, multifocal and generalised ischaemic lesions. May also detect IVH. Should be performed within first 5 days for prognosis.
LP: To exclude meningitis if clinically indicated.

MANAGEMENT
Prevention: Good antenatal care, detection and management of maternal medical conditions, prompt recognition and appropriate intervention for significant fetal distress.
Neonatal resuscitation: See Appendix 2.
Prevention of 2° CNS insults: Seizure control with anticonvulsants, correction of hypoglycaemia, hypotension, hyponatraemia (slowly), hypocalcaemia, hypomagnesaemia, control of brain oedema, prevention of fluid overload, appropriate oxygenation +/− ventilation, treatment of other affected organ systems.
Therapeutic cooling: Reduces mortality and major neurodevelopmental disability (up to 18 months) in term newborns with moderate–severe HIE.

Developmental follow-up: Close monitoring in consultation with neonatal consultant, community paediatrician and paediatric neurologist. Children with neurological sequelae will require multidisciplinary input from occupational, physical, SALT and appropriate educational placement.

COMPLICATIONS   HIE may result even if managed aggressively as most asphyxia occurs before and not after birth.

PROGNOSIS   The combination of EEG, MRI and neurological examination gives the best correlation with outcome.

1. *Stage 1*: 90% have a good outcome.
2. *Stage 2*: 40–50% have normal neurological outcome.
3. *Stage 3*: 90% have major neurological sequelae: microcephaly, global developmental delay, cerebral palsy and epilepsy.

DEFINITION   Contagious superficial infection of the skin. There are two forms:

- *Bullous impetigo (30% of cases)*: blistering form.
- *Non-bullous impetigo (70% of cases)*: crusted form.

AETIOLOGY
Bullous: Results from invasion by phage group II strains of *Staphylococcus aureus* onto either intact or disrupted skin. This occurs after colonisation of the URT, usually involving the nasopharyngeal tract.

Non-bullous: In both developing and developed countries, group A β-haemolytic streptococcus is the primary pathogen. However, in developed countries *Staph. aureus* is responsible in up to 50% of cases. Bacteria invade disrupted skin 2° to eczema, insect bites, abrasions, varicella lesions or other trauma.

ASSOCIATIONS/RELATED   High temperature or humidity, impaired skin barrier, immunocompromise.

EPIDEMIOLOGY   Most common skin infection in children.
Bullous: Affects neonates and older children.
Non-bullous: Affects 2–5-year-old children.

HISTORY AND EXAMINATION
Bullous: Usually has a history of disseminated 1–2 cm thin-roofed bullae that rupture spontaneously without a history of localised lymphadenopathy or cutaneous disruption. Lesions are most commonly found on the face.

Non-bullous: A tiny pustule or honey-coloured crusted plaque forms following a break in the skin and spreads rapidly with occasional associated pruritus. Regional lymphadenopathy occurs in 90% of cases. Lesions may be found on the face, trunk, extremities, buttocks and perineum.

PATHOPHYSIOLOGY
Bullous: An epidermolytic toxin is thought to disrupt epidermal cell attachments and allow *Staph. aureus* to invade intact skin.

Non-bullous: Organisms directly penetrate epidermis superficially. Dermal vessels dilate and upper dermis fills with migrating polymorphs. Collections of pus form in the stratum corneum; these pustules rupture rapidly.

INVESTIGATIONS   Diagnosis is based mainly on history and examination of lesions.
Bacterial culture: Nasal swabs to determine carriage of *Staph. aureus*.

MANAGEMENT
Local wound care: Application of wet dressings to affected areas to aid removal of the honey-coloured crusts in non-bullous impetigo.

Topical antibiotic treatment: Topical mupirocin is considered the treatment of choice for individuals with uncomplicated localised impetigo.

Systemic antibiotic treatment: Oral flucloxacillin +/− penicillin V (if non-bullous) should be used in infections that are widespread, complicated or have systemic manifestations.

Prevention of spread:

1. School/nursery exclusion until lesions are healed/treated and dry.
2. Nasal carriage of *Staph. aureus* (15–20%) can be eradicated with nasal cream containing mupirocin.

COMPLICATIONS   Acute post-streptococcal GN is a rare but serious complication of non-bullous impetigo 2° to group A β-haemolytic streptococcus infection. It occurs ~3 weeks after onset of skin lesions and is due to an antibody response to a kidney antigen that cross-reacts with a streptococcal antigen.

PROGNOSIS   Good with appropriate treatment.

DEFINITION   Ingestion of harmful substances by children unaware of the consequences.

AETIOLOGY

Wide variety: Iron tablets, alcohol, paracetamol, acids, alkalis, salicylates, OCPs, sleeping tablets, antidepressants. Between 2 and 4 years, chemicals such as lavatory cleaners and polish are likely causes.

ASSOCIATIONS/RELATED   Lack of accident preventive measures, poor supervision of children.

EPIDEMIOLOGY

Peak age: $2\frac{1}{2}$ years – age of the inquisitive toddler.

HISTORY

Elicit a thorough history: Exact time of ingestion, estimated amount and method of ingestion. Assess whether there are any inconsistencies in the history – warning signs of abuse. Check if child has a child protection plan or is known to social services. Determine any medical conditions affecting the child.

EXAMINATION

Depends on substance ingested: Vomiting, lethargy, diarrhoea, breathing difficulties, bleeding, confusion, coma, convulsions, hypotension, tachycardia, arrhythmias. Chemical burns around mouth and lips.

PATHOPHYSIOLOGY   Dependent on individual poison.

INVESTIGATIONS

Iron: AXR, serum levels of iron and glucose.
Alcohol. Blood glucose, alcohol.
Paracetamol: Plasma concentration 4 h post ingestion, LFTs, INR.
Acids/alkalis: Early upper GI endoscopy.
Salicylates: Glucose, U&Es, LFTs, INR, ABG, salicylate level may continue to rise for several hours thus requires repeated measurements.

MANAGEMENT

Resuscitate: Ensure stability of airway, breathing and circulation.
Assess toxicity of poison: Contact any Poison Centre in the UK, e.g. Guy's Hospital, for specialist advice or access the website TOXBASE from the emergency department.
Gastric decontamination: Lavage, activated charcoal – usually performed within 1 h of ingestion. If unconscious, there is significant risk of aspiration pneumonia. Avoid in acid/alkali ingestion.
Prevention: All inadvertant poisoning should be followed up by health visitor

1. Child-resistant packaging; however, do not rely on child-proof containers.
2. Take medications away from bedside or bags; locked cabinet is ideal.
3. Throw away old or unwanted drugs or return to pharmacist.
4. Ensure supervision if child is in kitchen or bathroom.

Specific measures:

1. *Iron*: desferrioxamine antidote
2. *Paracetamol*: N-acetylcysteine
3. *Salicylates*: alkaline diuresis $+/-$ renal dialysis may be required in severe cases
4. *Acid/alkali ingestion*: steroids may reduce inflammation.

General measures: Observation and monitoring of vital functions may be all that is required.

COMPLICATIONS

Iron: Metabolic acidosis, liver failure, hypoglycaemia, gastric strictures, and multiorgan failure.

Alcohol: Hypoglycaemia and respiratory failure.

Paracetamol: Gastric irritation, liver failure, multiorgan failure.

Acids/alkalis: Ulceration and subsequent stenosis of the upper GI tract.

Salicylates: Hearing impairment, hypoglycaemia, respiratory alkalosis followed by metabolic acidosis, cardiac depression, pulmonary oedema and/or hepatic encephalopathy (Reye syndrome).

PROGNOSIS   Recovery is expected in most cases if vital functions are not affected.

DEFINITION   Hereditary biochemical disorders resulting from a mutation in a gene important in amino acid metabolism.

AETIOLOGY

Phenylketonuria (PKU): Autosomal recessive mutation leads to *classical PKU*, complete or near-complete deficiency of phenylalanine hydroxylase, required for the degradation of phenylalanine down the tyrosine pathway, or *hyperphenylalaninaemia*, due to deficiency of the phenylalanine hydroxylase co-factor.

Homocystinuria: Autosomal recessive. Three types: most commonly due to cystathionine synthase deficiency (homocystinuria type 1).

Oculocutaneous albinism (OCA): Two genetically distinct autosomal recessive forms. *OCAI:* gene defect on the long arm of chromosome 11, encoding the enzyme tyrosinase. *OCAII:* most common form of generalised albinism due to a gene defect on chromosome 15 → absence in the protein required for transport of tyrosine across the melanosome membrane.

ASSOCIATIONS/RELATED   Chromosomal abnormalities, e.g. Prader–Willi and Angelman syndrome, that have deletions on chromosome 15 may also have OCAII.

EPIDEMIOLOGY

PKU: 1/15,000 live births.
Homocystinuria: 1/344,000 live births.
OCAI: 1/40,000 live births.
OCAII: 1/15,000 live births.

HISTORY

PKU: *Infants:* normal at birth, gradual development of cognitive impairment if untreated, lose 4 IQ points/month, severe vomiting. *Older children:* hyperactive, purposeless movements, rhythmic rocking and athetosis, severe learning disability.

Homocystinuria: Normal at birth. *Infants:* non-specific, failure to thrive, developmental delay and convulsions. *>3 years old:* subluxation of ocular lens → severe myopia. Later, astigmatism, glaucoma, retinal detachment, optic atrophy. Progressive cognitive impairment and thromboembolic episodes are common.

OCA: Lack of pigment evident at birth; photophobia, ↓ visual acuity, absent binocular vision. Blindness and skin cancer are major late sequelae in severe forms. OCAII is milder than OCAI.

EXAMINATION

PKU: Blonder than siblings, fair skin and blue eyes, may have seborrhoeic/eczematoid skin rash, unpleasant odour of phenylacetic acid (musty), hypertonic with hyperactive deep tendon reflexes. NB: clinical manifestations are rarely seen in countries where neonatal screening programmes exist.

Homocystinuria: Skeletal abnormalities: tall and thin with elongated limbs and arachnodactyly, high arched palate, genu valgum and pes cavus.

OCA: Lack of skin, eye and hair pigmentation, strabismus, presence of red reflex, pink translucent iris at birth that may change to blue or brown with age.

INVESTIGATIONS

Classic PKU: Guthrie test: elevated levels of phenylalanine after 48–72 hours of life, raised plasma phenylalanine, ↑ urinary levels of phenylalanine metabolites, normal tyrosine and co-factor levels.

Homocystinuria: Elevation of methionine and homocysteine in plasma and urine. Generalised osteoporosis is the main radiographic finding.

OCA: Genetic analysis.

MANAGEMENT

PKU: Lifelong phenylalanine-free diet to maintain blood levels below 0.6–0.8 mmol/l. Levels should be monitored 2–3× per week at onset, then once a week after 1 year.

Homocystinuria: Pyridoxine (100–500 mg/day) and folic acid (10–20 mg/day). All animal proteins should be withheld; plant sources are acceptable. Betaine is used to recycle homocysteine to methionine. Dipyridamole or low-dose aspirin for anticoagulation. OCP should be avoided.

OCA: Avoid sunlight: sun protection, tinted glasses, regular ophthalmic and dermatological review.

COMPLICATIONS

PKU: Learning difficulties. If diagnosis and treatment are delayed, permanent brain damage is likely to occur. There is CNS deterioration if the phenylalanine-free diet is stopped.

Homocystinuria: Raised homocysteine has been recognised as a risk factor for IHD and thromboembolic disease in adults, such as pulmonary embolus.

OCA: Skin cancer, nystagmus and strabismus. Most patients are registered blind.

PROGNOSIS

PKU: Excellent if treatment commences within 2–3 weeks of life. If delayed, outcome is variable. If delayed till 6 months, some improvement in IQ occurs but likely to have moderate to severe learning disability.

Homocystinuria: Good if treatment continues. Treatment prevents the development of complications but will not reverse damage that has already occurred.

OCA: Variable depending on the mutation.

DEFINITION   Inherited biochemical disorders such as glycogen storage disorders (GSD) and galactosaemia that occur as a result of genetic mutations leading to disorders in the synthesis and degradation of carbohydrates.

AETIOLOGY
GSD: A genetic mutation in any of the enzymes involved in the synthesis or degradation of glycogen. This leads to an abnormality in the quantity and/or quality of glycogen produced.
Galactosaemia: Mutation leads to disorder of galactose metabolism with abnormally high plasma levels.

ASSOCIATIONS/RELATED   Family history, consanguinity.

EPIDEMIOLOGY
GSD: 1/20,000–25,000 live births. Most common enzymatic defect is glucose 6-phosphatase deficiency (type Ia).
Galactosaemia: 1/30,000 (Ireland) to 1/70,000 (UK) live births.

HISTORY AND EXAMINATION
GSD: Clinical manifestations vary widely from harmless to lethal depending on subtype.
Von Gierke disease (Ia): Presents at about 3–4 months with growth retardation, doll-like facies (fat deposition), short stature, hepatomegaly, protruding abdomen, hepatomegaly, hypoglycaemia and lactic acidosis. Platelet dysfunction may lead to easy bruising and epistaxis.
Pompe disease (II): Presents with muscle weakness and cardiomyopathy.
Other subtypes have varying degrees of myopathies.
Galactosaemia: Neonates present with prolonged jaundice (initially unconjugated then conjugated), vomiting, hypoglycaemia and 2° convulsions. Later present with cataracts, hepatosplenomegaly, stunted growth, ascites and learning disability

PATHOPHYSIOLOGY
GSDs have been categorised:

1. Numerically in order of defect identification (Ia, Ib, II, III, IV, V, VI)
2. According to organ involvement and clinical manifestation of liver and muscle glycogenoses.

Galactosaemia: Associated with three enzyme deficiencies, the most common enzyme deficiency, defined as 'classic galactosaemia', is galactose-1-phosphate uridyl transferase, which is an autosomal recessive genetic condition.

INVESTIGATIONS   Definitive diagnosis requires demonstration of the enzymatic defect in the affected tissue.
GSD: Low glucose, elevated uric acid, lactate and triglycerides are indicative. Liver biopsy is diagnostic.
Galactosaemia: Universal screening now in place in the UK; reducing substances in the urine may be found in patients ingesting lactose (glucose and galactose).

MANAGEMENT
GSD: Aimed at maintaining normal blood glucose levels by continuous NG infusion of glucose initially until slow-release carbohydrates (corn-starch) can be introduced into the diet.
Galactosaemia: Requires complete elimination of galactose from diet. Breastfeeding is contraindicated.

COMPLICATIONS
GSD: Hepatic adenomas develop in late teens and may progress to hepatocellular carcinoma, renal disease (2° to hyperuricaemia), hypertension, bleeding tendency may result in iron deficiency anaemia.

Galactosaemia: Short stature, delayed puberty, infertility, developmental delay, learning difficulties.

PROGNOSIS

GSD: Complications occur mainly in adults whose disease was not adequately treated during childhood. Long-term complications are avoided by good metabolic/dietary control. Children are now surviving into adulthood.

Galactosaemia: If untreated, severe classic galactosaemia is rapidly fatal. Most patients reach adulthood if they follow a galactose exclusion diet.

DEFINITION   Chronic idiopathic inflammatory condition affecting the bowel encompassing two related but distinct disorders: ulcerative colitis (UC) and Crohn's disease (CD).

AETIOLOGY
General: Unknown aetiology, likely 2° to environmental factors (infections, medications) triggering a response in genetically susceptible patients (multiple genes identified). Genetic component: CD > UC. Smoking: ↑d CD risk and ↓d UC risk.

Ulcerative colitis (UC): Diffuse mucosal inflammation of the rectum extending proximally (variable length). Subdivision into distal (proctitis and proctosigmoiditis) and extensive disease (left-sided or extensive colitis and pancolitis).

Crohn's disease (CD): Patchy transmural inflammation affecting one or several segments of the intestinal tract (segmental/skip lesions). Defined by anatomical location or pattern of disease (inflammatory, fistulating or stricturing). Combined Montreal classification.

Indeterminate colitis (IC): 10% of children are unclassifiable as features of both conditions present.

ASSOCIATIONS/RELATED   FHx, smoking.

EPIDEMIOLOGY   5.2/100,000 (<16 years); 60% CD, 28% UC and 12% IC. Mean age (diagnosis): 11.9 years. Bimodal peaks at 10 and 40 years.

HISTORY AND EXAMINATION
General: UC characterised by exacerbation and remission episodes (50% relapse per year), skin manifestations rare, typically present with bleeding/diarrhoea/abdominal pain. CD are more heterogeneous and non-specific; classic triad now uncommon (abdominal pain/diarrhoea/weight loss).

Common symptoms: Abdominal pain (CD 72%, UC 62%, IC 72%), diarrhoea (CD 56%, UC 74%, IC 78%), rectal bleeding (CD 22%, UC 84%, IC 49%), weight loss (CD 58%, UC 31%, IC 35%), lethargy (CD 27%, UC 12%, IC 14%) and anorexia (CD 25%, UC 6%, IC 13%).

Other symptoms: Arthropathy, N&V, constipation, encopresis, psychiatric symptoms, 2° amenorrhoea.

Signs: Anal fistula, growth failure/delayed puberty, anal abscess/ulcer, erythema nodosum/rash, liver disease, toxic megacolon.

PATHOPHYSIOLOGY
UC: *Macro:* mucosal erythema, friability, ulceration and inflammatory pseudopolyps. *Micro:* distortion of crypt architecture, inflammatory cell infiltrate, goblet cell depletion and crypt abscesses.

CD: *Macro:* mucosal (oedema/fibrosis), deep ulceration (serpiginous or fissuring), fistulas. *Micro:* transmural inflammation, lymphoid aggregates, non-caseating granulomas

INVESTIGATIONS
General: ESPGHAN IBD Working Group consensus protocol.

Bloods: ↓Hb, ↑ESR/CRP, serum folate, B12, LFTs (abnormality requires investigation with ERCP, USS and biopsy for primary sclerosing cholangitis (PSC)), albumin.

Specific: Limited use of perinuclear antineutrophil cytoplasmic antibody (pANCA) with UC and anti-*Saccharomyces cerevisiae* antibody (ASCA) with CD; sensitivity – 60–80%.

Microbiology: Stool culture (infective causes), *Clostridium difficile* toxins A and B.

Radiology: AXR (toxic dilation), small bowel follow-through, technetium white cell scanning (highlights areas of inflammation).

Endoscopy: Ileocolonoscopy and upper GI endoscopy with histology of multiple biopsies from all segments.

MANAGEMENT

CD: *First line:* exclusive liquid enteral nutrition, corticosteroids, antibiotics (perianal disease), aminosalicylates (mesalazine/sulphasalazine), budesonide, IV steroids. *Second line:* azathioprine, parenteral nutrition. *Third line:* infliximab and surgery (isolated ileocaecal disease, strictures or fistulae). *Remission maintenance:* azathioprine/6-mercaptopurine, methotrexate, enteral supplementary therapy.

UC: *Induction of remission:* ASA/sulphasalazine (mild disease) or corticosteroids (moderate–severe disease). *Maintenance:* aminosalicylates/mesalazine. *Second line:* azathioprine/6-mercaptopurine. *Specific:* surgery with acute toxic megacolon/resistance to medical therapy, aminosalicylates and steroid enemas with distal disease.

COMPLICATIONS

UC: Toxic megacolon, perforation, colorectal carcinoma, PSE.

CD: Megaloblastic anaemia, gallstones, perianal disease (tags, fissures, fistulas, purulent discharge), strictures, obstruction.

PROGNOSIS   Good with early detection and treatment, mortality highest in first 2 years of diagnosis.

DEFINITION   Intraventricular haemorrhage usually arising in the germinal matrix and periventricular regions of the brain.

- *Grade I*: germinal matrix haemorrhage only.
- *Grade II*: blood within the lateral ventricle without ventricular dilation.
- *Grade III*: blood within the lateral ventricle with ventricular dilation.
- *Grade IV*: IVH with periventricular parenchymal haemorrhagic infarct.

AETIOLOGY

1. Prematurity (major factor).
2. *Factors that* ↑/↓ *BP*: hypovolaemia, hypotension, hypertension, pulmonary haemorrhage, mechanical ventilation, ↑pCO_2, ↓pO_2, prolonged labour, PDA.
3. *Others*: acidosis, hypothermia, HIE, severe RDS, pneumothorax, coagulopathy.

ASSOCIATIONS/RELATED   Maternal smoking.

EPIDEMIOLOGY
Most common in very low-birthweight infants: 30–40% of infants weighing <1500 g; 50–60% of infants weighing <1000 g.

HISTORY AND EXAMINATION   Highest incidence in first 72 h of life, 60% within 24 h, 85% within 72 h, <5% after 1 week postnatal age.
Signs and symptoms: May be asymptomatic (grade I or II), seizures, poor tone, apnoea, lethargy, shock and anaemia (grade III or IV).
Signs of raised ICP: Bulging fontanelle, Cushing response (↑BP, ↓HR).
Monitor head circumference: For progressive hydrocephalus.

PATHOPHYSIOLOGY   The germinal matrix tissue is located adjacent to the lateral ventricles. It is the site of origin of migrating neuroblasts from the end of the first trimester and has become highly cellular and richly vascularised by 24–26 weeks. The vessels are thin-walled and fragile and susceptible to damage from fluctuations in cerebral blood flow leading to haemorrhage. Haemorrhage in this area may destroy the migrating neuroblasts and impair subsequent brain development. The germinal matrix involutes by the 36th gestational week which is why preterm infants are most affected.

Periventricular parenchymal haemorrhagic infarct occurs due to compromised venous return rather than direct extension of bleeding from the germinal matrix.

INVESTIGATIONS
Bloods: FBC, clotting, capillary gas for acid/base balance.
USS: Used in the diagnosis and classification of IVH.

MANAGEMENT
Routine screening: USS indicated in infants <32 weeks gestational age within the first week of life and should be repeated in the second week.
Prevention: Maintain acid/base balance and avoid fluctuations in BP.
Supportive care: Ventilatory support and blood transfusion in large haemorrhage.
Treatment of ↑ICP: Diuretics (mannitol) may be required.
Interventional: External ventriculostomy or permanent ventricular–peritoneal shunt.

COMPLICATIONS   Hydrocephalus (10–15%), neurological impairment.

PROGNOSIS
Grade I and II: Rarely have harmful neurological consequences, as they originate in the germinal matrix (which disappears) and do not normally extend into the white matter.
Grade III: 30–45% incidence of neurological impairment.
Grade IV: 60–80% incidence of neurological impairment.

DEFINITION Invagination or telescoping of part of the intestine (intussuscepian) into an adjacent intestinal lumen (intussusceptum).

AETIOLOGY 90% are idiopathic. 2–10% have an identified lead point, most commonly Peyer's patches in the ileum 2° to a viral illness. Less commonly, lymph nodes, Meckel's diverticulum, intestinal polyp, appendiceal stump or adhesions from recent surgery.

ASSOCIATIONS/RELATED Viruses (adenovirus), Henoch–Schönlein purpura, familial adenomatous polyposis.

EPIDEMIOLOGY 1–4/1000. M : F = 2 : 1. 60% are <1 year, 80% <2 years. Most common cause of small bowel obstruction, rare in neonates.

HISTORY AND EXAMINATION Classic triad of symptoms (vomiting, colicky severe intermittent abdominal pain and PR bleeding). Vomiting is initially non-bilious then becomes bilious once intussusception more established. Pain episodes are characteristically 'inconsolable' with leg pulling, pallor and screaming. Infant may appear well between episodes. Characteristically bleeding is 'redcurrant jelly stools' (late sign as 2° to mucosal necrosis and sloughing). Examination may reveal normal infant, signs of dehydration with shock, abdominal distension, 'sausage-shaped, mass, blood PR.

PATHOPHYSIOLOGY Most common site of invagination is the terminal ileum into the caecum. Mesenteric constriction → venous return obstruction → engorgement and oedema → bleeding → prevention of arterial perfusion → intestinal infarction and perforation. Peyer's patches = oval or round lymphoid follicles located in the lamina propria layer of the mucosa and extending into the submucosa of the ileum.

INVESTIGATIONS
Bloods: CRP(?↑), U&Es (dehydration), FBC(?↑WCC, ↓Hb), G&S.
AXR: Dilated bowel may be present; 'crescent sign' – presence of a curvilinear mass on the right, especially in the transverse colon distal to the hepatic flexure, is pathognomonic.
USS: Confirmatory investigation, presence of a 'donut' or 'target' sign.

MANAGEMENT
General: IV access, fluid resuscitation (20 ml/kg/bouls), NGT placement, IV antibiotics for reduction and immediate confirmation of the intussusception with USS.
Therapeutic enema: Air, water or contrast enema for reduction. Usually three attempts as risk of perforation. Fluid between the bowel walls with a long-standing intussusception are poor prognostic factors for successful reduction. However, most centres will attempt a reduction as it is far less invasive.
Surgical reduction: If therapeutic air enema fails; may be by either the laparoscopic or open technique. Open access is through a right lower transverse incision. Reduction should be careful to avoid perforation and involve a retrograde milking technique. Laparoscopic reduction involves a gentle traction. Limited right hemicolectomy if the bowel is necrotic upon full reduction.

COMPLICATIONS Prolonged intussusception can lead to shock, peritonitis and intestinal perforation.

PROGNOSIS Highest risk of recurrence in the first 24 hours. Children with multiple episodes of intussusception should be investigated for a pathological lead point.

DEFINITION   Juvenile idiopathic arthritis is a group of chronic arthropathies of childhood. Seven subtypes are suggested by the International League of Associations for Rheumatology (ILAR).

1. *Systemic (sJIA)*: $\geq$1 joint with or preceded by fever lasting for $\geq$3 days with $\geq$1 of: rash, generalised lymphadenopathy, hepatomegaly, splenomegaly or serositis.
2. *Oligoarticular* ($\leq$4 joints affected in first 6 months of disease):
   (a) Persistent; followed by $\leq$4 joints involvement
   (b) Extended; followed by >4 joint involvement.
3/4. *Polyarticular* (>4 joints affected during first 6 months):
   3. Rheumatoid factor (RF)-negative
   4. RF positive.
5. *Enthesitis-related arthritis (ERA)*: arthritis and enthesitis (inflammation at insertion of tendon, ligament, joint capsule or fascia to bone) or $\geq$2 features of enthesitis: sacroiliac joint/lumbosacral pain, HLA-B27 positive, male onset >6 years, acute anterior uveitis (first-degree relative), Reiter syndrome (acute reactive arthritis following gastroenteritis/STI).
6. *Psoriatic arthritis*: arthritis with psoriasis or $\geq$2 features of psoriasis: dactylitis, nail pitting/onycholysis or psoriasis in first-degree relative.
7. *Undifferentiated*: no category or $\geq$2 of the categories above.

AETIOLOGY   An aberrant immune/inflammatory response. Activated T cells (Th1 proinflammatory cytokines), humoral immunity (ANA or RF) and innate immunity (in particular neutrophils) all have evidence to support being involved in the pathogenesis of different subtypes of JIA. HLA subtypes have been linked to all classified subtypes.

ASSOCIATIONS/RELATED
DD sJIA: Bacterial or viral infection, malignancy, vasculitis, connective tissue disease. Septic arthritis is an important differential in single joint involvement.

EPIDEMIOLOGY   JIA is the most common chronic rheumatic disease in children. In developed countries the prevalence is 16–150/100,000. sJIA comprises 10–20% of all JIA.

HISTORY
General: Acute joint swelling, pain, warmth and stiffness; typically worse in the morning and improves with activity, may later present with reduced range of movement, overgrowth or contractures. Children often do not complain of pain and instead tend to stop using the affected joint.
sJIA: Usually symmetrical, polyarticular and associated with severe myalgia, abdominal pain, daily high temperature spike with associated rash.

EXAMINATION   Paediatric Gait Arms Legs Spine (pGALS) system has been validated as a screening tool for the musculoskeletal system in children.

PATHOPHYSIOLOGY   All subtypes of JIA are characterised by persistent joint swelling caused by an accumulation of synovial fluid and thickening of the synovial lining.

INVESTIGATIONS   FBC, markers of inflammation (ESR, CRP, ferritin), RF, ANA, HLA type, slit lamp examination (anterior uveitis), X-ray, USS, MRI of joints.

MANAGEMENT   Holistic approach with involvement of multidisciplinary team: physiotherapy, occupational therapy and psychological support.
Symptomatic treatment: Analgesia; NSAIDs with gastric protection, steroids (oral, intra-articular or IV pulsed).
Disease-modifying antirheumatic drugs (DMARDS): Methotrexate, etanercept (anti-TNF-α).

COMPLICATIONS   As anterior uveitis is asymptomatic, failure to screen for this may lead to glaucoma, cataracts and blindness.

PROGNOSIS   A high proportion of affected children develop destructive joint disease (30–40% with polyarticular JIA), often requiring early joint replacement.

DEFINITION   A childhood acute febrile illness with small and medium vessel vasculitis.

AETIOLOGY   Epidemiological studies suggest that an infectious agent may induce the disease in genetically susceptible individuals.
Infectious hypothesis: Winter–spring seasonality, occurrence of community outbreaks.
Genetic susceptibility hypothesis: Japanese individuals are more likely to contract KD no matter where they live.
Superantigen hypothesis: Results have so far been inconclusive.

ASSOCIATIONS/RELATED   1% of cases have a positive family history. Siblings have a 10-fold risk of developing KD within the next year; in 50% of cases this is within the following 10 days.
Main differential diagnosis: Streptococcal disease (scarlet fever), viral infections (measles, EBV, enterovirus), staphylococcal scalded skin syndrome.

EPIDEMIOLOGY   KD is now the leading cause of acquired heart disease. Annual incidence rate is >1/1000 in <5 year olds (Japan) but $10\times$ lower in the US and $30\times$ lower in the UK. Peak age: 1–2 years. 80% of cases $\leq$5 years. $M : F = 1.5 : 1$.

HISTORY AND EXAMINATION:
Classic features: High fever $\geq$5 days and the presence of $\geq$4 of:

1. Erythema/oedema of hands and feet followed by desquamation
2. Diffuse maculopapular rash (usually within 5 days)
3. Bilateral, non-exudative conjunctivitis
4. Erythema of lips and oral mucosa, strawberry tongue
5. Cervical lymphadenopathy ($\geq$1.5 cm), usually unilateral.

Revised guidelines: Fever persisting $\geq$4 days if other clinical features are present.

PATHOPHYSIOLOGY   Marked cytokine cascade stimulation and endothelial cell activation leads to systemic vasculitis. Coronary artery aneurysms are caused by influx of neutrophils, lymphocytes and IgA plasma cells causing destruction of the internal elastic lamina. Fibroblastic proliferation/remodelling may subsequently lead to coronary artery stenosis.

INVESTIGATIONS
Bloods: ↑WCC, ↑CRP/ESR, ↑platelets (subacute phase).
Microbiology: Blood culture, throat, nose and rectal swab, ASOT.
2D-ECHO/coronary angiography: KD may be diagnosed if coronary artery aneurysm, fever and <4 classic features.

MANAGEMENT
Antibiotics: Until bacterial infection has been excluded.
IVIG: Decreases the risk of cardiac complications. High-dose (2 g/kg) IVIG should be administered $\leq$D10 (ideally $\leq$D7). Treatment $\leq$D5 appears no more likely to prevent cardiac sequelae than D5–7, but is associated with an increased need for IVIG retreatment. If $\geq$D10, IVIG should still be administered if the child is febrile or has raised inflammatory markers. Measles/varicella immunisation should be deferred for 11 months after high-dose IVIG.
Aspirin: High-dose aspirin anti-inflammatory therapy (7.5 mg/kg QDS) until day 14 followed by low-dose antiplatelet therapy (1–2 mg/kg TDS) for 6–8 weeks until ECHO has confirmed no coronary artery involvement. S/E: Reye syndrome; aspirin should be stopped if child develops influenza or chickenpox.
Steroids: Only considered if two infusions of IVIG have been ineffective.

COMPLICATIONS   Coronary artery aneurysms develop in 15–25% of untreated children and may lead to myocardial infarction, sudden death or ischaemic heart disease (2%).

PROGNOSIS   KD is usually self-limiting and resolves spontaneously without treatment within 4–8 weeks. Duration of fever and older age are poor prognostic factors. Mortality rates vary between 0.08% (Japan) and 3.7% (UK). Recurrence rate is 3% (Japan).

DEFINITION   Genetic defect of the sex chromosomes in males leading to a karyotype of 47XXY (80–90% of cases) or more rarely a mosaic of 46XY/47XXY.

AETIOLOGY

1. Extra X chromosome.
2. Non-dysjunction during meiosis and mitosis; 50–60% due to maternal non-dysjunction and 75% meiosis 1 errors.
3. Anaphase lags during meiosis and mitosis.

Rarely caused by structural chromosomal abnormalities.

ASSOCIATIONS/RELATED   ↑d maternal age, paternal non-dysjunction errors, genetic association.

EPIDEMIOLOGY   1–2/1000 males. Most common cause of hypogonadism.

HISTORY AND EXAMINATION
Prenatal: Detection with chromosomal analysis (amniocentesis).
Childhood: Possible speech, language and reading problems, but most XXY individuals have normal intelligence.
Puberty: Patients may lack 2° sexual characteristics 2° to ↓d androgen production; sparse facial/body/sexual hair, high-pitched voice, female fat distribution and ↓d muscle mass. Small and firm testes (<2 cm), microphallus and gynaecomastia due to ↑d oestrogen levels and oestrogen:testosterone ratio.
Adulthood: Usually present with infertility or gynaecomastia. Also suffer from erectile dysfunction and low libido. Usually tall, with disproportionately long arms and legs.

PATHOPHYSIOLOGY
Testicular biopsy: Seminiferous tubular hyalinisation, sclerosis and atrophy with focal hyperplasia of mostly degenerated Leydig cells. Germ cells are markedly deficient or absent.

INVESTIGATIONS
Bloods: ↑d LH and FSH, ↓d testosterone.
Chromosomal studies: Karyotype analysis confirms diagnosis (>20 cell analysis to detect mosaics).
Semen analysis: Assess whether conception is possible using intracytoplasmic sperm injection (ICSI).
Testicular biopsy: Infertility evaluation.
Bone mass density: Osteoporosis may develop in 25% due to lack of sex hormone regulation on osteoblast/osteoclast activity in the bone.
Echocardiography: Mitral valve prolapse assessment.

MANAGEMENT
Testosterone replacement: Regular IM injections or skin patches, commenced as patients enter puberty. This helps in developing 2° sexual characteristics but does not ↑ fertility. Dose ↑d until normal levels of oestrogen/testosterone/FSH/LH.
Surgical intervention: Persistent gynaecomastia treatment by mastectomy (↓d breast carcinoma).
Regular follow-up: Bone mass density (DEXA scan), treatment monitoring.
Psychosocial therapy: Speech, language, physical and occupational combined with psychological support.
Infertility: Artificial reproductive technologies combined with genetic counselling; microsurgical testicular sperm extraction with *in vitro* fertilisation.

COMPLICATIONS

1. ↑d risk of breast cancer with gynaecomastia (~×20).
2. Osteoporosis and related fractures.

3. Infertility is seen in practically all individuals with a 47XXY karyotype who require ICSI to reproduce. Patients with Klinefelter syndrome mosaicism (46XY/47XXY) may be fertile.
4. Mitral valve prolapse (55% of patients).

PROGNOSIS   Individuals have a normal lifespan with normal quality of life.

DEFINITION   Inability to metabolise the carbohydrate lactose due to lactase deficiency.

AETIOLOGY
Congenital: Autosomal recessive condition.
Primary: Natural non-persistence of lactase enzyme after early childhood. Persistence of lactase is due to polymorphisms in the gene encoding for lactase (common in N. Europe).
Secondary: Damage to the intestinal brush border following gastroenteritis.

ASSOCIATIONS/RELATED   Lactose intolerance is often confused with delayed non-IgE mediated cow's milk protein allergy. Lactose intolerance is not immune mediated and is due to an intolerance of cow's milk carbohydrate (sugar), not cow's milk protein.

EPIDEMIOLOGY
Congenital: Extremely rare (40 cases known in the world).
Primary: 5% (UK) to 17% in N. Europe increasing to >50% in Africa, Asia and South America. Rarely presents before 5 years of age.

HISTORY AND EXAMINATION
GI: Loose stools (frothy and explosive), bloating and cramping abdominal pain, flatus.
Congenital: Infantile diarrhoea, failure to thrive
Primary: GI symptoms increase with age due to progressive loss of lactase. There is a wide variety in the amount of lactose that individuals can tolerate.
Secondary: Preceding infective episode of diarrhoea.

PATHOPHYSIOLOGY   Disaccharide enzymes (for lactose, sucrose and maltose) are located at the brush border of the small intestine. The enzyme lactase breaks down lactose to glucose and galactose which can be absorbed into the bloodstream. For effective metabolism of lactose, only 50% lactase activity is required.
    Deficiency of lactase prevents hydrolysis of ingested lactose which results in an osmotic load in the gut and secretory diarrhoea. Abdominal pain and bloating are caused by bacterial fermentation of lactose in the colon.

INVESTIGATIONS
Hydrogen breath test: Detects hydrogen in breath 3–6 hours following ingestion of lactose. 20% will have a false-negative result due to hydrogen non-excretion.
Stools for reducing substances: Stools are acidic and contain undigested sugar.
Jejunal biopsies: Rarely needed to differentiate from coeliac disease.

MANAGEMENT   Lactose is contained in only mammalian milk.
Congenital: Life-long absolute avoidance of all traces of lactose. Lactose-free infant formulas and commercial lactose-free milk are available. Soya, rice, oat and pea milks are lactose free (recommend calcium-supplemented products). Rice milk is not recommended in children <4.5 years of age.
Primary: Low lactose diet is usually tolerated. These individuals may tolerate low lactose foods such as hard cheeses (Cheddar) and fermented yoghurts.
Secondary: Complete lactose avoidance is advised for 4–6 weeks to allow mucosal regeneration followed by gradual reintroduction of foods containing lactose.

COMPLICATIONS   Malabsorption, failure to thrive in congenital lactose intolerance if there is delay in diagnosis. Main complication is due to calcium deficiency in children with unsupervised cow's milk exclusion diets without appropriate milk alternative or calcium supplementation.

PROGNOSIS   Congenital lactose intolerance is a life-long condition. Primary lactose intolerance is variable depending on the individual and secondary lactose intolerance is transient.

DEFINITION   Ideopathic avascular necrosis of the capital femoral epiphysis of the femoral head.

AETIOLOGY
General: Unknown aetiology; probably multifactorial. 25% bilateral (doesn't occur synchronously in each hip). Possible theories: altered growth patterns (short stature, ↓d growth factors and delayed bone age), trauma (absent activity association, however), thrombosis and fibrinolysis defects (sickle cell disease and crisis, protein C and S deficiency).
Classification: Modified Elizabethtown; I-Sclerotic (A = no loss of height, B = height loss), II-Fragmentation (A = early, B = late), III-Healing (A = peripheral, B > 1/3 epiphysis), and IV-healed.

ASSOCIATIONS/RELATED   Sickle cell disease, socio-economic deprivation, low birthweight, ↑d parental age, later-born children, passive smoking.

EPIDEMIOLOGY   6–12/100,000. Peak: 7 years. M : F = 6 : 1.

HISTORY   Wide range of presentations.
Limp: Early sign, intermittent, abductor lurch, post-exercise. Classic presentation is with a painless limp.
Pain: Classically painless although may have mild intermittent pain in anterior thigh or hip pain 2° to necrosis of affected bone, possibly referred to the medial aspect of the ipsilateral knee/lateral thigh.

EXAMINATION
Look: Atrophy of the quadriceps muscles 2° to disuse on the affected side, leg length inequality, hip adduction flexion deformity, antalgic or Trendelenburg gait (2° to gluteus medius pain).
Feel: Nil objective signs (hidden joint).
Move: Restricted ROM, particularity internal rotation and abduction (2° impingement lesions). Late stages are characterised by global ↓ in all ROM.
Roll test: Supine position; roll the foot of the affected hip into internal and external rotation. +ve test invokes guarding or spasm, especially with internal rotation.
Clinical femoral head 'at-risk' signs (Catterall): ↑d age, ↑d weight, progressive loss of movement, adduction contracture, flexion with adduction.

PATHOPHYSIOLOGY   Femoral epiphysis rapid growth → vascular supply interruption → ischaemia → subchondral cortical bone infarction and avascular necrosis → eventual bone ossification with revascularisation. Remodelling at this stage determines prognosis. Articular cartilage is unaffected as synovial fluid provides nutrients.

INVESTIGATIONS
Bloods: FBC, CRP/ESR (? septic arthritis), Hb electrophoresis (? sickle cell).
Joint aspiration: Exclude septic arthritis.
X-ray (AP and frog-leg): Catterall head 'at-risk' signs; Gage sign, calcification lateral to the epiphysis, subluxation, epiphyseal angle, diffuse metaphyseal reaction.
Imaging: Bone scan, arthrography, MRI.

MANAGEMENT
General: Based on Catterall clinical/radiological grade and Elizabethtown stage.
Containment theory: Secure the injured femoral head within the socket and movement continued → post-regeneration is round and fully mobile.
Conservative: Only with healing stage (>8 years old) or if clinically good (<7 years old).
Surgical: To achieve containment and salvage the joint. Includes proximal femoral osteotomies, acetabular surgery, abduction osteotomies and cheilectomy. Avoidance of extensive and prolonged immobilisation.

COMPLICATIONS   Permanent femoral head deformity and early osteo-arthritis.

PROGNOSIS   Iowa long-term follow-up (40 years): 40% had a joint replacement, 10% disabling arthritis requiring a replacement, 10% had Iowa hip score <80.

DEFINITION   Malignant clonal disease characterised by proliferation of early B- and T-lymphocyte progenitors.

AETIOLOGY
General: Genetic lesions in the B- and T-lymphocyte progenitors. Karotype (80% are abnormal) = important predictor of outcome. Suggestion of *in utero* origin of the leukaemic clone (cord blood studies). B-cell precursor ALL is the most frequent.
Cytogenetic abnormalities: 25% B-cell precursor ALL have the *TEL-AML-1* fusion gene = t(12;21)(p13;q22). Both genes are required for haematopoiesis. *TEL-AML-1* has been detected in cord blood. Philadelphia chromosome t(9;22)(q34;q11) is characteristic of chronic myeloid leukaemia (CML) but is a significant abnormality with ALL. 50% of T-cell ALL have activating mutations involving *NOTCH1*.

ASSOCIATIONS/RELATED
Inherited genetic syndromes (5%): Trisomy 21, Fanconi anaemia, achondroplasia, ataxia telangiectasia, xeroderma pigmentosum, X-linked agammaglobulinaemia, ↑ risk in siblings.

EPIDEMIOLOGY   30/million/yr. Peaks 2–5 years old. 85% of childhood leukaemias.

HISTORY AND EXAMINATION
Symptoms of bone marrow failure: Anaemia (fatigue, dyspnoea), bleeding (spontaneous bruising, bleeding gums and menorrhagia if adolescent) and infections (bacterial/viral/fungal)
Symptoms of organ infiltration: Meningeal involvement with headache, visual disturbance and nausea, cranial nerve palsies, retinal haemorrhage or papilloedema on fundoscopy, lymphadenopathy, tender bones, mediastinal compression in T-ALL with dyspnoea, hepatosplenomegaly, testicular swelling.

PATHOPHYSIOLOGY   Malignant lymphoblasts subclassified using FAB (French American British) classification based on morphology L_1–L_3.

INVESTIGATIONS
Bloods: ↓ Hb: normochromic, normocytic +/− ↓ platelets, ↑WCC, ↑uric acid, ↑LDH, clotting.
Bone marrow aspirate/trephine biopsy: Hypercellular: >30% lymphoblasts, histochemical stains, flow cytometry, cytogenetics +/− specimen banking (if consented).
Cytogenetics: Karyotype abnormalities: chromosomal loss/gain, translocations. B-lineage ALL +ve with PAS stain, T-lineage ALL acid phosphatase.
Lumbar puncture: CSF analysis ?meningeal involvement.
Imaging (CXR): Mediastinal lymphadenopathy, thymic enlargement, lytic lesions.
Bone radiographs: 'Punched-out' lesions of the bones, e.g. skull, due to leukaemic infiltration.

MANAGEMENT
Chemotherapy: Paediatric ALL treatment protocols differ in medications/doses/schedules but share overall treatment strategy. Remission-induction phase → intensification (or consolidation) phase → continuation therapy. Remission-induction phase = ↓ leukaemic blast bone marrow by 99% (↓extramedullary disease and restores normal haematopoiesis). Intensification = eradication of drug-resistant residual leukaemic cells. Continuation therapy for 2–2.5 years.
Allogenic stem cell transplantation: If Philadelphia +ve, poor initial response to treatment, WCC >200 × 10^9 or B-cell with t(8,14).
CNS-directed radiation: Only with high-risk patients.
Supportive care: Antiemetics, central venous access, blood products/growth factors, mouth care.

COMPLICATIONS

General: Venous thromboembolism (0–36%) 2° to chemotherapy protocols.

Chemotherapy: Cardiotoxicity, fertility problems, 2° malignancy (intracranial tumours, non-Hodgkin lymphoma) and relapse.

PROGNOSIS   60–80% 5-year survival (age dependent).

Poor prognosis: Philadelphia translocation t(9,22); 0–15% disease free at 5 years, age (<2, >10 years), male sex, WCC >100 × 10^9/L, t(4,11), T-cell ALL, CNS involvement at presentation, lack of response to treatment.

Good prognosis: t(12,21).

DEFINITION   Malignant clonal disease characterised by a block in differentiation and unregulated proliferation of myeloid progenitor cells.

AETIOLOGY
General: Occurs 1° or 2° to myeloproliferative or myelodysplasia/previous chemotherapy. 80% of children have clonal chromosomal abnormalities. Symptoms 2° leukaemic blast cells suppressing normal haemopoietic elements in the bone marrow and invading extramedullary sites.
Cytogenetic abnormalities: 11q23 abnormalities most common (*MLL* gene rearrangement in 20%), others include M2 = t(8;21), M3 = t(15;17), M4Eo = inv(16). Specific abnormalities linked to outcome.
FAB (French American British) classification: 8 morphological variants: M0–M7. M1/2 (30–40%), M3 (10%), M4 (20–25%), M5 (20%) and M6/7 (10%).

ASSOCIATIONS/RELATED   Trisomy 21 (2%). Sweet syndrome (acute febrile neutrophilic dermatitis). Constitutional trisomy 8. Shwachman–Diamond syndrome. Fanconi anaemia. Toxins exposure (ethanol/pesticides and dietary topoisomerase II inhibitors).

EPIDEMIOLOGY   4–10/million, 60–70 new cases/year (UK), 17% of all acute childhood leukaemias. M = F.

HISTORY
Bone marrow failure: Anaemia (lethargy, dyspnoea), bleeding (DIC or thrombocytopenia in case of M3 promyelocytic leukaemia), infections (bacterial/viral/fungal).
Tissue infiltration: Gum swelling/bleeding, CNS involvement (headaches, nausea, diplopia), bone pain.
Systemic: Malaise, weakness, pyrexia. Concurrent coagulopathy may be present (M3 and M5) leading to ↑d haemorrhage risk.

EXAMINATION
Bone marrow failure: Pallor, cardiac flow murmur, ecchymoses and infection (pyrexia, mouth infections, e.g. *Candida*, herpes simplex, skin infections, e.g. *Pseudomonas*, respiratory, perianal infections, e.g. *E. coli* and *Streptococcus faecalis*, perineal infections).
Tissue infiltration: Skin rashes, gum hypertrophy, deposit of leukaemic blasts may rarely be seen in the eye ('chloroma'), hepatosplenomegaly, adenopathy and lymphadenopathy.

PATHOPHYSIOLOGY   FAB subtypes reflect the morphology and histochemistry of the predominant AML clone.

INVESTIGATIONS
Bloods: ↓Hb, ↓Plts, ↑↓WCC, ↑uric acid, ↑LDH fibrinogen/D-dimers (if DIC is suspected in M3). Patients have a conserved clonotypic immunophenotype ('molecular fingerprint') that may be useful for disease monitoring.
Blood film: AML blasts show cytoplasmic granules or Auer rods.
Bone marrow aspirate/biopsy: Hypercellular with >30% blasts (immature cells). Histochemical stains, flow cytometry, cytogenetics +/− specimen banking (if consented).

MANAGEMENT   More intensive than ALL as remission is more difficult to achieve and maintain.
Emergency: DIC with M3: FFP and platelet transfusions (see DIC).
Chemotherapy: Paediatric AML treatment protocols differ in medications/doses/ schedules but share overall treatment strategy. Remission induction and CNS prophylaxis → consolidation → intensification   phase +/− maintenance   phase. Induction therapy aim = ↓ leukaemic blast bone marrow % <5% (↓ extramedullary disease and restores normal haematopoiesis).
Allogenic stem cell transplantation: From a HLA-matched sibling in the first remission.

Supportive care: Central venous access, blood products/growth factors, infection treatment and prophylaxis, counselling.

Future: Possible immunotherapy with monoclonal antibodies.

COMPLICATIONS   Leucostasis (pulmonary/CNS infarcts 2° ↑↑WCC and WBC thrombi); chemotherapy side effects; graft versus host disease (GVHD), relapse, rejection (transplant).

PROGNOSIS   34–56% survival from time of diagnosis.

DEFINITION   Arthralgia and arthritis leading to ataxia 2° to either an acute suppurative process or transient sterile inflammation of the hip synovium.

AETIOLOGY
Septic arthritis (SA): Joint infection 2° to pyogenic bacteria from either bacterial translocation from osteomyelitis (via transient transphyseal vessels) or haematological spread. Most common organism: *Staphylococcus aureus*. Less common: *Streptococcus pyogenes (group B)*, *Strep. pneumonia*, *E. coli* and *Proteus*. All joints can potentially develop SA.
Transient synovitis (TS/irritable hip): Unknown aetiology, unilateral in presentation, preceding viral infection common, especially URTI (30%), ligamentous or minor capsular injury 2° trauma (5%). Viral aetiology suspected 2° to Hx and ↑d serum interferon levels in affected children although nil viral antibodies have been detected.

ASSOCIATIONS/RELATED   URTI, pharyngitis, bronchitis, otitis media & osteomyelitis.

EPIDEMIOLOGY
SA: 6/100,000.
TS: Most common cause of acute hip pain in children aged 3–10 years. M : F = 2 : 1.

HISTORY
General: Often identical presentation with TS and SA. Non-specific signs/symptoms with infants. Septicaemia with SA.
Pain: Unilateral hip or groin pain +/– radiation to the knee or medial thigh. Rest pain (SA).
Limp: Painless limp or antalgic gait (TS) or painful (SA) also non-weight bearing
Pyrexia: Mild pyrexia (37.5–38 °C) with TS > 38 °C = ?SA.

EXAMINATION
Look: Leg may be held in flexion and internal rotation, no leg length inequality.
Feel: Pain elicited on palpation.
Move: Pain on passive movement and mild restriction in range of movement, particularly internal rotation and abduction.
Leg roll: Patient supine, involved leg is rolled from side to side – involuntary muscle guarding occurs on one side when compared to the other.

PATHOPHYSIOLOGY   Intracapsular inflammation with synovial proliferation +/– exudates or transudate distended joint capsule leading to laxity, subluxation and dislocation.

INVESTIGATIONS
Exclude septic arthritis.
Bloods: FBC (↑d neutrophils/WCC), ↑d CRP and ESR.
Microbiology: Blood and urine cultures.
AP and frog-leg lateral XR: Medial joint space may be slightly wider in the affected hip, ↑d teardrop distance (excess fluid), possible accentuated pericapsular shadow, Waldenström sign. Also for exclusion of differential diagnosis (occult fracture, osteoid osteoma).
Ultrasonography: Intracapsular effusion detection and aspiration guidance.
Aspiration: Cell count and gram stain. >50,000 cells with >90% polymorphonuclear leucocytes, SA is likely even with nil organism cultured. Under GA with image intensifier guidance. ↑d synovial fluid proteoglycans (TS).
Kocher criteria: Four major predictors: history of pyrexia, non-weight bearing, ESR >40 mm/h, WCC >12,000. Predicted possibility of septic arthritis (number of predictors): 1 (3%), 2 (40%), 3 (93%) and 4 (93%).

MANAGEMENT
SA: Organism identification (BC/aspiration culture), IV antibiotics +/– joint lavage (arthrotomy under GA). Possible CVC (PICC/long line) for prolonged antibiotic therapy.
TS: Conservative; rest (exercise avoidance), heat therapy, NSAIDs.

COMPLICATIONS

SA: <2 years = ↑d complications. Chondrolysis, limb deformity (AVN/dislocations/premature closure of proximal femoral physis or triradiate cartilage), osteoporosis, overgrowth of the greater trochanter, 2° infections.

TS: No definite long-term sequelae; possible link with development of Perthes disease of the hip.

Prognosis

TS self-limiting, SA excellent with prompt diagnosis and treatment.

DEFINITION   Chronic disease of the hepatic cells → decrease in overall liver function.

AETIOLOGY
Chronic active hepatitis:

1. Autoimmune disease of parenchyma (autoimmune hepatitis) or biliary tree (primary sclerosing cholangitis)
2. *Viral hepatitis*: HBV, HCV
3. *Drugs*: NSAIDs, antibiotics (nitrofurantoin), anticonvulsants, paracetamol.

Wilson disease: Genetic disease of copper metabolism which → deposition of copper in the liver, brain, kidneys and cornea.
Cystic fibrosis (see chapter).

ASSOCIATIONS/RELATED   Family history, origin from developing countries (HBV/HCV).

EPIDEMIOLOGY
HBV: 5% of the world's population has chronic HBV infection. Age at infection determines the rate of progression from acute to chronic infection: ~90% in the perinatal period, 20–50% in children aged 1–5 years, and < 5% in adults.
HCV: 1% worldwide chronic infection, with development of cirrhosis and hepatocellular carcinoma in a number of cases, after an interval of 10–15 years.
Autoimmune hepatitis: 0.1–1.2/100,000. M:F = 1:4. Peak ages: 10–20 years and 45–70 years.
Wilson disease: 1/30,000 live births.

HISTORY AND EXAMINATION   Presentation may be acute or insidious.
General: Failure to thrive, lethargy, loss of fat and muscle bulk.
GI: Distended abdomen (ascites/hepatosplenomegaly), scrotal swelling, dilated abdominal veins (portal hypertension).
Autoimmune hepatitis: Skin rash, lupus erythematosus, arthritis, haemolytic anaemia or nephritis.
Wilson disease: Kayser–Fleischer rings in the corneas at >7 years, neurological features > 12 years such as speech changes, tremor, difficulty with fine motor tasks and gait.

PATHOPHYSIOLOGY
HBV/HCV: Death of hepatocytes at an interface between parenchyma and connective tissue, with infiltration of plasma cells and lymphocytes.
Autoimmune hepatitis: Inflammatory cell infiltrate with hepatocellular necrosis.
Wilson disease: Autosomal recessive disorder with multiple mutations on chromosome 13 → a reduced synthesis of caeruloplasmin (copper-binding protein) and defective excretion of copper in bile.

INVESTIGATIONS
HBV/HCV: Serology and surface/core antigen screen.
Autoimmune hepatitis: Hypergammaglobulinaemia (IgG >20 g/l), autoantibodies, smooth muscle cell autoantibodies, antinuclear antibodies, liver/kidney microsomal antibodies.
Wilson disease: ↓ Serum caeruloplasmin, ↓ serum copper, ↑ urinary copper, ↑ hepatic copper.

MANAGEMENT
HBV: Immunisation for at-risk infants. Supportive management + α-interferon.
HCV: α-interferon. No vaccine is available.
Autoimmune hepatitis: 90% of children respond to prednisolone and azathioprine.
Wilson disease: Penicillamine reduces hepatic and CNS copper deposition, zinc reduces copper absorption, pyridoxine prevents peripheral neuropathy. All may require liver transplantation in end-stage liver disease.

COMPLICATIONS   Coagulation defects, electrolyte disturbances, hypoglycaemia.

PROGNOSIS   Depends on the underlying pathology. The prognosis is greatly improved with adequate and prompt treatment of the underlying condition. Autoimmune hepatitis has the best prognosis due to its high response to therapy.

DEFINITION   Acute failure of the hepatic cells to maintain normal function, also called fulminant hepatitis.

AETIOLOGY   Acute liver failure is caused by damage to the hepatic cells by:

1. *Infection*: acute viral hepatitis (A, B); EBV may precipitate infectious mononucleosis hepatitis.
2. *Drugs/inadvertent poisoning*: paracetamol, isoniazid, halothane and *Amanita phalloides* (poisonous mushrooms).
3. *Reye syndrome*: there is convincing evidence that aspirin given to patients <14 years of age is associated with an acute non-inflammatory encephalopathy with associated liver damage (especially with concomitant varicella infection).

ASSOCIATIONS/RELATED   See Aetiology.

EPIDEMIOLOGY   Uncommon in children. EBV is common in adolescents (age 15–20) as it is transmitted through exchange of bodily fluids of close contacts.

HISTORY AND EXAMINATION
General: May present within hours with jaundice, encephalopathy, coagulopathy, hypoglycaemia or other electrolyte disturbances.
Encephalopathy:

1. *Young children*: there may be a history of alternating periods of irritability and confusion with drowsiness
2. *Older children*: may have a history of aggression and being unusually difficult

PATHOPHYSIOLOGY
Reye syndrome: Microvesicular fatty infiltration of the liver.

INVESTIGATIONS
Bloods: ↑ Bilirubin (although may be normal in the early stages), deranged clotting, ↑ transaminases (ALT, AST), ↑ALP, ↑ plasma ammonia, and ↓ glucose.
ABG sampling: For frequently associated acid/base imbalance.
Viral serology: To detect hepatitis strain.
CT/MRI brain: May show cerebral oedema in encephalopathy.
Other: EEG may show acute hepatic encephalopathy.

MANAGEMENT   Treatment of complications, including the following:
Hypoglycaemia: Dextrose infusion.
Sepsis: IV broad-spectrum antibiotics.
Coagulation defect: FFP and H2-blockers/proton pump inhibitors to prevent gastric bleed. Vitamin K is avoided unless necessary as may mask deterioration in clotting factors, which is used as an indication for liver transplantation.
Cerebral oedema: Fluid restriction and diuresis with mannitol.
Liver transplantation: With worsening clinical, biochemical and clotting profile; prothrombin time is the best marker of liver failure.

COMPLICATIONS   Cerebral oedema, haemorrhage from gastritis or coagulopathy, sepsis, pancreatitis.

PROGNOSIS   Although acute liver failure is uncommon, it has a high mortality.
Poor prognostic signs:

1. Liver starting to shrink in size
2. Rising bilirubin with falling transaminases
3. ↑ Coagulation defect
4. Progression to encephalopathy and coma.

A patient who progresses to coma and does not receive a liver transplant has 70% mortality.

DEFINITION   Lymphomas are neoplasms of lymphoid cells, originating in lymph nodes or other lymphoid tissues. Hodgkin lymphoma is characterised histopathologically by the presence of the Reed–Sternberg cell, and T-cell dysfunction.

AETIOLOGY   Likely to be due to environmental triggers in a genetically susceptible individual (may be due to defect in cell-mediated immunity). EBV genome has been detected in ~50% of Hodgkin lymphomas, but its role in its pathogenesis is unclear.

ASSOCIATIONS/RELATED   Higher socio-economic groups. Past history of infectious mononucleosis.

EPIDEMIOLOGY
Incidence: 1/100,000/year. Non-Hodgkin (85%) > Hodgkin (15%).
Age of presentation: Late childhood/adolescence. M : F = 2 : 1.

HISTORY
Enlarged lymph nodes: Painless enlarging mass, often in neck, occasionally axilla or groin.
Constitutional B symptoms: Fevers >38 °C, night sweats, weight loss >10% bodyweight in 6 months.
Others: Pruritus, cough or dyspnoea with intrathoracic disease, SVC obstruction (blackouts, dyspnoea, feeling of fullness in the head).

EXAMINATION

1. Non-tender firm lymphadenopathy (cervical, axillary or inguinal).
2. Splenomegaly, occasionally hepatomegaly.
3. Skin excoriations.
4. *Signs of intrathoracic disease*: SVC obstruction (facial oedema, ↑JVP).

PATHOPHYSIOLOGY
Histological subtypes

1. Nodular sclerosing (70%)
2. Mixed cellularity (20%)
3. Lymphocyte predominant (5%)
4. Lymphocyte depleted (5%)

Reed–Sternberg cell: Large cell with abundant pale cytoplasm and two or more oval lobulated nuclei containing prominent 'owl-eye' eosinophilic nucleoli.

INVESTIGATIONS
Bloods: ↓Hb (normochromic, normocytic), leucocytosis, eosinophilia, lymphopenia (with advanced disease), ↑ESR, ↑CRP, ↑LDH, ↑AST/ALT (with liver involvement).
Lymph node biopsy: Immunophenotyping, cytogenetics.
Bone marrow aspirate and trephine biopsy: Involvement seen only in very advanced disease.
Imaging: CXR, CT (thorax, abdomen, pelvis), gallium scan, PET scan.
Staging (Ann Arbor):

- *I*: single lymph node region
- *II*: two or more lymph node regions on one side of the diaphragm
- *III*: lymph node regions involved on both sides of the diaphragm
- *IV*: extranodal involvement (liver or bone marrow)
- *A*: without B symptoms; *B*: with B symptoms; *E*: localised extranodal extension; *S*: spleen involved.

MANAGEMENT
Stage I, IIA: Radiotherapy: *mantle* for above the diaphragm, *inverted Y* for below the diaphragm (para-aortic lymph nodes and groin) +/− chemotherapy.
Stage III, IV: Cyclical chemotherapy +/− radiotherapy.
Stem cell transplantation: For relapsed disease.

COMPLICATIONS
Late malignancy 2° to chemotherapy: AML (1% at 10 years), NHL or solid tumours.
Inverted Y irradiation: Infertility, early menopause, skin cancer.
Mantle irradiation: Thyroid disease, accelerated CAD, pulmonary fibrosis.

PROGNOSIS
Stage I, II: 80–90% cured.
Stage III, IV: 50–70% cured.
Poor prognostic factors: B symptoms or if lymphocyte-depleted histological subtype.

DEFINITION   Lymphomas are neoplasms of lymphoid cells originating from lymph nodes or other lymphoid tissues. NHLs are a diverse group, 85% B cell, 15% T cell, and NK cell neoplasms, ranging from indolent to aggressive disease, which can be referred to as low-, intermediate- and high-grade NHL.

AETIOLOGY   Environmental triggers in a genetically susceptible individual result in DNA mutations or translocations → uncontrolled proliferation of lymphoid cells.

ASSOCIATIONS/RELATED
Inherited or acquired immunodeficiency syndromes:

1. HIV and high-grade B-cell lymphomas
2. EBV and post-transplant lymphoproliferative disease
3. Prior treatment with chemo- or radiotherapy.

Infective causes:

1. HTLV-1 → adult T-cell leukaemia/lymphoma
2. EBV → Burkitt lymphoma
3. *Helicobacter pylori* → MALT lymphoma.

EPIDEMIOLOGY
Incidence: 1/100,000/year. Non-Hodgkin (85%) > Hodgkin (15%).
Onset: Late childhood/adolescence. $M:F = 2:1$.

HISTORY
Localised: Stage I, II, relatively unusual; cough, sore throat with enlarged neck glands or tonsils, or in the ileocaecal region presenting as intussusception.
Aggressive/rapidly enlarging:

1. *Mediastinal T-cell tumour*: respiratory or SVC obstruction
2. *Infiltrative, large retroperitoneal B-cell tumour*: vomiting, abdominal pain
3. *Dissemination (stage IV)*: presents as ALL with masses.

EXAMINATION
General: Non-tender, firm lymphadenopathy (cervical, axillary or inguinal), hepatosplenomegaly, signs of bone marrow involvement (anaemia, infections or purpura).
Specific:cutaneous T-cell lymphomas:

1. *Mycosis fungoides*: well-defined, thickened, indurated, scaly, plaque-like lesions
2. *Sézary syndrome*: erythroderma, peripheral lymphadenopathy, and cellular infiltrates of atypical lymphocytes (Sézary cells).

PATHOPHYSIOLOGY   The REAL classification is based on a combination of morphology, immunophenotype, genetic features and clinical features.

INVESTIGATIONS
Bloods: ↓Hb 2° to bone marrow involvement: neutropenia and thrombocytopenia (may also be due to hypersplenism), ↑ESR, ↑CRP, ↑LDH (used as a prognostic marker), ↑ALT/AST with liver involvement, ↑Ca^{2+}.
Blood film: Lymphoma cells may be visible in some patients.
Lymph node biopsy: Immunophenotyping, cytogenetics.
Bone marrow aspirate/biopsy.
Imaging: CXR, CT (thorax, abdomen, pelvis).
Staging: NHL has traditionally been staged according to extent of disease spread using the Ann Arbor system (see Hodgkin lymphoma). In NHL prognosis is more closely related to histological type (REAL classification).

MANAGEMENT

T-cell NHL: Chemotherapy and CNS prophylaxis as for ALL. There is improved prognosis in T-cell stage III with the UK ALL X protocol giving a 90% 4-year survival.

B-cell NHL: Aggressive pulsed chemotherapy regimen for stage IV disease using alkylating agents and methotrexate is improving survival. Surgery is only indicated for emergency tumour obstruction of airways, bowel or bladder.

COMPLICATIONS

2° to treatment: Bone marrow suppression, nausea and vomiting, mucositis, infertility, tumour lysis syndrome, 2° malignancies.

PROGNOSIS Depends on histological type, other factors include age, performance status, stage, extranodal sites and LDH level. There is a 90% 5-year survival rate if localised, falling to 20% if there is CNS involvement.

DEFINITION   Failure of normal embryological rotation of the small intestine around the superior mesenteric artery (SMA) during embryological development, predisposing to intestinal obstruction, volvulus and ischaemia.

AETIOLOGY
General: Normal rotation takes place around the SMA as the axis in three stages: stage I (herniation), stage II (return to the abdomen with 270° counter-clockwise rotation), stage III (fixation).
Non-rotation: Midgut only rotates 180°.
Incomplete rotation (malrotation): Duodenal loop lacks 90° and the caecocolic loop 180° of the normal 270° rotation.

ASSOCIATIONS/RELATED   Gastroschisis, congenital diaphragmatic hernia, duodenal atresia, jejunoileal atresia, Hirschsprung disease, gastro-oesophgeal reflux, intussusception.

EPIDEMIOLOGY   1/500. Common adult postmortem finding. M : F = 2 : 1 (neonatal), 1 : 1 >1 year.

HISTORY
Acute mid-gut volvulus: Usually presents <1 year old with sudden onset of bilious (bright green) vomiting, abdominal distension and severe pain.
Chronic mid-gut volvulus: Recurrent abdominal pain and malabsorption syndrome. Between volvulus episodes, may appear normal.
Acute duodenal obstruction: Usually presents in infancy with forceful vomiting, abdominal distension and gastric waves. 2° to compression or kinking of the duodenum by Ladd bands.
Chronic duodenal obstruction: Usually presents in infancy–preschool with bilious vomiting. Patients may also have failure to thrive and intermittent abdominal pain.

EXAMINATION
Acute obstruction: Tachycardia, abdominal distension, tinkling bowel sounds.
Infarction/necrosis: Shock (↑HR, pallor, ↑CRT, ↓ responsiveness), pyrexia and signs of acute peritonitis.

PATHOPHYSIOLOGY   See Aetiology.

INVESTIGATIONS
Bloods: ↑WCC, ↓Hb (GI bleeding), U&Es (abnormal due to vomiting/abdominal secretions). Acidosis with ↑d lactate may be present although with complete obstruction of mesenteric vessels may be absent.
AXR: Variable appearance with dilated loops of bowel or gasless abdominal field.
UGI contrast: If patient is stable, should be performed on all infants with bright green (bilious) vomiting. Cork-screw appearance with volvulus or a duodenal-jejunal flexure to the right of the midline with malrotations (normal DJ = left of midline & level of pylorus).

MANAGEMENT
Preoperative management: Correction of fluid and electrolyte deficits + broad-spectrum antibiotics, NG tube insertion to decompress proximal bowel. UGI contrast series if stable or immediate surgical intervention if not.
Ladd procedure: Reduction of volvulus (if present), division of mesenteric bands, placement of small bowel on the right and large bowel on the left of the abdomen, and appendectomy. Traditionally via a transverse supraumbilical incision in an infant. Non-acute malrotations may be corrected with the laparoscopic approach.

COMPLICATIONS   Bowel strangulation and necrosis and perforation leading to septic shock. Loss of viable small bowel may lead to short bowel syndrome with malabsorption.

PROGNOSIS   Good with prompt surgical intervention. Depends on how much bowel is preserved and degree of short bowel syndrome.

DEFINITION   Autosomal dominant inherited connective tissue disease.

AETIOLOGY   Commonly caused by mutations in the glycoprotein fibrillin gene (FBN1) on chromosome 15q21.1, and occasionally caused by mutations with transforming growth factor-β genes: TGF-βR1 and TGF-βR2 located on chromosome 9 and on chromosome 3p24.2-p25, respectively. >500 fibrillin gene mutations have been identified, wide spectrum of genetic and phenotypic abnormalities, poor genetic-phenotypic correlation, therefore likely undiscovered genetic abnormalities.

ASSOCIATIONS/RELATED   First-degree relatives affected.

EPIDEMIOLOGY   1/10,000, gender and race are equal.

HISTORY AND EXAMINATION
General: Usually tall, thin individual with ↓ upper:lower segment ratio and arm span > height.
Musculoskeletal: Muscle hypotonia, hyperextensible lax joints with frequent dislocation (delayed motor milestones), arachnodactyly, Steinberg sign, scoliosis, kyphosis, pes planus, high arched palate, pectus excavatum.
Ocular: Poor or loss of vision (upwards lens dislocation), myopia and retinal detachment.
Cardiovascular: May develop aortic root dilation and aortic regurgitation (early diastolic murmur), mitral valve prolapse and regurgitation (ejection click and pansystolic murmur), arrhythmias.
Respiratory: Spontaneous pneumothoraces.
Dermatological: Striae atrophicae (shoulders, hips and lower back)

PATHOPHYSIOLOGY
Electromicroscopy (fibrillin): Significant ↑ fraying of microfibrils. Fibrillin is a major component of microfibrils which constitute the structural components of some connective tissues (suspensory ligament of the lens) and also is a substrate for elastin (aortal wall).

INVESTIGATIONS   Diagnosis remains clinical, despite Ghent criteria (1996).
Molecular/genetic studies: Identification of FBN1 mutation (poor sensitivity and specificity as an investigation for Marfan); linkage studies (direct family genetic analysis) may improve sensitivity/specificity
Other: Cardiovascular (ECHO and ECG), ocular, musculoskeletal, MRI/CT (presence of dural ectasia).

MANAGEMENT   Multidisciplinary approach.
General: Endocarditis prophylaxis, annual follow-up (including ECHO, contact sports avoidance).
Medical: β-Blockers (delays aortic dilation), ACE inhibitors (↓ central arterial pressure and conduit arterial stiffness), animal studies on use of matrix metalloproteinase and TGF-β antagonism. Hormonal therapy for early induction of puberty to ↓ ultimate height (possible ↓d scoliosis).
Surgical: Aortic aneurysm and dissection, aortic and mitral regurgitation. Prophylactic surgery if the aortic diameter at the sinus of Valsalva is >5 cm/aortic ratio >1.5, aortic root:descending aorta ratio >2.
Ophthalmic: Refractive lens for myopia, laser treatment of detached retina, removal of lens in some cases.
Orthopaedic: Arch support for pes planus, surgery in severe cases of scoliosis/pectus excavatum.
Counselling: Genetic (50% pathological mutation inheritance), high-risk pregnancy with prepartum aortic root >4 cm/previous cardiovascular disease/surgery. Prophylactic surgery may be required.

COMPLICATIONS   1° cause of morbidity and mortality is aortic dissection.

PROGNOSIS
Mortality: Untreated, 30–40 years of age; with good management many have normal life expectancy. Neonatal presentation is associated with a more severe course.

DEFINITION   Infectious RNA viral illnesses.

AETIOLOGY
Measles: Transmitted by droplets or direct contact. Incubation period: 7–14 days. Infectious 2 days before symptoms and 4 days after onset of rash.
Mumps: Transmitted by direct contact, droplet spread. Incubation period: 14–21 days. Infectious up to 7 days after the onset of parotid swelling.
Rubella: Transmitted by droplet spread or via the placenta to the fetus. Incubation period: 14–21 days. Infectious 6–14 days after onset of rash.

ASSOCIATIONS/RELATED   Malnutrition, immunocompromise, not being immunised, contact with affected individuals. The MMR vaccine has been shown not to be associated with autistic spectrum disorder.

EPIDEMIOLOGY
Measles: 4/100,000; has dropped significantly from 800,000/year (1960s) to 3000/year (1990s) (UK figures) due to MMR vaccine. *Peak age*: <1 year (before immunisation) or older children not immunised. Most common in developing countries.
Mumps: 3–4/100,000. *Peak age*: 5–9 years.
Rubella: 3–4/100,000. *Peak age*: >15 years.

HISTORY AND EXAMINATION
Measles: Prodrome of fever, conjunctivitis, coryza, cough and Koplik spots (grain-like white spots opposite lower molars and buccal mucosa). Rash appears 3–4 days later, usually behind the ear, and spreads to the whole body. Rash is initially maculopapular, but subsequently becomes blotchy and confluent. May desquamate in the second week.
Mumps: Up to 40% are asymptomatic. Prodrome of fever, muscular pain, headache and malaise. Pain/swelling of one or both parotid glands.
Rubella: Lymphadenopathy, malaise, fever, headache, coryza, maculopapular rash (small, pink) on face spreading within 24 h to chest, upper arms, abdomen and thighs.

PATHOPHYSIOLOGY   Entry is via the oropharynx with viral replication, viraemia and subsequent involvement of glands and other tissues.
Measles: Morbillivirus (paramyxovirus).
Mumps: Paramyxovirus.
Rubella: Rubivirus.

INVESTIGATIONS   Usually a clinical diagnosis. Confirm by serology and/or viral culture.

MANAGEMENT
Supportive: Antipyrexials and encourage oral intake.
Immunisation: MMR vaccine at 13 months with second preschool dose at 3–5 years.
Prevention of spread: Children should avoid school/day-care until no longer infectious.
Notification: Measles, mumps and rubella are diseases notifiable to a consultant in communicable disease control (CCDC).

COMPLICATIONS
Measles: *Common*: otitis media, pneumonia, diarrhoea; *rare*: encephalitis (1/5000), SSPE (1/100,000).
Mumps: Viral meningitis (10%), encephalitis (1/5000), orchitis (more commonly affects adults), oophoritis, pancreatitis, deafness.
Rubella: Arthropathy (common), encephalitis, thrombocytopenia, myocarditis, congenital rubella syndrome (75–90% transmission during first trimester).

PROGNOSIS
Measles: Mortality rate has fallen but is still 750,000/year (UNICEF), usually due to pneumonia or diarrhoea (developing countries). Encephalitis has 15% mortality and

results in seizures, deafness, hemiplegia and severe learning difficulties in 40%. SSPE is a severe illness that may rarely affect children ~7 years after the initial illness.

Mumps: The disease is usually self-limiting and has a good prognosis.

Rubella: Not a debilitating disease in adults. Congenital rubella syndrome, however, may → developmental delay, hearing impairment, CHD, neurological, ophthalmic and endocrinological complications.

DEFINITION   Outpouching of the ileum along the antimesenteric border containing heterotopic tissue of the stomach (acid-secreting parietal cells), pancreas or normal intestinal mucosa.

AETIOLOGY
General: Partial or incomplete involution of the vitelline duct (omphalomesenteric duct) during embryogenesis. True diverticulum containing all three layers of the intestinal wall and its own blood supply.
Rule of 2s: 2% of the population, 2 inches (3–5 cm) long, 2 feet (60 cm) from the ileocaecal valve, 2% are symptomatic, 2 types of ectopic tissue (gastric or pancreatic), clinical presentation commonly aged 2 and males are 2–3× more likely to be affected.

ASSOCIATIONS/RELATED   Intussusception.

EPIDEMIOLOGY   2% of the population. M : F = 2 : 1. Symptomatic: M : F = 3 : 1.

HISTORY AND EXAMINATION   Most children are asymptomatic. 4.2–16% of children with MD estimated to be symptomatic.
Intermittent painless rectal bleeding: 2° to ulceration of the ileal mucosa by ectopic acid production. Characteristically bright red blood. Normal abdominal examination.
Signs and symptoms of anaemia: Lethargy, pallor and failure to thrive.
Intussusception: MD may be a lead point.
Meckel diverticulitis: Characterised by peritoneal irritation which may localise to the RIF; may be identical presentation to acute appendicitis.

PATHOPHYSIOLOGY   During embryogenesis the vitelline duct runs between the terminal ileum, the umbilicus and the yolk sac; usually regresses by 7/40. Failure to atrophy; can cause either a remaining fibrous band running from the diverticulum to the umbilicus, an umbilical cyst, an ileo-umbilical fistula or MD. MD is the most common and is formed when the entire duct except the portion adjacent to the ileum is obliterated.

INVESTIGATIONS   Depend on clinical presentation. Possible anaemia (↓Hb, ↓MCV). Stool sample for obvious or occult blood with MC&S. A radionucleotide scan (Meckel scan) can also be performed with IV technetium-99m; binds to ectopic gastric mucosa with pre-scan suppression with an H2-Antagonist (e.g. cimetidine). Sensitivity of scan is 50–90% so only a positive scan is helpful with the diagnosis.

MANAGEMENT
General: Often an incidental finding at operation; during an appendicectomy, operative reduction of an intussussception or laparotomy/laparoscopy for other pathology. Should be excluded with a normal appendicectomy. Surgical removal of an incidental MD is generally not recommended due to procedure-associated morbidity; pathological MD should be removed.
Surgical: Ileal resection and 1° anastomosis. Ileal resection recommended as opposed to simple diverticulectomy as ectopic tissue may extend beyond the MD. Can be performed by either the open or laparoscopic approach. Laparoscopic approach involves delivery of the MD via the umbilicus with extracorporeal anastomosis. Laparoscopy is also recommended for the investigation of PR bleeding possibly 2° to MD.

COMPLICATIONS   Anastomotic complications (stricture, leak) with surgical intervention. Rarely may contain sarcomas/carcinoid/adenocarcinoma tumours.

PROGNOSIS   Excellent with surgical outcome.

DEFINITION Respiratory distress in the neonate 2° to passage of meconium (fetal intestinal contents) stained amniotic fluid into the respiratory system.

AETIOLOGY Fetal hypoxic stress → *in utero* meconium passage from neural stimulation of a mature GI tract. Head or cord compression may also cause peristalsis and relaxation of the anal sphincter. Meconium is rarely found in the amniotic fluid <34/40. Meconium-stained fluid may be aspirated into the lungs, causing obstruction and chemical pneumonitis.

ASSOCIATIONS/RELATED Low birthweight, postmaturity, cord compression, placental insufficiency, maternal hypertension, pre-eclampsia, oligohydramnios, maternal drug abuse (tobacco and cocaine).

EPIDEMIOLOGY Meconium staining: 10–15% live births; of these, 1–9% experience meconium aspiration syndrome.

HISTORY AND EXAMINATION

Meconium aspiration: Fetal tachycardia, bradycardia or absence of fetal accelerations on cardiotocography *in utero* identifies high-risk infant. At birth the neonate may exhibit signs of postmaturity with evidence of weight loss and heavily stained yellow nails, skin and umbilical cord.

Respiratory distress: Diagnosed at birth, or within 4 hours; consists of tachypnoea, tachycardia, recession; intercostal/subcostal/sternal/substernal, nasal flaring, grunting in respiration against a partially closed glottis, harsh diminished breath sounds, chest may has a overinflated appearance (?° to air trapping). In severe cases the neonate may become cyanosed.

PATHOPHYSIOLOGY

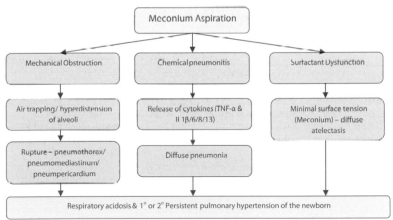

INVESTIGATIONS

CXR: Hyperinflation, flattening of the diaphragm, cardiomegaly, gross patchy shadowing.

Blood gas: ↓pO₂ (right → left shunting of blood through the foramen ovale 2° to pulmonary hypertension).

MANAGEMENT Neonates born through meconium-stained liquor require a paediatrician to be present at birth.

Good condition: No further management.

Poor condition: Airway suction under direct vision, directly/via an ET tube/meconium aspirator. +/− intermittent positive airway ventilation.

Subsequent management on NICU: Supportive respiratory therapy with antibiotics, ventilatory assistance, exogenous surfactant therapy. Inhalation of nitric oxide and extracorporeal membrane oxygenation (ECMO) may be required.

COMPLICATIONS   See Pathophysiology.

PROGNOSIS   Ultimate prognosis depends on the extent of asphyxial insult to the neonate which depends on the degree of meconium aspiration.

DEFINITION   Infection of the subarachnoid space associated with an inflammatory response of the meninges.

AETIOLOGY

Bacterial
Neonatal to 3 months: Group B streptococcus (GBS) early (90% day 1–5) or late (10% 6 days–3 months), *E. coli, Listeria monocytogenes.*
1 month to 6 years: *Neisseria meningitidis* (meningococcus), *Streptococcus pneumoniae, Haemophilus influenzae* type B (Hib).
>6 years: *N. meningitidis* (14–25 years), *Strep. pneumoniae*, mumps (pre-MMR).
Mycobacterium tuberculosis: Can cause TB meningitis at all ages. Most common in children 6 months–6 years.

Viral
Enteroviruses (80%), cytomegalovirus (CMV), arbovirus. Herpes simplex virus (HSV) is more likely to cause encephalitis (see chapter).

ASSOCIATIONS/RELATED
Impaired immunity: Young age, HIV, defects of complement system leading to meningococcal susceptibility (see chapter on primary immune deficiency), asplenia 2° to sickle cell disease (*Strep. pneumoniae* and Hib susceptibility).
Environmental factors: Crowding, poverty and close contact with affected individuals (transmission by respiratory secretions).

EPIDEMIOLOGY
Viral meningitis: The most common meningitis. Incidence 3000/year in the UK.
Bacterial meningitis: There are 2000/year new cases of bacterial meningitis in the UK. *N. meningitidis* (meningococcus) is the most common UK cause of bacterial meningitis. Has ↓ since the introduction of vaccine Men C, but Men B in now the most common cause of disease. *Strep. pneumoniae* (pneumococcal) meningitis is the second most common UK cause of bacterial meningitis and incidence is rising. *E. coli* accounts for 20% of UK neonatal meningitis. Hib meningitis has ↓90% since the introduction of the Hib vaccination. GBS: 340 cases/year UK. TB meningitis: >300 cases documented in the UK in 2007. Enteroviruses: more common in autumn and summer

HISTORY
Prodromal features of infection: Otitis media/tonsillitis/respiratory/GI symptoms.
Infants: Non-specific symptoms such as fever (or hypothermia), irritability, lethargy, seizures, shrill cry or poor feeding.
Children: Fever, headache, leg pain, neck stiffness, alteration in consciousness (from lethargy to coma), nausea, vomiting, photophobia, anorexia, rash or seizures.
TB meningitis: Can occur 3–6 months after the initial TB infection.

EXAMINATION
Neck stiffness: From meningeal irritation.
Kernig sign: In the supine position, extension of leg is painful when knee and hip are flexed.
Non-blanching rash: Purpuric or petechial (may initially be blanching). Characteristic of meningococcal infection.
↑ICP: Papilloedema, ↓consciousness, focal neurology (e.g. 6th nerve palsy), Cushing reflex (↑BP, ↓HR), decerebrate posturing.

PATHOPHYSIOLOGY   Bacteraemia precedes infection and bacteria enter the CSF via the choroid plexus and rapidly multiply as local complement and antibody levels are low. Inflammation follows with disruption of the blood–brain barrier, oedema and neutrophil infiltration.

INVESTIGATION
Bloods: ↑WBC, ↑CRP, U&E, glucose, clotting studies, group and save.
MC&S: Blood, stool, throat swab, mid-stream urine, urinary pneumococcal antigen.
CT scan: If signs suggestive of ↑ICP to avoid coning on LP.
LP: Contraindicated if focal neurological signs, ↑ICP or petechiae/purpura.
CSF (bacterial meningitis): Neutrophils, ↑ protein (1–5 g/l), ↓ glucose (<50% serum level). MC&S (gram stain, acid-fast bacilli in TB meningitis) for diagnosis.
CSF (viral meningitis): Lymphocytes (initially neutrophils), normal/mildly elevated protein, normal glucose, PCR for diagnosis.

MANAGEMENT
Resuscitation: Stabilise airway, breathing and circulation.
Start empirical parenteral antibiotic treatment before the results of investigations as meningococcal septicaemia is often rapidly fatal.
Bacterial meningitis: Third-generation cephalosporin: ceftriaxone or cefotaxime IV. In infants <3 months, ampicillin should be started empirically for *L. monocytogenes*. TB meningitis requires 6–9 months therapy with isoniazid, rifampicin, pyrazinamide and streptomycin. **Culture and sensitivity will indicate subsequent antibiotic therapy.**
Corticosteroids: Studies of patients with Hib meningitis have shown some improvement in morbidity (deafness or neurological deficit) with corticosteroid treatment alongside antibiotics. Data are lacking in pneumococcal and meningococcal meningitis.
Supportive care: Analgesics, antipyretics.
Notification: Meningitis is a notifiable disease (CCDC).
Contact prophylaxis: 2/7 of rifampicin for meningococcal infection.

Prevention
Immunisations: BCG vaccine, Men C, pneumococcal, Hib. There is no vaccine for Men B as yet.
Intrapartum antibiotics: IV penicillin (or clindamyin if allergic) during labour if mother has had GBS-positive high vaginal swab (HVS) or prolonged rupture of membranes and signs of maternal chorio-amnionitis.

COMPLICATIONS
During illness: Convulsions, cerebral oedema, circulatory shock, DIC.
Neurological sequelae: Hearing loss (10%), visual impairment, cerebral palsy, subdural effusion, hydrocephalus, cerebral abscess, learning disability; children must have audiology/neurological follow-up for early detection and management of complications.

PROGNOSIS
Bacterial: Overall mortality 5–10%; neurological complications 10–20%. *Meningococcal meningitis*: mortality 5%, with septicaemia 18–50%, usually have favourable neurological outcome if they survive the acute illness. *Pneumococcal meningitis*: mortality 16%, 50% adverse neurological sequelae. *E. coli meningitis*: neonatal mortality is 20%, high adverse neurological sequelae. *TB meningitis*: mortality 15–30%, 25% adverse neurological sequelae.
Viral: 95% have complete recovery with no neurological sequelae. Some may experience headaches, hearing impairment or tinnitus (ringing in the ears). *TB meningitis*: mortality 30%, especially if treatment is delayed, 10–30% severe neurological impairment.

DEFINITION   Mesenteric lymph node inflammation associated with systemic illness and abdominal symptoms.

AETIOLOGY

General: Acute or chronic problem. Infection causes inflammation and enlargement of mesenteric lymph nodes and possibly an oedematous mesentery, suppuration may be present. Involved nodes may be intra-abdominal or retroperitoneal, ileocolic vascular distribution most common. Bowel wall usually unaffected.

Causative organisms: Viruses (upper respiratory tract viruses most common cause), bacterial URTI/gastrointestinal (group A β-haemolytic streptococcus, *Yersinia enterocolitica*, *Helicobacter jejuni*, *Campylobacter jejuni*, and *Salmonella* or *Shigella* species).

ASSOCIATIONS/RELATED   Most common differential diagnosis for acute appendicitis. URTIs & tonsillitis.

EPIDEMIOLOGY   Affects children of all ages. True incidence unknown.

HISTORY   Often diagnosis of exclusion. Most common finding at a negative appendicectomy. URTI or gastrointestinal infection; symptoms of coryza, pharyngitis or gastroenteritis may still be present (mainly diarrhoea). Gastrointestinal; vague abdominal pain may vary intermittently.

EXAMINATION

General: May be identical to acute appendicitis. Cervical lymphadenopathy. Signs of URTI/tonsillitis or high pyrexia (>38.5°) with vague abdominal signs.

Specific. Peritoneal irritation may be present (guarding and percussion tenderness).

PATHOPHYSIOLOGY

Macroscopic: LNs are enlarged and often soft. Oedema of the adjacent mesentery.

Microscopic: Non-specific hyperplasia, necrotic changes may be present with suppurative mesenteric adenitis.

INVESTIGATIONS

Bloods: ↑WCC, U&Es (may be dehydrated), ↑CRP. May not aid the differentiation between appendicitis.

USS of RIF: May confirm the diagnosis with the visualisation of an inflamed appendix (non compressible tubular structure in the RIF)/presence of free intraperitoneal pus/enlarged lymph nodes. With mesenteric adenitis the nodes are in clusters of >5 and >1 cm in diameter. Operator dependent.

CT scan: Rarely performed in UK (radiation dose high) but has excellent positive predictor value for mesenteric adenitis and high negative predictive value for appendicitis.

MANAGEMENT   All children with the diagnosis in doubt should be admitted and observed for possible acute appendicitis. This should include regular observations, repeated examination (preferably by the same clinician) and repeated blood investigations if indicated. Mesenteric adenitis is a self-limiting disease whereas acute appendicitis will progress and more symptoms will become apparent.

COMPLICATIONS   None with mesenteric adenitis; complications may be associated with the original underlying diagnosis.

PROGNOSIS   Mesenteric adenitis is a benign self-limiting disease.

DEFINITION Autosomal dominant multisystem disorder characterised by progressive muscle wasting, muscle weakness and myotonia (abnormal sustained contraction of muscle).

AETIOLOGY

Genetic defect: Caused by expansion of CTG nucleotide triplet repeats at the 3'UTR of the myotonic dystrophy gene on chromosome 19. This gene codes for DMPK.

Genetic anticipation: The disease has earlier onset or ↑ severity in the offspring than in parents as a result of further triplet repeat expansion in successive generations.

ASSOCIATIONS/RELATED Family history, antenatal history; polyhydramnios.

EPIDEMIOLOGY 2/10,000 live births (UK). Severe congenital type is much rarer and almost always inherited via the mother.

HISTORY
Depends on number of CTG repeats:

1. Unaffected individuals (5–27 repeats)
2. Mild myotonic dystrophy (50–100 repeats): cataracts, slight muscle weakness in adulthood
3. Classic myotonic dystrophy (100–1000 repeats): myotonia, muscle wasting, frontal balding, hypogonadism, cardiomyopathy, cardiac arrhythmias, DM, respiratory impairment, adverse reactions to anaesthesia
4. Congenital myotonic dystrophy (1000–4000 repeats):

At birth: hypotonia, respiratory and feeding difficulties, marked facial weakness. Myotonia is not a feature of the condition at this stage. *If infant survives*: gradual improvement in muscle strength and tone, delayed motor development, persistence of facial weakness, severe learning disability (60–70% of cases), classic features of myotonic dystrophy by the age of 10.

EXAMINATION

Peripheral weakness: Hands (unable to release grip), forearms and feet as opposed to proximal weakness (hip, shoulder) in other dystrophies.

Myopathic facies: Facial muscle weakness and wasting; bilateral ptosis, wasting of frontalis and temporalis muscle, and weakness of sternomastoids, all of which result in lack of facial expression.

PATHOPHYSIOLOGY Disturbance in muscle fibre maturation with incomplete differentiation.

Infants: Small undifferentiated muscle fibres.

Children: Type 1 fibre atrophy; central nuclei, sarcoplasmic masses, ring fibres.

INVESTIGATIONS

Bloods: CPK may be raised.

Muscle biopsy: See Prognosis.

EMG: Characteristic 'diver bomber' spontaneous electrical discharge by age 3.

DNA mutation analysis: Sizing of the repeat array by PCR and/or Southern blotting.

MANAGEMENT
Multidisciplinary approach.

Physiotherapy: Strength and flexibility training.

SALT: Difficulties swallowing and dysarthria due to muscle weakness.

Occupational therapy: Specially designed utensils for hand weakness, wrist braces.

Medical: Myotonia may be treated with quinine or procainamide. Support respiratory and GI problems. Monitor for deformities.

Surgical: Cataract operations.

Orthopaedic: Ankle–foot arthroses for foot-drop.

Genetic counselling: For antenatal diagnosis.

Psychological support: For parent and child.

COMPLICATIONS Joint contractures, foot deformities, early-onset dementia.

PROGNOSIS Depends on the number of CTG repeats, extent of learning disability and early appropriate multidisciplinary involvement. The older the child is when muscle weakness is first noticed, the slower the progression and less serious the consequences. Most do not survive past 50 years of age.

DEFINITION
Drowning: Death from asphyxia <24 h after submersion in water.
Near-drowning: Survival >24 h after submersion episode.

AETIOLOGY
2° causes: Seizures, head or spine trauma, cardiac arrhythmias, alcohol/drug ingestion, syncope, apnoea, suicide, hypoglycaemia.
<1 year: Bathtubs/buckets of water. Consider child abuse in all cases.
1–5 years: Residential swimming pools.
15–19 years: Ponds, lakes, rivers, oceans.

ASSOCIATIONS/RELATED   Inability to swim, failure to observe water safety rules, unsupervised swimming.

EPIDEMIOLOGY
UK incidence: 1.5/100,000/year, mortality 0.7/100,000/year. ∼500 children die from drowning in the UK per year.
Worldwide: Second/third cause of accidental death in children in the UK, Australia and USA. *Peak age*: toddlers <4 years of age and 15–19 years. M : F = 12 : 1 boating injuries, M : F = 4 : 1 non-boating injuries, bathtubs F > M.

HISTORY   Most patients are found after having been submerged in water for an unobserved period. Relevant factors in the history include time under water, associated trauma, drug/alcohol use, water contamination, water temperature, rescue manoeuvres, response to resuscitation.

EXAMINATION   Hypothermia, ↑/↓HR, ↑RR, ↓GCS. Cardiorespiratory arrest.

PATHOPHYSIOLOGY   Following submersion in water, 90% aspirate water or gastric contents (wet drowning), 10% develop laryngospasm (dry drowning). In both cases resultant hypoxia and metabolic acidosis result in:
CNS: Hypoxic neuronal injury and subsequent cerebral oedema.
Cardiovascular: Cardiac dysrhythmias +/− myocardial damage that may → cardiogenic shock and hypovolaemia 2° to ↑ capillary permeability and intracompartmental fluid shifts.
Respiratory: Aspiration causes disruption of surfactant, pulmonary oedema, and may result in acute respiratory distress syndrome (ARDS).
The **mammalian diving reflex** is protective and occurs if suddenly immersed in cold water. It produces apnoea, bradycardia and vasoconstriction of non-essential vascular beds with shunting of blood to the coronary and cerebral circulation.

INVESTIGATIONS
Bloods: ABG, FBC, U&E, LFTs, CK, drug/alcohol screen, blood cultures.
Bronchoalveolar lavage (BAL): If intubated to assess likelihood of 2° pneumonia.
Monitoring: Cardiac, pulse oximetry, invasive BP monitoring.
Trauma series: Cervical spine/chest/pelvic X-ray.
CT head: If deteriorating GCS/focal neurology.

MANAGEMENT   Rescue and basic life support (BLS) at the scene are the most important factors in determining outcome. Transfer to emergency department.
Cervical spine immobilisation.
Airways: Consider ET intubation, NG tube to prevent vomiting.
Breathing: 100% O$_2$ via reservoir bag. Consider mechanical ventilation if poor respiratory effort, ↓GCS, severe hypoxia, acidosis or significant respiratory distress.
Circulation: Fluid resuscitation +/− inotropes if BP not responsive, central venous access arterial line. Strict fluid balance. Electrolyte correction.

Disability: AVPU (initial paediatric assessment; Alert, Verbal, Pain, Unresponsive), GCS (full assessment of neurological disability). May require IV mannitol or hypertonic saline for cerebral oedema and ↑ICP.

Exposure: Consider spinal injuries in all diving accidents. Correct hypothermia as may exacerbate bradycardia, acidosis and hypoxaemia. Remove wet/cold clothing, external warming (bear-hugger, radiant lamp), active care rewarming if temperature <32 °C (warmed ventilator gases, gastric/bladder lavage). Resuscitation should not be discontinued until core temperature >32 °C.

Sepsis: Prophylactic antibiotics and steroids not indicated. If BAL positive then treat.

Prevention: Adult supervision, fencing around lakes/pools, community BLS education.

COMPLICATIONS Cerebral oedema/↑ICP, 2° pulmonary infection, rhabdomyolysis, ARDS, acute renal/hepatic failure, DIC.

PROGNOSIS 70% of children survive if BLS is provided. Only 40% survive without early BLS despite hospital measures, ~30% have neurological impairment.

Good prognostic factors: Immersion time <15 min, rapid recovery to consciousness, CPR <25 min at the scene, ↑GCS (motor response to pain in emergency department).

Poor prognostic factors: Acidosis (pH <7 in emergency department), hypoxia. No implication whether salt or fresh water immersion.

DEFINITION Severe gastrointestinal disease characterised by massive epithelial destruction leading to intestinal barrier failure.

AETIOLOGY Exact aetiology unknown, likely to be multifactorial. Current hypothesis involves the combination of immature intestinal epithelial barrier and mucosal immune system leading to bacterial translocation with intestinal inflammation. Cycle of localised intestinal mucosal injury leads to infiltration of indigenous bacteria and causes local immunocytes to secrete proinflammatory mediators (chemokines, prostanoids and nitric oxide). This response causes further damage to the intestinal barrier with ↑d bacterial translocation and therefore ↑d release of proinflammatory mediators. This cycle eventually causes intestinal necrosis +/− perforation and generalised sepsis.

Bell's classification: I (suspect; non-specific septic signs), II (definite; blood investigation derangement and XR changes), III (advanced; shock, peritonitis, pneumoperitoneum).

ASSOCIATIONS/RELATED Prematurity, low birthweight, formula feeding, perinatal stress, bacterial colonisation of the intestines, UAC/UVC insertion, congenital heart disease (↓ cardiac output), maternal cocaine use, respiratory distress syndrome.

EPIDEMIOLOGY 0.5% of all live births. 3–5% of infants <1500 g. Majority of surgical neonatal admissions to neonatal unit.

HISTORY AND EXAMINATION Depends on the stage of the disease.

Stage I: Temperature instability, brachycardias and apnoeas, lethargy, poor feeding, bilious (bright green) aspirates, GI bleeding, mild ileus on XR.

Stage II: As above, with metabolic acidosis, thrombocytopenia, ↑d GI bleeding, abdominal tenderness, abdominal wall erythema, possible mass, definite AXR signs.

Stage III: As above, with shock, inotropic support, neutropenia, DIC, generalised peritonitis, marked abdominal distension, pneumoperitoneum on AXR.

PATHOPHYSIOLOGY See Aetiology.

INVESTIGATIONS

Bloods: Depends on stage; ↓Hb, ↓platelets, ↑WCC, metabolic acidosis, electrolyte derangement, coagulopathy.

AXR: Pneumatosis intestinalis, ileus, portal venous gas, persistent 'fixed' dilated loops of bowel or pneumoperitoneum 'football sign' (in the supine position, air collects anterior to the abdominal viscera, the falciform ligament is also outlined).

USS: Operator dependent but may visualise intramural gas and the presence of NEC mass.

MANAGEMENT

Conservative: Initial management of all stages I and II; NBM (>1/52), NGT decompression, intravenous broad-spectrum antibiotics (gram +ve and −ve cover), blood and platelet transfusions, electrolyte imbalances correction.

Surgical: With failure of conservative management (progression of symptoms +/− ↑ing inotropic or ventilatory support). Laparotomy via supraumbilical transverse incision. Resection of necrotic bowel with formation of a stoma and mucous fistula +/− 1° anastomosis. Extensive disease may be left as balance of resection versus short gut syndrome. May require second-look laparotomy. Surgical drain may be placed in very unwell neonates as a stabilisation prior to theatre.

COMPLICATIONS Strictures, fistulas, abscesses, recurrent NEC, 'short gut' syndrome, malabsorption, TPN associated cholestasis and enterocyst formation.

PROGNOSIS 20–40% of neonates who develop NEC require surgical intervention. Average mortality is 20–50% in this group. 15% have pancolitis and therefore significant mortality.

DEFINITION   Excess amount of bilirubin in the neonatal circulation causing a yellow discolouration of the skin and sclera.

AETIOLOGY
Physiological unconjugated hyperbilirubinaemia 2° to:

1. *Instability of fetal haemoglobin*: neonates have ↑RBC volume but ↓RBC survival
2. *Defective bilirubin metabolism*: immature hepatic function results in defective hepatic uptake and conjugation of bilirubin
3. *Defective bilirubin excretion*: neonates have absent gut flora.

'Breast milk jaundice': Physiological prolonged unconjugated hyperbilirubinaemia; peaks in the second week and resolves very slowly (<3/12). 2° to a factor in breast milk that inhibits uridine diphosphoglucuronic acid (UDPGA) glucuronyl transferase.
Unconjugated haemolytic hyperbilirubinaemia:

1. *Immune mediated*: haemolytic disease of the newborn which may be 2° to ABO or rhesus incompatibility
2. *Hereditary*: spherocytosis, elliptocytosis, glucose-6-phosphate dehydrogenase deficiency
3. *Acquired*: congenital infection, bacterial sepsis.

Unconjugated non-haemolytic hyperbilirubinaemia:

1. ↑*d haemoglobin load*: haemorrhage, polycythaemia
2. Galactosaemia, hypothyroidism.

Conjugated hyperbilirubinaemia:

1. *Bile duct obstruction*: biliary atresia, choledochal cyst
2. *Neonatal hepatitis*: TPN-related hepatitis, congenital infection, α1-antitrypsin deficiency, cystic fibrosis.

ASSOCIATIONS/RELATED   Previous affected sibling, prematurity, breastfeeding.

EPIDEMIOLOGY   50% of all neonates to various degrees, 33% of breastfed neonates >2/52.

HISTORY
General presentation: May be asymptomatic in physiological jaundice or unwell (vomiting, lethargy, poor feeding, behavioural changes, tachypnoea, instability of temperature, pale stools and dark urine)
Age of onset: Important in determining likely pathological cause; <24 h (pathological), >24 h (probably physiological but beware sepsis and galactosaemia), >2/52 (investigate).

EXAMINATION   Clinically jaundiced at bilirubin of 80–120 μmol/L. Correlation between the level to which the jaundice extends and the serum bilirubin level. Sclera is best place to detect jaundice as there are variations in skin colour. Examine also for pallor, presence of hepatosplenomegaly, signs of sepsis and petechiae.

PATHOPHYSIOLOGY   See Aetiology.

INVESTIGATIONS
Early jaundice (<24 h): FBC, blood film, maternal and infant ABO and Rhesus typing, direct Coombs (antiglobulin) test, infection screen (blood cultures, TORCH screen).
Jaundice at >24 h: If normal history and examination, monitor only.
Persistent jaundice (>2 weeks): Total serum bilirubin and conjugated fraction should be obtained. TFTs, LFTs, urine for reducing agents in G6PD, direct antiglobulin test.
Conjugated hyperbilirubinaemia: Requires urgent investigation; USS biliary tree +/− liver biopsy isotope scanning HIDA/DISIDA and referral to a paediatric liver centre.

MANAGEMENT

General: Treat the cause if present.

Treatment of jaundice: Independent of disease process if bilirubin levels are high or are increasing rapidly to prevent bilirubin encephalopathy (kernicterus).

Intensive phototherapy: Place the neonate under a series of 450 nm wavelength lights on a radiant warmer bed. Converts the stereoisomer, making it soluble and allowing renal excretion. Eye protection masks during therapy.

Exchange transfusion: If intensive phototherapy fails to lower bilirubin level, or in conjunction with phototherapy with extremely elevated bilirubin levels in all age groups. All neonates with bilirubin levels over the 'exchange transfusion level' should have hearing screening. Can be performed via an umbilical vein catheter.

COMPLICATIONS   Bilirubin neurotoxic effects: seizures, athetoid cerebral palsy sensorineural deafness and learning difficulties.

PROGNOSIS   Good with physiological jaundice as usual spontaneous resolvement.

DEFINITION   Characterised by hypoalbuminaemia, proteinuria and oedema.

AETIOLOGY   All causes of glomerulonephritis (GN) can cause nephrotic syndrome.
Primary: Described by histology; minimal change disease (MCD), focal segmental glomerulosclerosis (FSGS) and membranous nephropathy (MN).
Secondary: SLE, post-infectious (group A β-hemolytic streptococcus, syphilis, malaria, TB, varicella, hepatitis B, HIV, EBV), collagen vascular disease, HSP, hereditary nephritis (Alport syndrome), sickle cell disease.

ASSOCIATIONS/RELATED   See Aetiology.

EPIDEMIOLOGY
Developed countries: 2–7/100,000/year (UK). MCD is the cause of nephrotic syndrome in 90% of children; most common in boys <5 years. *Peak age*: 2–4 years.
Developing countries: Infectious causes of GN: malaria (40%), HBV infection (6%) and group A β-haemolytic streptococcal infection (rare).

HISTORY AND EXAMINATION
General: Anorexia, lethargy, oliguria, hypertension.
GI: Diarrhoea, poor feeding, abdominal pain.
Oedema: Swelling of face, ascites, oedema of legs/scrotum.
Symptoms of complications: Infections, renal vein thrombosis, loin pain, haematuria.

PATHOPHYSIOLOGY
Proteinuria: Structural damage to the glomerular membrane and reduction of its negatively charged components prevent the action of repelling negatively charged proteins, which are therefore excreted in excess.
Hypoalbuminaemia: $2°$ to proteinuria and ↑ breakdown of albumin in the kidney.
Oedema: Hypoalbuminuria leads to ↓ intravascular colloid osmotic pressure.

INVESTIGATIONS
Bloods: U&E, ↓ albumin, ↑ESR/CRP, lipid profile ($2°$ hyperlipidaemia).
Post-infectious nephropathy: *Plasmodium falciparum* (thick and thin blood films), ASOT, HBV/EBV/HIV serology, HIV PCR.
Urine dipstick: 3/4 + protein, microscopic haematuria.
MSU: MC&S.
24-h urine collection: Creatinine clearance and 24-h protein excretion.
Renal USS: Other renal diseases may cause proteinuria, e.g. polycystic kidney disease.
Renal biopsy: Reserved for older children with haematuria, ↑BP, renal impairment, steroid resistant patients.
Doppler USS, renal angiogram, CT, MRI: If renal thrombosis is suspected.

MANAGEMENT
Symptomatic treatment: Limit oedema with low-sodium diet and diuretics.
Monitor: BP, U&E, Ca^{2+}, weight, fluid balance.
Treatment of initial presentation: Longer duration (6 months) of initial prednisolone treatment is associated with fewer relapses and lower total prednisolone dose over the first 2 years.
Treatment of relapse: Prednisolone daily until in remission, then a slow gradual reduction of dosage.
Treatment of steroid-resistant patients: Alternate-day prednisolone with long-term cyclosporin or cyclophosphamide. Steroid-sensitive patients (85–90% cases) respond after 4 weeks, steroid-resistant (10–15% cases) have no remission after 4 weeks.
Treatment of hypertension: ACE inhibitors are the drug of choice.
Prevention of complications: Penicillin prophylaxis to prevent pneumococcal peritonitis and septicaemia, mobilisation/TED stockings to prevent thrombosis.

COMPLICATIONS

Renal failure: 2° to hypovolaemia, diuretics or renal vein thrombosis.

↑ **Infection susceptibility:** Peritonitis, pneumococcal infections due to urinary loss of Ig.

Hypercoagulability: Renal vein thrombosis and DVT 2° to hypovolaemia, urinary loss of antithrombin III, protein C and S, ↑ synthesis of fibrinogen in the liver, immobility 2° to leg oedema and steroid therapy.

Hyperlipidaemia: ↑ Synthesis of triglycerides and cholesterol with albumin in the liver.

PROGNOSIS   Before the introduction of steroids, 60% of children with the relapsing form of nephrotic syndrome died. Steroids have revolutionised the prognosis of this condition but prognosis is affected by complications and S/E of treatment.

DEFINITION   Disorders involving ectodermal tissue that cause defects in the skin and neurological system.

AETIOLOGY   AD transmission 50%, *de novo* mutation 50%.
Neurofibromatosis type 1 (NF1) (von Recklinghausen disease): Mutation on chromosome 17 that codes for tumour suppressor protein neurofibromin.
NF2 (acoustic neuroma): Mutation on c22.
Tuberous sclerosis type 1 (TS1): Mutation on c9 that codes for tumour suppressor protein hamartin.
TS2: Mutation on c16 that codes for tumour suppressor protein tuberin.

ASSOCIATIONS/RELATED   Family history (first-degree relatives).

EPIDEMIOLOGY
NF: 1/4000 live births, **NF1:** 80%, **NF2:** 20%. **TS:** 1/6000 live births.

HISTORY AND EXAMINATION
NF1 and 2:
Café-au-lait spots – well-circumscribed brown/cream lesions:

- Prepubertal: ≥6 with >5 mm diameter
- Postpubertal: ≥6 with >15 mm diameter.

Freckling: Axillary or inguinal.
NF1.
Skin: >2 neurofibromata (nodules) distributed over peripheral and cranial nerves, focal neurological deficit may occur 2° to nerve compression by neurofibromata.
Eyes: Lisch nodules; iris hamartomas; dome-shaped, clear yellow/brown lesions.
Bony lesions: Sphenoid dysplasia (thinning of long bone cortex, long bone bowing), pseudoarthroses (false joint resulting from a fracture within a long bone that has not healed).
NF2: Deafness/tinnitus, headaches, possible facial weakness and cerebellar ataxia, few cutaneous lesions.
TS:
Skin: Depigmented 'ash-leaf' lesions that fluoresce under UV light (Wood's light), acne-like rash; 'adenoma sebaceum' in butterfly distribution over bridge of the nose and cheeks, periungual fibromata, Shagreen patch.
Developmental delay: Moderate to severe learning disability.
Neurological: Infantile spasms, epilepsy.
Renal: Renal angiolipomatas, flank pain, haematuria, hypertension.
Other: Cardiac rhabdomyomata, retinal hamartomas.

PATHOPHYSIOLOGY
NF1: Neurofibromata are well-differentiated tumours consisting of elongated spindle-shaped cells and pleomorphic fibroblast-like cells.
NF2: Bilateral tumours of the 8th cranial nerve cause pressure damage to neighbouring nerves.
TS: Multisystem involvement of small benign 'tuber-like growths' of connective tissue that grow in the brain, kidneys, heart, eyes, lungs and skin.

INVESTIGATIONS
NF1: Slit lamp examination for Lisch nodules.
MRI/CT brain: Glial nodules.
X-rays: Pseudoarthrosis, scoliosis.
Skull X-ray: 'Railroad track' calcification.
TS: Urine analysis (haematuria), ECHO (cardiac rhabdomyomata), ECG (arrhythmias), MRI brain (tumours).

MANAGEMENT

NF1 + 2:

Medical: Regular follow-up for monitoring BP, ophthalmology assessment, testing of 8th nerve and skeletal complications.

Surgical: Laser removal of nodules, orthopaedic or neurosurgical intervention.

TS: Antiepileptic medications, antihypertensives, neurosurgical intervention.

Genetic counselling: Antenatal diagnosis with amniocentesis/CVS.

Educational: TS patients often require statementing for special school attendance.

Support: For parents and child, linking with associations, charities and other families.

COMPLICATIONS

NF1: Gliomas (benign, occasionally sarcomatous), scoliosis, spinal cord tumours, phaeochromocytoma, pulmonary hypertension and renal artery stenosis.

NF2: Meningiomas, neurofibromas and schwannomas.

TS: Cardiac rhabdomyomas may cause hydrops fetalis, renal cysts, brain tumours; cortical tubers, subependymal nodules and giant cell astrocytomas.

PROGNOSIS

NF1: Most just have café-au-lait spots with no neurological symptoms and live healthy long lives. Lifespan may be reduced by complications.

NF2: Depends on complications; higher morbidity and mortality than NF1.

TS: Depends on the severity of symptoms, learning disability, epilepsy and renal/CNS complications.

DEFINITION   The involuntary passage of urine during sleep after the age when continence is anticipated.

AETIOLOGY

General: May be 1° (never achieved night-time continence) or 2° (recurrence having been dry for >6/12). International Children's Continence Society terminology: monosymptomatic (absence of daytime voiding symptoms) and non-monosymptomatic (subtle daytime symptoms).

Developmental: Immature bladder control (with daytime frequency), disorder affecting arousal from sleep.

Environmental: Stress, family break-up, maternal separation, moving house, birth of a younger sibling, hospital attendance.

Abuse: Sexual, physical, emotional.

Structural: ↓d bladder capacity, congenital anomalies (ectopic ureter/posterior urethral valves/urethral diverticulum/congenital stricture).

Medical: Urinary tract infections, constipation, epilepsy, occult spina bifida, diabetes mellitus/insipidus, hyperthyroidism, neurogenic bladder.

ASSOCIATIONS/RELATED   Familial, developmental delay, large families, institutional upbringing.

EPIDEMIOLOGY   M:F = 2:1. ↓d incidence with ↑d age: 7 year olds (M 9%, F 6%), 10 year olds (M 7%, F 3%).

HISTORY

General: Fluid/diet intake, voiding diary (objective documentation of voiding patterns/bowel movements), FHx, parental/child attitudes.

Medical: Symptoms of low functional bladder capacity (frequency/nocturia), urgency, daytime incontinence, ? clothes/bedding change, thirst, polyuria.

Social assessment: Family stresses? Indication of sexual abuse?

EXAMINATION   Hard stool in the abdomen, patulous anus (wide gaping anal orifice), absence of anal wink, cutaneous stigmata of spinal dysraphism (dimple above cleft/midline pigmentation/hair tuft), full neurological examination (for presence of a possible neuropathic bladder).

PATHOPHYSIOLOGY   See Aetiology.

INVESTIGATIONS

Urine: MC&S and specific gravity (↑ with ↓ fluid intake).

Imaging: Bladder USS (pre-voiding capacity/wall thickness/residual volume).

MANAGEMENT

General: Exclusion and treatment of any underlying structural (surgical) or medical cause.

Supportive: Parental and child encouragement. Non-punitive approach important.

Behavioural therapy (>5 years): Star charts for dry nights; 20% response. Achieving good bladder and bowel habits. Easy access to toilet (esp. at school). Good fluid intake. ↑d physical activity. Regular voiding (2 hourly).

Enuresis alarms (>6 years): 60% response. Use audio to waken child once wet. ↑s awareness and ensures good bladder habits. Will respond in first month if successful, 3–6/12 continuous therapy, discontinue once dry for several months.

Medication: Desmopressin (synthetic antidiuretic hormone); ↓ O/N urine production (Cochrane review evidence). Oxybutynin and tolterodine (anticholinergic medications); ↑ bladder capacity and ↓ detrusor overactivity. Imipramine and other tricyclics have good results but seldom used (S/E; mood changes and sleep disturbances).

Therapy sequence: Supportive/behavioural therapy → enuresis alarms → desmopressin → other medications.

COMPLICATIONS   Low self-esteem, depression, ↓ social interactions.

PROGNOSIS   Spontaneous resolution with no treatment in 15% per year. Majority of patients will have improvement or resolution with combination therapy. 1% of adults continue to require medications. Also dependent on underlying co-morbidity.

DEFINITION   Body Mass Index (BMI) >85th centile (overweight) or >95th centile (obese) for sex and age.

AETIOLOGY   Accumulation of adipose tissue when total energy intake > total energy expenditure. Multifactorial.

Diet: Quantitative terms and relative fat content.

Psychosocial: Lifestyle, poor physical activity (sedentary lifestyle = ↓ energy expenditure), food preferences, personal/family structure and stability.

Genetic predisposition: Leptin deficiency (obesity, hyperphagia and insulin resistance). Concordance rates for obesity are ↑d in monozygotic versus dizygotic twins.

Genetic syndromes: Prader–Willi syndrome, Lawrence–Moon–Biedl syndrome, muscular dystrophy (late presentation), Turner syndrome, trisomy 21.

Hormonal diseases: GH deficiency/resistance, hypothyroidism, PCOS, prolactin-secreting tumours, precocious puberty.

Acquired syndromes: Cushing syndrome.

ASSOCIATIONS/RELATED   Obese parents or siblings, maternal diabetes.

EPIDEMIOLOGY   10% of 5–17 year olds are overweight with 2–3% being obese (WHO International Obesity Task Force). Underlying disease ~5% of cases.

HISTORY AND EXAMINATION   Dietary history including details of physical activities. Psychosocial history. Screen for potential complications, in addition to specific syndromes associated to obesity. Detailed examination for stigmata of disease.

PATHOPHYSIOLOGY

Leptin deficiency: Leptin conveys a signal from adipose tissue to hypothalamic nuclei that integrate whole-body fuel metabolism, informing those nuclei about the magnitude of fuel reserves. With ↓d leptin there is an incorrect perception of insufficient energy availability and therefore activation of pathways to restore fuel depots occurs.

INVESTIGATIONS

Nutritional assessment: BMI and triceps skinfold thickness.

Bloods: Cholesterol and triglyceride level. Endocrine assays for specific conditions, e.g. adrenal disease.

Urine: Glucosuria (type II diabetes).

Radiology: USS/CT/MRI head for specific conditions/syndromes.

MANAGEMENT

General: Exclusion of underlying medical condition. Early intervention is important. Confidentiality, self-esteem building and development of a positive body image are important factors. Parental involvement versus patient's independence. Multicomponent interventions that address lifestyle within the family and social settings.

Therapeutic aims:

1. Gradual reduction of excessive weight (growth needs should be included).
2. Dietary counselling with vitamin and micronutrient supplementation. Availability of healthy food.
3. Behaviour modification.
4. Stepwise physical activity program; ↑ activity and ↓ inactivity.
5. Adherence to the plan which requires strong support for the child and family.
6. Fat intake <30% of diet (WHO).

Surgical: Various bariatric surgical procedures have been used in adults. Possibility of adolescent application but not currently recommended.

COMPLICATIONS

Psychosocial: Peer discrimination, bullying, ↓d college acceptance, social isolation.

Growth: Advanced bone age, increased height, early menarche.

Respiratory: Sleep apnoea, pickwickian syndrome (obesity hypoventilation syndrome).

Orthopaedic: Slipped capital femoral epiphysis, Blount disease (idiopathic varus bowing of tibia).

Metabolic syndrome X: Characterised by insulin resistance and atherogenic dyslipidemia 2° to ↑ triglycerides/↓ HDL cholesterol and hypertension.

Hepatobiliary: Hepatic steatosis, gallstones.

PROGNOSIS   Obese children are likely to be obese in adulthood. Patients with metabolic syndrome X are at significant risk of atherosclerosis. There is also an increasing incidence of Type II diabetes.

DEFINITION Congenital malformation of the oesophagus with failure of continuity of the oesophageal lumen resulting in an upper and lower oesophageal pouch. A tracheo-oesophageal fistula (TOF) is an abnormal communication between the oesophagus and the trachea often associated with oesophageal atresia (OA).

AETIOLOGY
General: Aetiology unclear. Spitz classification of survival involves the birth-weight and presence or absence of major cardiac anomalies.
Classification: Proximal OA with distal TOF (86%), isolated OA (7%), H-type TOF without atresia (4%), OA with proximal TOF (1%) and OA with proximal and distal TOF (<1%). Long gap oesophageal atresia = gap > 6–8 vertebrae (>3–3.5cm).

ASSOCIATIONS/RELATED 50% have associated anomalies: VACTERL anomalies (vertebral, anorectal, cardiac, tracheal, (o)esophageal renal, limb anomalies), CHARGE association (coloboma, heart defects, atresia choanal, retarded growth and development, genital hypoplasia and ear deformities) and SCHISIS association (exomphalos, cleft lip and palate, genital hypoplasia). Also Potter syndrome (bilateral renal agenesis) and trisomy 18 (very poor prognosis).

EPIDEMIOLOGY 1/4500 live births, M : F = 1.26 : 1.

HISTORY
Prenatal: Presence of polyhydramnios is indicative of a high intestinal obstruction which may be OA. A small or absent stomach bubble ↑s the likelihood of OA +/– TOF.
Postnatal: All infants with a history of polyhydramnios should have a NGT (8–10 F) passed at birth. Infants can also have excess mucus, or present with coughing, choking and cyanosis with the first feed.

EXAMINATION Abdominal distension with associated TOF, 'scaphoid' (sunken and non-distended) abdomen if none. Thorough examination for exclusion of other anomalies: murmurs, genital, anorectal, limb, etc.

PATHOPHYSIOLOGY Upper pouch is blind ending with a hypertrophied muscular wall that typically extends to the level of the second to fourth thoracic vertebra. Distal oesophageal pouch has a small-diameter, thin muscular wall and extends a variable distance above the diaphragm.

INVESTIGATIONS
Plain XR: CXR confirms diagnosis with coiled NGT in upper pouch; distal bowel gas indicates presence of distal TOF.
Specific: ECHO (cardiac anomalies, position of aortic arch), RUSS.

MANAGEMENT
Initial: Immediate transfer to a neonatal surgical centre. During transfer, nurse neonate head up and prone; prevents regurgitation of gastric contents into the trachea via a TOF if present. Suction and irrigation applied to the upper pouch using a replogle tube. NBM. Avoid 'bag and mask' if distal TOF.
Surgical (short gap): Single-stage correction with anastomosis of the upper and lower pouch with TOF ligation as appropriate. If the anastomosis is under tension then the infant may be paralysed and ventilated for 5/7. Chest drain usually left at the anastomotic site.
Surgical (long gap): Multiple techniques including initial placement of a PEG +/– ligation of the TOF and then infant growth before further surgical intervention. Secondary surgery involves oesophageal replacement with a gastric transposition or gastric tube and small or large bowel thoracic transposition.
Surgical approach: Repair can be performed via the traditional thoracotomy (open) approach or minimal access thoracoscopic approach.

COMPLICATIONS

Surgical: Anastomotic leakage, oesophageal dysmotility, gastro-oesophageal reflux disease, oesophageal stricture at the site of the anastomosis and fistula recurrence. Long-gap OA is associated with a significantly higher morbidity.

Other: Tracheomalacia, failure to thrive and complications associated with co-morbidity.

PROGNOSIS Overall survival rates are currently >90%. Risk factors for mortality are very low birth-weights (<1500 g) and major cardiac abnormalities. The majority of long-gap OA patients will require multiple operations (either oesophageal dilatations or fundoplications etc.).

DEFINITION   Extra-articular disease consisting of a tibial tubercle apophyseal traction injury causing pain and inflammation.

AETIOLOGY
General: Traumatic mechanism. Coincides with the year following a rapid growth spurt. Bilateral in 25%.
Mechanism: Stress from quadriceps contraction is transmitted through the patellar tendon onto a small portion of the partially developed tibial tubercle apophysis, possibly resulting in a partial avulsion fracture through the ossification centre. 2° heterotopic bone formation occurs in the tendon near its insertion point, forming the visible lump.

ASSOCIATIONS/RELATED   Sports especially those with high knee impact (e.g. repetitive jumping). Should be differentiated from tibial fracture, underlying tumour, quadriceps tendon avulsion, chondromalacia patellae, osteomyelitis of the proximal tibia and patellar tendonitis.

EPIDEMIOLOGY   Most common knee disorder in adolescence; post-rapid growth spurt; girls 10–11 years, boys 13–14 years. M>F ($\uparrow$d sporting activities in boys).

HISTORY   Pain just below the knee where the patellar tendon inserts, usually present for several months before presentation. Memorable history of trauma. Pain is exacerbated by running, jumping, ascending and descending stairs, relieved by rest.

EXAMINATION
Look: Soft tissue swelling over the proximal tibial tuberosity.
Feel: Tenderness over the proximal tibial tuberosity at the site of patellar insertion.
Move: Pain is reproducible on extending the knee against resistance, stressing the quadriceps or squatting with the knee in full flexion. Hamstrings and quadriceps are usually tight and frequently weak. Knee joint examination is normal as this is an extra-articular condition

PATHOPHYSIOLOGY   See Aetiology.

INVESTIGATIONS
X-ray knee: Shows fractures of the tibial tubercle, possibly a separate ossicle.

MANAGEMENT
Rest: Avoidance of offending activity and other sports with strain on quadriceps. Aim is the achievement of pain-free state.
Medical: NSAIDs (pain relief/$\downarrow$inflammation).
Orthopaedic devices: Infrapatellar strap and in severe cases a knee immobiliser splint may be used.
Surgical: Excision of the mobile ossicle is rarely required (skeletally mature adults).
Rehabilitation: Quadriceps-stretching and hip extension exercises should be advised after the acute symptoms have resolved so as to reduce tension on the tibial tubercle.

COMPLICATIONS   Non-union of the tibial tubercle, patellar tendon avulsion, continuing pain, bony prominence.

PROGNOSIS   Benign self-limiting disease

DEFINITION

Acute otitis media (AOM): Inflammation of the middle ear chamber.

Chronic secretory otitis media (CSOM): Also known as 'glue ear' or 'otitis media with effusion (OME)', is middle ear effusion without perforation for >3 months.

AETIOLOGY

AOM: Viruses (65%): rhinovirus (50%), RSV (13%), influenza, parainfluenza, enteroviruses and adenovirus (2%). Bacteria (35%): *Streptococcus pneumoniae* (30%), Non-typeable *Haemophilus influenzae* (i.e. not Hib) (20%), *Moraxella catarrhalis* (20%).

CSOM: Obstruction of Eustachian tube 2° to adenoidal hypertrophy, allergic rhinitis or craniofacial anomalies (cleft palate, Down syndrome).

ASSOCIATIONS/RELATED

AOM: Exposure (nursery, crowded living space), low birth-weight, parental smoking.

CSOM: Most likely to occur in children <2 years with recurrent otitis media.

EPIDEMIOLOGY

AOM: 50% by 2 years and >80% by 3 years. 5% of all children suffer ≥6 episodes, and 10% meet the definition of recurrent AOM (3 episodes/6 months or 4 episodes/year). Incidence declines after 6 years.

CSOM: 70% of 4-year-olds, 20% of 5-year-olds, and 1% of 7-year-olds have glue ear, but often do not have hearing problems and do not present to health professionals.

HISTORY

AOM: Ear pain (pulling at ear) preceded by URTI, fever, irritability, hearing loss. In infants, anorexia, vomiting and diarrhoea may be the only presenting features.

CSOM: May be asymptomatic. May have poor listening skills, inattention and behavioural problems, indistinct speech.

EXAMINATION

AOM: Otoscopy shows a bright red, bulging tympanic membrane with loss of normal light reflex. Occasionally, acute perforation occurs and pus is visible in the external auditory canal.

CSOM: The tympanic membrane is dull/retracted and white fluid can be visualised behind it, developmental assessment (delayed speech and language skills).

PATHOPHYSIOLOGY In AOM there is initial hyperaemia of the tympanic membrane followed by serous fluid exuding into the middle ear that may later become purulent. The drum then looks dull and bulges. In uncomplicated infections the fluid becomes serous again and finally resolves. In CSOM the serous fluid persists.

INVESTIGATIONS

Simple AOM: Swab can be taken if there is discharge from the ear for MC&S.

Recurrent AOM/CSOM: Depending on the history, the child may warrant baseline screening for immune deficiency (FBC and immunoglobulins).

CSOM: Audiology assessment (tympanometry).

MANAGEMENT

AOM acute presentation:

- *Analgesics*; paracetamol (antipyretic and analgesic), topical analgesics (local anaesthetics). Decongestants and antihistamines are of unproven value
- *Antibiotics*: oral antibiotics do not decrease pain at 24 hours but do at 2–7 days, however S/E such as vomiting, diarrhoea or rash were also increased. Antibiotics are most beneficial in children <2 years, with bilateral otitis media and discharging ears. Topical antibiotics (quinolones) are more effective than systemic antibiotics if there is eardrum perforation and purulent discharge. Aminoglycosides should be avoided if the eardrum is perforated due to ototoxicity.

AOM prophylaxis: Pneumococcal vaccination in infancy shows only marginal benefit in preventing otitis media. Not effective when given to older children.

CSOM (NICE guidelines):

- No benefit treating with antihistamines, decongestants or combinations. There is conflicting evidence for the use of antibiotics. Oral steroids $+/-$ antibiotics lead to quicker resolution of CSOM in the short term (2 weeks) but not in the long term. Insufficient evidence regarding the effectiveness of intranasal steroids
- Children with persistent bilateral OME documented over a period of 3 months with a hearing level in the better ear $\leq$25–30 dB HL should be considered for ventilation tubes $+/-$adenoidectomy. Hearing aids may be offered as an alternative to surgery.

COMPLICATIONS

AOM: Perforation of the middle eardrum may lead to hearing impairment depending on the size of the tear. Children should be advised to avoid water in the ear canal, e.g. swimming. Most cases resolve spontaneously but may occasionally require surgery (tympanoplasty).

CSOM: Perforated eardrum and chronic discharge for >6 months. Need to exclude cholesteatoma: a collection of epidermal and connective tissues within the middle ear which grows independently and can be locally invasive.

Rare complications: Mastoiditis, meningitis, subdural, extradural, brain abscess.

PROGNOSIS Most cases of AOM and CSOM resolve satisfactorily without intervention.

DEFINITION   Failure of closure or reopening of the ductus arteriosus postnatally.

AETIOLOGY   The ductus arteriosus (DA) allows the blood leaving the right ventricle to bypass the pulmonary circulation and enter the descending aorta distal to the origin of the left subclavian artery. Remnant of the distal sixth aortic arch; typically left aortic remnant (normal) or right (associated with other abnormalities). Fetal patency is ensured by ductal prostaglandin E2 (PGE2) production. PGE2 antagonism causes premature closure. Normal closure at 15 hours; first breath = abrupt contracture of the ductal muscular wall. True anatomical closure occurs after several weeks. PDA if patent >3/12.
Reasons for patency: Prematurity, perinatal distress, excessive fluid therapy, hypoxia.

ASSOCIATIONS/RELATED   Chromosomal abnormality, congenital rubella, fetal alcohol syndrome, maternal amphetamine abuse, maternal phenytoin, FHx.

EPIDEMIOLOGY   ≤40% in <1500 g, 8/1000 (premature), 1/2000 (term), F : M = 2 : 1.

HISTORY   Dependent on PDA size and degree of left-to-right shunting.
Small: Asymptomatic.
Medium: ↓d exercise tolerance, left-to-right shunt may be associated with a hoarse cry, cough, lower respiratory tract infections (LRTI), atelectasis or pneumonia.
Large: Symptoms of congestive cardiac failure with dyspnoea and failure to thrive. Neonatal apnoeas and bradycardias.

EXAMINATION
Premature: Rough systolic murmur (left sternal border), ↑d precordial activity and bounding peripheral pulses.
Small: Normal pulses, BP, continuous 'machinery' murmur and thrill below left clavicle due to pressure gradient between aorta and pulmonary artery throughout cardiac cycle and thrill, loud S2 when both components close together.
Medium: Wide pulse pressure, bounding peripheral pulses, signs of LRTIs.
Large: Absent thrill, murmur present in systole only as pressures in the aorta and pulmonary artery are equal in diastole, loud and single S2, collapsing pulse.
CHF: Tachycardia, tachypnoea, respiratory distress, displaced apex, cool peripheries.

PATHOPHYSIOLOGY
Functional closure: Postnatal contraction of muscular media = ductal shortening.
Permanent closure: Folding of the endothelium and proliferation of the subintimal layers.

INVESTIGATIONS
CXR: Cardiomegaly with ventricular prominence, ↑d pulmonary vasculature.
ECG: Usually normal; possible left atrial/ventricular hypertrophy.
Doppler Echo: Confirms patency, direction of flow.

MANAGEMENT
Preterm infants: 1° conservative (asymptomatic); fluid restriction, prostaglandin inhibitor (indomethacin/ibuprofen) or surgical ligation (symptomatic).
Older children: Minimal access closure with cardiac catheterisation >1 year or open thoracotomy. Recommended as ↑d PDA-associated bacterial endocarditis risk.

COMPLICATIONS
Preterm: Intraventricular haemorrhage, bronchopulmonary dysplasia, CHF.
Older children: Bacterial endocarditis, pulmonary hypertension, Eisenmenger syndrome, pulmonary or systemic emboli, aortic rupture.

PROGNOSIS   Untreated: mortality rate = 20% (<20 years), 42% (<45 years), 60% (<60 years). 0.6% per year undergoes spontaneous closure. Following PDA closure, patients experience no further symptoms and have no further cardiac sequelae.

DEFINITION Persistently raised pulmonary vascular resistance which → shunting of blood away from the lungs via the ductus arteriosus and foramen ovale.

AETIOLOGY May be primary (idiopathic) or secondary to:

- Severe surfactant deficiency
- Meconium aspiration syndrome (MAS)
- Pulmonary hypoplasia (congenital, oligohydramnios)
- Diaphragmatic hernia
- Congenital pneumonia
- HIE

ASSOCIATIONS/RELATED IUGR, fetal distress, Down syndrome.

EPIDEMIOLOGY 1/500–700 live births; occurs in term and preterm infants.

HISTORY AND EXAMINATION Should be suspected in all infants when hypoxaemia is out of proportion to the severity of parenchymal lung disease on CXR. Hypoxia is universal in all causes of PPH and does not respond to 100% O_2 (hyperoxia test).
Signs of respiratory distress: Tachycardia, tachypnoea, recession: intercostal/subcostal/sternal/substernal and cyanosis.
Signs of cardiogenic shock: May occur 2° to myocardial ischaemia and papillary muscle dysfunction with mitral and tricuspid regurgitation; presents with signs of ↓end-organ perfusion: oliguria, lethargy, hypotension.

PATHOPHYSIOLOGY After birth pulmonary vascular resistance normally declines rapidly as a consequence of pulmonary vessel vasodilation 2° to lung inflation, ↑PaO_2, ↓$PaCO_2$ and ↑pH. Three main mechanisms lead to failure or compromise of pulmonary vessel vasodilation.

1. *Maladaptation of the pulmonary circulation due to injury*: this leads to an abnormal response to lung inflation.
2. *Chronic fetal hypoxia*: causes pulmonary artery constriction via leukotriene activation.
3. *Obstruction of the vasculature*: 2° to polycythaemia.

INVESTIGATIONS
Bloods: ABG, Hb, WCC, blood glucose and clotting screen.
CXR: Oligaemic lungs.
ECHO: To exclude CHD and extent of right → left shunt through patent foramen ovale.

MANAGEMENT
Antenatal: At-risk infants should be identified in the antenatal period. Correct any predisposing conditions (hypoglycaemia and polycythaemia).

Dilation of pulmonary vasculature
Ventilation: Lung inflation and oxygen are the two most potent natural pulmonary vasodilators. Tight control of pH, PaO_2, $PaCO_2$ is required. HFO ventilation may improve gas exchange in these children.
Surfactant: + Additional dose especially in surfactant deficiency and MAS.
Inhaled nitric oxide (NO): A selective pulmonary vasodilator leads to smooth muscle relaxation. Monitor levels of methaemoglobin.
Metabolic acidosis: Correction of acidosis causes pulmonary vasodilation and improves cardiac output as acidosis has a negatively inotropic effect.
Cardiovascular support: Inotropes may be required to optimise cardiac output and BP.
ECMO: A very effective rescue strategy for those who fail other treatments.

COMPLICATIONS Severe hypoxia has deleterious effects on all organs but especially the brain (HIE), gut (NEC) and kidneys (ARF).

PROGNOSIS With appropriate treatment, complications are avoided and prognosis is usually the same as that of the underlying pathology.

DEFINITION   Unretractile foreskin 2° to either a physiological or pathological process.

AETIOLOGY

Physiological phimosis: The foreskin is not fully developed at birth; preputial adhesions cause the glans to adhere to the foreskin. It is rare for the neonate's foreskin to be completely retractile (4%). Unretractile foreskin may be normal until adolescence. Ballooning of the foreskin is a normal process that aids the breakdown of adhesions. Foreskin protects the glans whilst the neonate is incontinent of urine (ammoniacal).

Pathological phimosis: Most likely to be 2° to balanitis xerotica obliterans (BXO) which is a progressive fibrotic condition of unknown aetiology (may also affect the urethral meatus).

ASSOCIATIONS/RELATED   Preputial pearls (retained smegma), lichen sclerosus et atrophicus (LSA).

EPIDEMIOLOGY

Physiological: 50% of cases at 1 year of age, 90% by 3 years of age, and 99% by age 17.
Pathological: BXO = 0.6% (<15 years).

HISTORY AND EXAMINATION

General: Forceful retraction should not be attempted. Often the child will self-retract, allowing inspection.

Physiological: May have a history of ballooning and spraying of urine. Distal erythema (2° to urine ammonia irritation). Should have a spout of mucosa as the foreskin is retracted.

Pathological: There is a white fibrotic ring at the distal foreskin. Absence of normal mucosal spout. Associated with pain +/− haemorrhage.

Balanitis: Often misdiagnosed. True balanitis involves oedema, erythema and generation of purulent material from the distal phimotic foreskin.

PATHOPHYSIOLOGY

BXO: Oedema and homogenisation of collagen in the upper dermis, inflammatory infiltration of lymphocytes and histiocytes in the mid-dermis, atrophy of the stratum malpighi and hydropic degeneration of the basal cells.

HIV: Possible protective role of circumcision in HIV transmission; HIV binds to the Langerhans cells on the inner surface of the foreskin. ↓ incidence of cervical carcinoma 2° to ↓d HPV transmission. Nil evidence for UTI/penile carcinoma prevention.

INVESTIGATIONS   Normally none required.

MANAGEMENT

Conservative: No attempts should be made to retract a foreskin. Variable results for the use of topical steroids for physiological phimosis. Gentle retraction with tissue drying in older boys may aid retraction and prevent ammonia irritation.

Preputial plasty: Small non-traumatic dorsal slit procedure to widen the meatus.

Circumcision: Only treatment for BXO. Usually performed under a GA with the sleeve dissection method. In neonatal ritual procedures, devices such as the Plastibell™ may be used.

COMPLICATIONS

Pathological: May lead to progressive phimosis and possible urinary retention.

Circumcision: Haemorrhage, infection, meatal stenosis, glans injury, urethrocutaneous fistula, anaesthetic risks.

PROGNOSIS

Physiological: Majority will retract with time.

Pathological: Advanced BXO may affect the urethral meatus and extend proximally which may require extensive reconstructive surgery.

DEFINITION   Infection of the lung parenchyma.

AETIOLOGY
Neonates: Organisms from the female genital tract: group B haemolytic streptococcus, *Escherichia coli* and gram-negative bacilli, *Chlamydia trachomatis*.
Infants–preschool children:

- *Viral (most common)*: parainfluenza, influenza, adenovirus and RSV. RSV can be particularly dangerous to ex-preterm infants and infants with underlying CLD of prematurity.
- *Bacterial*: *Streptococcus pneumoniae* (90% of bacterial pneumonia). *Staphylococcus aureus* is uncommon but causes severe infection.

Older children–adolescents: As above, but also atypical organisms such as *Mycoplasma pneumoniae* and *Chlamydia pneumoniae*. TB should be considered at any age.
Aspiration pneumonia: Enteric gram-negative bacteria +/− *Strep. pneumoniae*, *Staph. aureus*.
Non-immunised: *Haemophilus influenzae*, *Bordetella pertussis*, measles.
Immunocompromised (inherited or acquired):

- *Viral*: CMV, VZV, HSV, measles and adenoviruses.
- *Bacterial*: Pneumocystis carinii, TB.

ASSOCIATIONS/RELATED
CLD: Ex-preterm, CF, sickle cell disease.
Congenital cardiac abnormality: Especially with large left → right intracardiac shunt.
Chronic aspiration: Cerebral palsy, TOF, GORD.
Kartagener syndrome: Ciliary dysfunction, bronchiectasis and dextrocardia.

EPIDEMIOLOGY   29/10,000 children <5 years of age. 12/10,000 children <14 years of age. Decreasing since the introduction of the conjugate pneumococcal vaccine in all children.

HISTORY AND EXAMINATION
General: Fever, tachycardia, tachypnoea, cough, sputum (yellow, green or rusty in *Strep. pneumoniae*), vomiting particularly post-coughing, poor feeding, diarrhoea, preceding URTI (especially viral infections)
Signs of consolidation: ↓ Breath sounds, dullness to percussion, ↑ tactile/vocal fremitus, bronchial breathing, coarse crepitations.

PATHOPHYSIOLOGY
Stages of lobar pneumonia:

1. Congestion with vascular engorgement, intra-alveolar bacteria
2. *Red hepatisation*: alveolar spaces fill with neutrophils, fibrin and RBCs
3. *Grey hepatisation*: RBC disintegrates with fibrin and suppurative inflammation
4. *Resolution*: exudate in alveolar spaces is degraded and removed by macrophages.

Bronchopneumonia:

1. *Macro*: patchy areas of consolidation with grey/yellowish appearance
2. *Micro*: neutrophil inflammatory infiltrate in bronchi, bronchioles and adjacent alveoli.

INVESTIGATIONS
CXR: Focal consolidation suggests a bacterial cause; diffuse consolidation bronchopneumonia suggests a viral cause.
Bloods: ↑WCC, ↑ESR/CRP, U&Es (SIADH), mycoplasma serology.
Urine: Pneumococcal antigen.
Microbiology: Blood and sputum MC&S.
Blood film: RBC agglutination by *Mycoplasma* (cold agglutinins; see Haemolytic anaemia).

Immunofluorescence/PCR: Can detect RSV on nasopharyngeal aspirate.

MANAGEMENT

Supportive treatment: Maintain oxygen saturations >92%, IV resuscitation in dehydration or shock.

Antibiotics: Determined by presentation, i.e. viral/bacterial aetiology, severity and CXR appearance; normally oral amoxicillin or erythromycin. If severe, IV cefuroxime +/− erythromycin, metronidazole for aspiration pneumonia.

Respiratory failure: CPAP/BiPAP; may require PICU transfer.

Immunisation: Hib and pneumococcal (all infants), influenza (at-risk infants).

COMPLICATIONS Pleural effusion, empyema, lung abscess, septic shock, ARDS, ARF.

PROGNOSIS Most resolve within 1–3 weeks; however, children with an underlying respiratory, cardiac, immune or neurological abnormality may respond more slowly to treatment, and have a higher mortality.

DEFINITION Introduction +/− accumulation of air into the pleural space caused by a tear in the visceral or parietal pleura.

AETIOLOGY

Pneumothorax: Caused by overinflation resulting in alveolar rupture. It may be spontaneous, idiopathic or secondary to underlying pulmonary disease, trauma or aspiration syndromes.

Tension pneumothorax: Accumulation of air in the pleural space is sufficient to ↑ the intrapleural pressure above atmospheric pressure. A unilateral tension pneumothorax causes impaired ventilation in the collapsed affected side and impaired ventilation in the normal side due to mediastinal shift.

ASSOCIATIONS/RELATED Vigorous resuscitation at birth with positive pressure ventilation, respiratory distress syndrome, meconium aspiration syndrome, pulmonary hypoplasia, assisted ventilation therapy, asthma, pneumonia with empyema, cystic fibrosis, Marfan syndrome.

EPIDEMIOLOGY 1–2% of all live births. 10% are bilateral. Much more frequent in the neonatal period than in other times of life. M > F. Term/post-term infants > preterm.

HISTORY AND EXAMINATION

General: May be symptomatic or asymptomatic depending on size and whether tension pneumothorax.

Asymptomatic: Hyper-resonance and diminished breath sounds over the involved side of the chest. Chest signs may be absent in younger children.

Symptomatic: Usually sudden deterioration; asymmetry of chest wall expansion, respiratory distress (tachypnoea, tachycardia, subcostal recession, nasal flare, use of accessory muscles, grunting, ↑d pallor and cyanosis), trachea and cardiac apex deviation (tension pneumothorax).

PATHOPHYSIOLOGY

Pneumothorax: Air from a ruptured alveolus → interstitial spaces of the lung → causes interstitial emphysema → may track down along the peribronchial and perivascular connective tissue sheaths to the base of the lung. With large volumes of escaped air there is subsequent formation of a pneumothorax, pneumomediastinum or subcutaneous emphysema.

INVESTIGATIONS

CXR: Used for BTS classification of pneumothorax. In tension pneumothorax management should not be delayed by obtaining CXR.

ABG: May show respiratory compromise with hypoxia, hypercapnia +/−respiratory acidosis.

MANAGEMENT

Prevention: Infants requiring ventilatory support should be ventilated with the lowest pressures that provide adequate chest movement and satisfactory ABGs.

Emergency aspiration: In tension pneumothorax with a large-bore cannula in the second intercostal space mid-clavicular line or 4–6th intercostal space mid-axillary line.

Chest drain insertion: In symptomatic pneumothorax or in infants with underlying respiratory disease.

Conservative management: In an asymptomatic infant without any underlying respiratory disease (<20%).

COMPLICATIONS Usually no complications with adequate management.

PROGNOSIS Overall good prognosis. Can be fatal in neonates if not recognised promptly.

DEFINITION
Early onset of puberty:

- *Females*: development of 1° pubertal changes <8 years or menarche <10 years.
- *Males*: development of 1° pubertal changes <9 years.

AETIOLOGY
Central precocious puberty: Physiological normal pubertal development that is chronologically early. It results from hypothalamic GnRH-stimulated episodic gonadotrophin secretion (↑LH > FSH).

1. *Idiopathic*: there is often no demonstrable underlying pathology (especially in females).
2. *CNS dysfunction 2° to*:
   - Hypothalamic hamartoma: most common type of CNS tumour that causes precocious puberty. It is a congenital malformation consisting of nerve tissue mass containing GnRH neurosecretory neurons
   - Destruction from tumours: craniopharyngioma, ganglioneuroma
   - Destruction from space-occupying lesions: arachnoid cysts
   - Hydrocephalus
   - Infection: brain abscess, encephalitis, meningitis
   - Head trauma.

Peripheral precocious puberty: Pubertal development resulting from stimulation by a hormone other than hypothalamic GnRH, i.e. gonadotrophin-independent. May result from:

1. *Inappropriate sex steroid synthesis 2° to:*
   - Congenital adrenal hyperplasia
   - Tumours: adrenal, ovarian (granulosa cell), testicular (Leydig cell)
   - McCune–Albright syndrome: characterised by hyperpigmented lesions similar to café-au-lait spots, polyostotic fibrous dysplasia and several endocrine disorders such as precocious puberty, toxic multinodular goitre and amenorrhoea-galactorrhoea.
2. *Exogenous sex steroids*: OCPs, topical oestrogens and overuse of vaginal oestrogen (used in labial adhesions).

ASSOCIATIONS/RELATED Family history (especially idiopathic central precocious puberty).

EPIDEMIOLOGY F > M. Females are more likely to have idiopathic cause. Up to 8% of white and 25% of black girls in the United States exhibited breast development or pubic hair and therefore this group suggested that definitions should be decreased to <7 for Causacian girls and <6 for Afro-Caribbean girls. Males are more likely to have organic cause. Central is more common than peripheral.

HISTORY AND EXAMINATION
General: Early development of stages of puberty (Tanner stages; see Delayed puberty). Must perform full cranial and peripheral nerve examination to identify intracranial pathology.
Specific: Signs specific to individual syndromes, e.g. hyperpigmented lesions in McCune–Albright syndrome.

PATHOPHYSIOLOGY   See Aetiology.

INVESTIGATIONS
Bloods: LH/FSH/testosterone/oestrogen/LHRH levels.
Radiology:

1. CT +/− MRI brain if neurological cause suspected

2. USS of the uterus and ovaries or testes
3. Wrist X-ray: for assessment of bone age.

MANAGEMENT   A specialist paediatric endocrinologist should be involved. Organic causes should be investigated and managed appropriately. In idiopathic central precocious puberty, indications for treatment include the child's age of onset and rate of pubertal development.

COMPLICATIONS   Early bone maturation and reduced eventual adult height. May be associated with psychological problems. May indicate the presence of an intracranial/gonadal tumour or other serious problem.

PROGNOSIS   Mortality and morbidity ranges from mild to severe depending on aetiology: removal of exogenous sex steroids versus large unresectable cerebral tumours.

DEFINITION Early partial sexual development, often characterised by transient and minimal pubertal development in the absence of other stigmata of puberty. There are three categories.

Premature thelarche: Isolated development of the breasts in infancy.

Premature adrenarche: Pubic hair development before 8 years in females and 9 years in males.

Isolated premature menarche: Premature vaginal bleeding.

AETIOLOGY

Premature thelarche: Due to period of relatively high but decreasing activity of the hypothalamic–pituitary–ovarian axis from age 6 months to 2 years.

Premature adrenarche: Caused by early maturation of the normal pubertal adrenal androgen secretory mechanism.

Isolated premature menarche: Spontaneous regression of an ovarian cyst, hypothyroidism, McCune–Albright syndrome; characterised by pigmented lesions similar to café-au-lait spots, polyostotic fibrous dysplasia and several endocrine disorders including toxic multinodular goitre, amenorrhoea-galactorrhoea and precocious puberty.

ASSOCIATIONS/RELATED Polycystic ovarian syndrome (POS), obesity.

EPIDEMIOLOGY

Premature thelarche: Relatively common in girls <2 years of age.

Premature adrenarche: More common in Asian and Afro-Caribbean children.

Isolated premature menarche: Uncommon.

HISTORY AND EXAMINATION

Premature thelarche: Unilateral or bilateral enlargement of the breasts may occur physiologically between the ages of 6 months and 2 years. It is non-progressive and not associated with areolar development.

Premature adrenarche: Pubic hair development is usually self-limiting. It may be associated with a slight ↑ in growth rate.

Isolated premature menarche: May occur physiologically in the postnatal period. Must be distinguished from bloody foul-smelling discharge (trauma, foreign body, sexual abuse) and bleeding from the urinary tract. Obtain detailed history and examination to determine other causes (see Aetiology).

PATHOPHYSIOLOGY See Aetiology.

INVESTIGATIONS

General: May not be necessary with premature thelarche.

Pathology: LH/FSH/oestrogen levels, GnRH testing, ACTH testing (defects in steroidogenesis).

Radiology: USS of ovaries and uterus, bone age radiography.

Culture: Urine, vaginal discharge (premature menarche).

MANAGEMENT A specialist paediatric endocrinologist should be involved. Normally no intervention is required and management consists of investigation to exclude evidence of complete precocious puberty and regular follow-up.

COMPLICATIONS

Premature thelarche: Can progress to precocious puberty.

Premature adrenarche: May progress to polycystic ovarian syndrome (POS) or develop clinical features and hormonal evidence of excessive androgen synthesis in adolescence.

Isolated premature menarche: Depends on the cause.

Psychosocial impact: Difficulties associated with not developing at the same speed as peers.

PROGNOSIS Usually good. Most children go on to have normal puberty and no deficit in final adult stature.

DEFINITION Inherited defects in the innate or acquired (humoral/cell-mediated) immune system.

Innate immune deficiency:

1. *Neutropaenia*: $<2 \times 10^9$/l; significant infections usually $<1 \times 10^9$/l.
2. Chronic granulomatous disease (CGD)
3. Complement deficiency.

Humoral (antibody) deficiency:

1. Transient hypogammaglobulinaemia of infancy (THI)
2. IgA deficiency (IgAD)
3. Common variable immunodeficiency (CVID) (mixed humoral/cell mediated)
4. X-linked 'Brutons' agammaglobulinaemia (XLA).

Cell-mediated immunodeficiency:

1. Severe combined immunodeficiency (SCID)
2. Wiskott–Aldrich syndrome
3. Di George syndrome.

AETIOLOGY
Neutropenia: May be congenital (Kostmann syndrome), cyclical or 2° to bone marrow suppression (chemotherapy).
CGD: X-linked/AR.
Complement deficiency: AR or 2° to consumption (SLE).
SIgAD: AD or acquired after viral infection.
CVID: Gene–environmental interaction. Variable genetic subtypes.
SCID: 50% X-linked recessive, 50% AR gene mutations.
XLA: Mutation in X-linked tyrosine kinase gene expressed in early B lymphocytes.
WAS: X-linked.
Di George: Microdeletion on chromosome 22q11.

ASSOCIATIONS/RELATED
SIgAD, CVID + WAS: Autoimmunity and malignancy.

EPIDEMIOLOGY
SIgAD: 1–2/1000, most common inherited immunodeficiency.
THI: Not known.
CGD: 0.2/100,000.
Complement deficiency: C2 (most common): 1/10,000.
SCID: 1–2/75,000; most severe of all immunodeficiencies.
XLA: 1/90,000 males only.
WAS: 0.15/100,000 males only.
Di George: 1/5000 (25% have abnormal immunological investigation)

HISTORY AND EXAMINATION
Neutropenia: May be life-threatening. Early presentation with bacterial infections.
CGD: Skin and deep-seated abscess formation (liver), chronic granulomata and symptoms similar to inflammatory bowel disease.
Complement deficiency: Neisserial infections (in particular meningococcal).
SIgAD: Recurrent sinopulmonary/GI infections.
THI: May present as SIgAD.
CVID: May progress from SIgAD and THI. Similar infections to SCID but milder and later onset (>6 years). Autoimmune disorders and malignancies common.
SCID: Failure to thrive, diarrhoea, lymphadenopathy, hepatosplenomegaly, recurrent bacterial, viral, fungal and opportunistic (PCP) infections in early infancy.
XLA: Recurrent bacterial infections ≥6 months of age due to ↓ maternal antibodies.

WAS: Severe eczema, easy bruising, recurrent bacterial, viral, fungal infections.
Di George: Midline facial clefts, CHD, hypocalcaemia, recurrent infections.

PATHOPHYSIOLOGY
CGD: Impaired bacterial killing due to reduced production of cytotoxic oxygen radical.
Complement deficiency: Deficiency in complement pathway results in ↓ opsonisation, ↓ encapsulated cell lysis and ↓ clearance of immune complexes.
SIgAD: Failure of maturation of IgA B cells; immature forms are present in normal numbers.
THI: Delay in maturation of the immune system leading to low Ig after 6 months of age.
CVID: Defect in B cell class switching, variable Ig, immune dysregulation.
SCID: Deficiency and defects in T-cell and B-cell function lead to impaired cell-mediated and Ig-mediated immunity. Absent or immature lymph nodes, tonsils, adenoids.
XLA: Lack of mature B cells; there is virtually no serum Ig, but cell-mediated immune function is normal. T-cell numbers and function are normal.
WAS: T-cell dysfunction, microthrombocytopenia leads to bleeding diathesis.
Di George: Absent thymus leads to failure of development of T-cell populations.

INVESTIGATIONS
Baseline immunodeficiency screen: FBC; differential WCC, platelet, blood film, immunoglobulin IgA, IgM, IgG, antibody response to vaccines (tetanus).
Second line consider: Lymphocyte subsets, C3, C4, functional complement analysis (CH100, AP50), IgE, nitroblue tetrazolium reduction (NBT) for CGD.
CXR: Absent thymus (SCID/Di George syndrome).

MANAGEMENT
Immunisation: If functional B and T cells.
Prophylactic antibiotics: Azithromycin (3 days every 2 weeks), co-trimoxazole (PCP).
Prophylactic antifungals: Itraconazole/fluconazole (CGD, T cell dysfunction).
Granulocyte colony stimulating factor (G-CSF): For severe neutropenia.
Immunoglobulin: IVIg or SCIg is mainstay of treatment in antibody deficiency.
BMT: SCID, WAS, CGD (may be required in Di George).
Gene and enzyme therapy: May be used in some forms of SCID.
Complications: Failure to thrive, bronchiectasis, opportunistic infections (*Candida*, EBV) can be fatal.

PROGNOSIS
SIgAD: Good, except if progress to CVID (risk of autoimmunity/malignancy).
THI: Usually resolves by school age. If does not resolve, may progress to CVID.
XLA: Children who receive Ig before the age of 5 years have the best outcome.
SCID: 95% success if HLA-matched BMT is performed at <3 months.

DEFINITION   Acyanotic obstructive heart disease associated with right ventricular outflow obstruction 2° to a malformation in the pulmonary valve.

AETIOLOGY
General: May be valvular (80%), subvalvular (infundibular) or supravalvular. ↓d pulmonary valve orifice size = ↑d outflow obstruction. Changes 2° to obstruction; RVH and pulmonary arterial dilation. Graded according to the peak gradient pressure: mild <50 mmHg, moderate 51–79 mmHg, severe >80 mmHg.
Congenital valvular stenosis: Common variants: dome-shaped pulmonary valve; fused leaflets form a conical windsock-like structure. Uncommon variants: unicommissural, bicuspid and tricuspid valves.
Acquired valvular stenosis: 2° to rheumatoid fever, endocarditis and malignant carcinoid.

ASSOCIATIONS/RELATED   Noonan syndrome, ASD, VSD, PDA, patent foramen ovale, tetralogy of Fallot and familial (siblings 2–3%).
Epidemiology
10% of all congenital heart defects. M = F.

HISTORY
Mild stenosis: Incidental detection of a murmur in childhood although may also be asymptomatic until adulthood.
Moderate stenosis: Dyspnoea and fatigue may appear as ↑d severity and decompensation.
Severe stenosis: Exercise intolerance, angina on exertion and heart failure. Rarely, severe stenosis may present with cyanosis due to R-L shunting through the foramen ovale or an associated ASD.

EXAMINATION
Mild to moderate stenosis: Child is usually acyanotic with a right ventricular heave +/− systolic thrill (suprasternal notch), HS; S1 with ejection systolic click and S2 split widely. Ejection systolic murmur heard loudest at the left upper sternal border, radiating to the back; the severity of stenosis is directly related to timing and duration of the murmur but not the intensity.
Severe stenosis: Signs of cyanosis and heart failure with tricuspid insufficiency; giant 'a' waves in JVP, hepatomegaly and a pulsatile liver. Fourth heart sound.

PATHOPHYSIOLOGY   See Aetiology.

INVESTIGATIONS
CXR: Normal heart size, post-stenotic pulmonary arterial dilation, ↓d pulmonary blood flow. May show signs of CHF (right ventricular and atrial enlargement, cardiomegaly).
ECG: Normal in mild stenosis but in severe stenosis may show right axis deviation, right ventricular hypertrophy and signs of right heart strain.
Doppler echo: Diagnostic, determines severity of stenosis (pressure gradient) and associated cardiac anomalies, enables management pathway associated with grade.

MANAGEMENT
Mild: Conservative; annual follow-up +/− echo.
Moderate: Depends on whether symptomatic evaluation of risk:benefit ratio.
Severe: Surgical intervention; minimal invasive technique (balloon pulmonary valvuloplasty) or open approach (valvotomy with inflow occlusion, hypothermia and cardiopulmonary bypass). Open approach only if minimally invasive not feasible.

COMPLICATIONS   RVH and CHF with severe pulmonary stenosis.

PROGNOSIS   Mild usually does not progress, but the moderate-to-severe disease does. Prognosis is good following surgical intervention; 25% of neonates need second intervention and 10% of older children. Life expectancy is similar to general population and most patients remain asymptomatic.

DEFINITION Hypertrophy and hyperplasia of pyloric sphincter muscle causing gastric outflow obstruction. Also called infantile hypertrophic pyloric stenosis (IHPS).

AETIOLOGY Multifactorial; both hereditary and environmental factors are involved. Identical twins have 87% concordance. Theories include deficiency of neurons containing nitric oxide synthase, abnormal myenteric plexus innervations, infantile hypergastrinaemia, exposure to macrolide antibiotics and persisting duodenal hyperacidity.

ASSOCIATIONS/RELATED 30% are first-born males. Male sex (M : F = 4 : 1). 7% FHx (parental). More common with Caucasian infants.

EPIDEMIOLOGY 1–2/500 live births.

History
Usually presents at 2–6/52 (up to 6/12). 95% of patients between 2–12/52.
Characteristic history:

1. Progressive non-bilious vomiting within 30 minutes of a feed; may become projectile. Occasionally associated with coffee-ground vomiting 2° to gastritis or Mallory–Weiss tear at the gastro-oesophageal junction
2. Persistently hungry following projectile vomiting
3. Constipation
4. Failure to thrive.

EXAMINATION
Systemic: Weight loss +/− signs of dehydration, ↑d CRT, ↓ skin turgor, sunken fontanelle, ↓ urinary output, may be jaundiced (5%).
Gastrointestinal: Visible peristalsis from left-to-right left upper quadrant during a feed. An 'olive-sized' pyloric mass deep in the right upper quadrant palpated during a feed or more likely immediately after a vomit. The palpation of the pyloric tumour can be aided by the use of a test feed (usually performed via an NGT).

PATHOPHYSIOLOGY Marked hypertrophy and hyperplasia of the two (circular and longitudinal) muscular layers of the pylorus occurs, leading to narrowing of the gastric antrum. The pyloric canal becomes lengthened and the whole pylorus becomes thickened. The mucosa usually is oedematous and thickened. In advanced cases, the stomach is markedly dilated.

INVESTIGATIONS
Bloods: U&Es for hypochloraemic hypokalaemic alkalosis 2° to vomiting: $\downarrow K^+$, $\downarrow Cl^-$, $\downarrow Na^+$, $\uparrow HCO_3^-$, ↑urea, +ve base excess and may have mild, unconjugated hyperbilirubinaemia.
USS abdomen: Can be used to aid diagnosis. Surgeon's choice compared to clinical examination. A pyloric muscle diameter >3–4 mm and pyloric channel >18 mm in length are considered diagnostic.

MANAGEMENT
Preoperative: Fluid resuscitation and correction of electrolyte imbalance. Requires extra intravenous fluids to correct the deficit caused by dehydration with potassium correction. Important that the electrolyte imbalances are corrected prior to an anaesthetic (due to respiratory complications).
Operation: Ramstedt pyloromyotomy; a longitudinal incision through the serosa with blunt splitting of sphincter muscles at the pylorus without incising the pyloric mucosa.
Operative approach: Traditionally access to the pylorus was through a right upper quadrant incision. The operation is now performed routinely via a supraumbilical incision for cosmetic reasons and some centres are also performing the pyloromyotomy via a laparoscopic approach.

COMPLICATIONS Recurrence is uncommon. Gastric or duodenal perforation can occur intraoperatively although morbidity <1%.

PROGNOSIS Excellent post-surgery. Initial postoperative vomiting common but settles within 24–48 hours.

DEFINITION   A significant deterioration in renal function occurring over hours or days, resulting in ↑ plasma urea, creatinine and oliguria. Complete recovery of renal function usually occurs within days/weeks.

AETIOLOGY
Pre-renal:

1. Hypovolaemia (haemorrhage, GI losses, DKA, burns, diarrhoea, septic shock)
2. Cardiac failure (severe coarctation, hypoplastic left heart, myocarditis)
3. Hypoxia (pneumonia, RDS).

Intrinsic renal:

1. Acute tubular necrosis (ATN) (80% of instrinsic renal causes) due to circulatory compromise or nephrotoxic drugs (paracetamol, aminoglycosides)
2. Acute GN (see chapter)
3. Acute interstitial nephritis (infection, drugs: NSAIDs, frusemide, penicillin)
4. Small/large vessel obstruction (renal artery/vein thrombosis, vasculitis, HUS, TTP).

Post-renal (obstructive):

1. *Neuropathic bladder*: may be acute in transverse myelitis, spinal trauma
2. Stones (bilateral pelviureteric junction or ureteral)
3. Urethral prolapse of bladder ureterocoele
4. *Iatrogenic*: catheters, stents, nephrostomy or surgery.

ASSOCIATIONS/RELATED   Acute illnesses and multiorgan failure.

EPIDEMIOLOGY   0.8/100,000 children.

HISTORY   Vomiting, anorexia, oliguria, convulsions, previous sore throat and fever (post-streptococcal GN), bloody diarrhoea and progressive pallor (HUS), drug history.

EXAMINATION   Assess intravascular volume status: volume depleted (cool peripheries, tachycardia, postural hypotension) or overloaded (oedema, weight gain, pulmonary oedema)? Is patient septic? Is patient obstructed? Examine abdomen for palpable bladder.

PATHOPHYSIOLOGY
Acute tubular necrosis:

* *Macro*: enlarged kidneys with pale cortex
* *Micro*: swelling and necrosis of the tubular cells, interstitial oedema with macrophage and plasma cell infiltration.

INVESTIGATIONS
Bloods: ↓Hb (hypovolaemia/haemorrhage), ↑WCC, ↑CRP, blood cultures (sepsis), ↑ urea, ↑ creatinine, ↑K^+, ↑ phosphate, ↓Ca^{2+}, ↓Mg^{2+}, LFTs, venous capillary blood gas, clotting (DIC), ASOT (post-streptococcal GN).
Blood film: HUS/TTP (RBC fragmentation).
Urine: Urinalysis for blood, protein (GN), glucose (interstitial nephritis), microscopy for casts (GN), urine Na^+, urea, creatinine, osmolality to differentiate between pre-renal and intrinsic renal failure.
ECG: Signs of hyperkalaemia; tall tented T waves → small or absent P waves → ↑P–R interval → widened QRS complex → sine wave pattern → asystole.
CXR: Signs of pulmonary oedema.
Renal USS: In ARF, kidneys appear normal or increased in size and echogenicity, may detect stones or clot in renal vein thrombosis (RVT).
Renal biopsy: If diagnosis has not been determined.

Monitor: Daily U&E, temperature, PR, RR, BP, O_2 saturation, strict input/output (need to catheterise), daily weights.

MANAGEMENT

Resuscitate: Especially in pre-renal causes of ATN.

Fluids: Allow insensible losses (400 ml/m^2) + ml for ml replacement of urine output in acute phase.

Treat the cause.

Dialysis: Indications for acute dialysis:

1. Severe extracellular fluid volume overload; ↑BP, pulmonary oedema not responding to diuretics
2. Severe ↑K$^+$; not responding to medical treatment
3. Severe systematic uraemia
4. Severe metabolic acidosis, not controllable with IV sodium bicarbonate
5. Removal of toxins (drugs, poisons).

COMPLICATIONS   Heart failure and pulmonary oedema (volume overload), GI bleeding (gastric ulceration and platelet dysfunction), muscle wasting due to hypercatabolic state, uraemic encephalopathy.

PROGNOSIS   Depends on the causative factor. Recovery of renal function following ARF is most likely following pre-renal causes, HUS, ATN, acute interstitial nephritis or uric acid nephropathy.

DEFINITION   Characterised by ↓GFR, persistently ↑ urea and ↑ creatinine concentration.

AETIOLOGY
Age <5 years: Congenital abnormalities: hypoplasia, dysplasia, obstruction (posterior urethral valve), malformations.
Age >5 years:

1. *Hereditary disorders*: Alport syndrome (thickened glomerular basement membrane), autosomal recessive polycystic disease
2. All causes of GN and tubulointerstitial nephritis may → CRF (see GN chapter)
3. VUR
4. Systemic disease (HSP, SLE).

ASSOCIATIONS/RELATED   See Aetiology.

EPIDEMIOLOGY   CRF prevalence not known but prevalence of end-stage renal failure (ESRF) 15–40/million (UK); more common in Asian children.

HISTORY
Clinical presentations: Antenatal diagnosis, failure to thrive, delayed puberty, malaise, anorexia, anaemia, incidental (blood test/urinalysis).

EXAMINATION   Examine flanks for palpable kidneys (polycystic disease), pallor, oedema, pigmentation, scratch marks, hypertension, growth retardation and rickets.

PATHOPHYSIOLOGY   Progressive fibrosis of the glomeruli, tubules and small vessels → renal scarring.

INVESTIGATIONS
Bloods: ↓Hb, MCV (usually normocytic) ↓Na$^+$, ↑K$^+$, ↑ urea, ↑ creatinine, ↓Ca^{2+}, ↑ phosphate, ↑ALP, ↑PTH (2° hyperparathyroidism).
Urine: 24-h collection for protein and creatinine clearance.
X-rays: For signs of osteomalacia and hyperparathyroidism.
Renal USS: For anatomical/hereditary abnormalities, measure size (small shrunken kidneys consistent with CRF), exclude obstruction/stones.
Renal biopsy: For changes specific to the underlying disease, contraindicated in shrunken kidneys.

MANAGEMENT
Monitor: Child's clinical (physical examination, growth, BP) and biochemical status.
Factors to treat:

1. **A**naemia
2. **B**P control
3. **C**a^{2+} maintenance: 1-hydroxylated vitamin D analogues, e.g. alfacalcidol
4. **D**iet: high-energy intake with enteral/parenteral nutrition if oral intake is poor, restrict K$^+$ in hyperkalaemia or acidosis, restriction of phosphate intake combined with use of phosphate binders to prevent 2° hyperparathyroidism
5. **D**rugs: avoid nephrotoxic drugs, adjust doses of other drugs, e.g. frusemide in oedema.

Continuous ambulatory peritoneal dialysis: Dialysate is introduced and exchanged through a catheter, inserted via a SC tunnel into the peritoneum. Preferred method in children.
Haemodialysis: Blood is removed via an arteriovenous fistula surgically constructed in the forearm to provide high flow. Uraemic toxins are removed by diffusion across a semi-permeable membrane in an extracorporeal circuit.
Transplantation: In end-stage renal failure. Requires long-term immunosuppressants to ↓ rejection.

COMPLICATIONS
Haematological: Anaemia, abnormal platelet activity (bruising, epistaxis).
Cardiovascular: Accelerated atherosclerosis, ↑BP and pericarditis.
Neurological: Peripheral and autonomic neuropathy, proximal myopathy.
Renal osteodystrophy: Osteoporosis, osteomalacia, 2°/3° hyperparathyroidism.
Endocrine: Amenorrhoea.
Peritoneal dialysis: Peritonitis (e.g. *Staphylococcus epidermidis*).
Haemodialysis:

1. *Acute*: hypotension due to excessive removal of extracellular fluid
2. *Long-term*: atherosclerosis, sepsis (2° peritonitis with *Staph. aureus* infection)
3. *Amyloidosis*: → periarticular deposition, arthralgia (e.g. shoulder) and carpal tunnel syndrome.

Transplantation/immunosuppression: Opportunistic infections (e.g. *Pneumocystis carinii*), malignancies (lymphomas and skin), and side effects of immunosuppressant drugs.

PROGNOSIS   Depends on complications. Timely dialysis/transplantation improves survival.

DEFINITION Respiratory compromise in a premature neonate 2° to surfactant deficiency.

AETIOLOGY Surfactant deficiency leads to high alveolar surface tension, alveolar collapse and intrapleural right-to-left shunting. May be 1° surfactant deficiency (prematurity and intrapartum hypoxia, acidosis, hypothermia and hypotension) or 2° (intrapartum asphyxia, pulmonary infections or haemorrhage, meconium aspiration pneumonia).
Respiratory compromise also worsened by small lung volumes 2° to immaturity and soft thoracic cage (with attempts to generate a large negative intrathoracic pressure, the ribs and sternum 'cave in' and the abdominal contents are displaced downwards – leads to the characteristic 'see-saw' breathing).

ASSOCIATIONS/RELATED Prematurity, maternal diabetes, caesarean section delivery infants, second-born twins, FHx.

EPIDEMIOLOGY 50% of infants born at 28–32/40 gestation. Majority of neonates <28 weeks, rarely term neonates.

HISTORY AND EXAMINATION
Progressive signs of respiratory distress: Tachypnoea, expiratory grunting (from partial closure of glottis), subcostal and intercostal retractions, cyanosis, nasal flaring; with extremely premature infants apnoea +/− hypothermia may develop. May progress rapidly to fatigue, apnoea and hypoxia.

PATHOPHYSIOLOGY
Macroscopic: Lungs appear airless and ruddy (liver-like).
Microscopic: Diffuse atelectasis of the distal airspaces with distension of some of the distal airways and perilymphatic areas.

INVESTIGATIONS
Blood gas:

1. Respiratory acidosis 2° to alveolar atelectasis +/− overdistension of terminal airways
2. Metabolic acidosis due to lactic acidosis 2° to poor tissue perfusion
3. Hypoxia due to right-to-left shunting.

CXR: Bilateral diffuse reticular granular or ground-glass appearance, air bronchograms and poor lung expansion
Echo: ?PDA.

MANAGEMENT
Prevention:

- Identification of at-risk infants, neonatologist/NICU early involvement
- Amniocentesis for estimation of fetal lung maturity by lecithin:sphingomyelin ratio and presence of phosphatidylglycerol in at-risk infants
- Antenatal steroids stimulate fetal surfactant production (used when preterm delivery is anticipated).

Treatment:

- Surfactant replacement therapy via ETT; ↓d mortality by 40%, should be given prophylactically at delivery (intubation)
- Correction of hypoglycaemia, hypothermia and electrolyte imbalances
- *Ventilation*: either continuous positive airway pressure (CPAP) via nasal cannula or conventional mechanical ventilation. High-frequency oscillatory ventilation (HFOV) may have to be used. Regional variation in ventilatory protocols
- Prophylactic antibiotics after blood cultures
- Gentle/minimal handling, enteral or parenteral nutrition.

COMPLICATIONS

Acute: Alveolar rupture leading to pneumothorax, intracranial haemorrhage and periventricular leucomalacia (ischaemic necrosis of periventricular white matter), PDA, pulmonary haemorrhage, NEC or GI perforation.

Chronic: Chronic lung disease of prematurity, retinopathy of prematurity (2° to oxygen therapy), neurological impairment.

Prognosis

Previously extremely poor (60% mortality) but improving with antenatal steroids, surfactant therapy and improvements in ventilation. Better prognosis >1500 g.

DEFINITION   Serious vasoproliferative disorder of the retina affecting extremely premature infants.

AETIOLOGY
General: Exact aetiology unknown. Possible theories include a neovascular response 2° to either gap junction development by mesenchymal spindle cells exposed to hyperoxic extrauterine conditions or retinal vasoconstriction 2° to hyperoxia leading to ischaemia with release of angiogenic factors (VEGF).
General risk factors: Very low birthweight and gestational age.
Other risk factors: Severe co-morbidity, prolonged exposure to high concentrations of supplemental oxygen, persistent acidosis, period of mechanical ventilation, PDA, intraventricular haemorrhage.
Classification system: Demarcation of disease location into zones of the retina (1, 2 and 3), extent of disease based on the clock hours (1–12), and severity of disease into stages (0–5).

ASSOCIATIONS/RELATED   See above.

EPIDEMIOLOGY   50–70% of infants <1250 g have ROP, 10% stage 3. Patients of Afro-Caribbean descent appear to have less severe disease. M = F.

HISTORY   All at-risk neonates should be screened: gestational age <32 weeks, birthweight <1500 g, Screening begins at 4/52 (non-corrected age) and continues until the retina is seen to be fully vascularised.

EXAMINATION   Experienced ophthalmologist. International classification system.

PATHOPHYSIOLOGY   Formation of retinal vasculature at 16/40; retinal vessels grow out of the optic disc as a wave of mesenchymal spindle cells. In preterm infants normal retinal vascular maturation is interrupted. The blood vessels constrict and atrophy, which disrupts the blood supply to the retina and causes ischaemia. Angiogenic factors (e.g. vascular endothelial growth factor) are released from the mesenchymal spindle cells and the ischaemic retina, leading to new vessel proliferation. New vessels are tortuous, fragile and may haemorrhage which results in fibrosis and subsequently retinal detachment.

INVESTIGATIONS   Diagnosis is based on findings on clinical examination.

MANAGEMENT
Prevention: Likelihood is reduced with careful control of pO_2 in the ventilated child and use of O_2 concentrations of <40%.
Neonatal screening: Studies have shown that ablative therapy to destroy the avascular areas of the retina performed in threshold disease improves outcome.
Ablative surgery
Cryotherapy (freezing): Requires general or local anaesthesia. Proven therapy with CRYO-ROP trial. *Complications*: intraocular hemorrhage, conjunctival haematoma or laceration, and bradycardia.
Laser therapy: Preferred option to cryotherapy as the ocular tissues are less traumatised, general anaesthesia is avoided and there are fewer complications. *Complications*: cataracts, intraocular haemorrhages.

COMPLICATIONS   Severe visual impairment, myopia, amblyopia and strabismus.

PROGNOSIS   Patients should receive yearly ophthalmology follow-up as the long-term visual sequelae need early detection and intervention.

DEFINITION   A systemic inflammatory disorder affecting the heart, joints, CNS, skin and SC tissue, characterised by an exudative and proliferative inflammatory lesion of the connective tissue.

AETIOLOGY   Follows 0.3% of group A β-streptococcal infection, usually of the URT.

ASSOCIATIONS/RELATED   Malnutrition, overcrowding, socio-economically disadvantaged groups.

EPIDEMIOLOGY   Still common in developing countries; however, is extremely rare (<1/million prevalence) in developed countries due to ↑ use of penicillin.
Peak age: 5–15 years. M = F.

HISTORY AND EXAMINATION   Rheumatic fever occurs ~20 days after streptococcal throat infection. Diagnosed by modified Duckett Jones criteria (2 major or 1 major and 2 minor):

Major:	Minor:
carditis	fever
migratory polyarthritis	arthralgia
erythema marginatum (serpiginous, flat, non-scarring, painless rash)	previous rheumatic fever or carditis
	positive ESR/CRP
SC nodules	leucocytosis
sydenham chorea (rapid unco-ordinated jerky movements primarily of hands, feet and face)	prolonged PR interval

Presentation:

- May be of sudden onset, typically beginning with a polyarthritis 2–6 weeks after streptococcal pharyngitis, and usually characterised by pyrexia and toxicity
- May be of insidious onset with mild carditis, usually as a result of a subclinical infection.

PATHOPHYSIOLOGY
Joints: Non-specific oedema and hyperaemia of inflamed synovial membranes.
Cardiac: Acute interstitial valvulitis causing valvular oedema, thickening, fusion and retraction of leaflets and cusps. This results in valvular stenosis or regurgitation. Aschoff bodies are found in the myocardium.
Skin: Nodule biopsies resemble Aschoff bodies.

INVESTIGATIONS   No investigation is pathognomic; diagnosis is confirmed using the modified Duckett Jones criteria.
Bloods: ↑ESR/CRP, ↑WCC, ASOT.
Throat swab: MC&S.
Local inflammation: ↑WCC with negative cultures in synovial fluid (usually clear/yellow).
ECG: PR prolongation in acute carditis.
ECHO: Mitral regurgitation, myocarditis, pericarditis.

MANAGEMENT
Eradicate streptococcus: Penicillin or macrolide (if penicillin allergic).
Arthritis: Analgesics such as codeine or NSAIDs in mild cases, aggressive use of anti-inflammatory drugs may be required in severe cases.
Carditis: NSAIDs to suppress inflammation. In severe carditis with heart failure, corticosteroids (prednisolone) may be started.
Antistreptococcal prophylaxis: Penicillin V orally for 25 years to prevent recurrence.
Prevention: Throat swab should be taken from children who have high temperature and tonsillar exudate to determine group A strep. If throat swab positive, child should receive antibiotic (penicillin/macrolide) for 10 days.

COMPLICATIONS   Recurrent streptococcal infections, damage to the heart valves (especially mitral and aortic stenosis), endocarditis, heart failure, arrhythmias and pericarditis.

PROGNOSIS

Duration of illness: In 75% of cases the acute attack lasts 6 weeks, 90% have resolved by 12 weeks and only 5% of patients have symptoms that persist for >6 months.

Risk factors for chronic rheumatic heart disease (CRHD): Severity of initial carditis, the presence or absence of recurrence, and amount of time since the episode of rheumatic fever.

Incidence of CRHD: At 10 years after initial presentation, incidence of CRHD is 34% in patients without recurrences but 60% in patients with recurrent rheumatic fever.

DEFINITION   'Safeguarding' is a relatively new term which encompasses child protection but also includes prevention/minimising risk of harm, working to agreed local policies and procedures and incorporating full partnership with other local agencies.

Child in Need (Section 17 Children Act 1989): Children whose vulnerability is such that they are unlikely to reach or maintain a satisfactory level of health or development, or their health and development will be significantly impaired, without the provision of services, plus those who are disabled.

Child suffering or likely to suffer significant harm (Section 47 Children Act 1989): Maltreatment of children via neglect, emotional, physical or sexual abuse.

1. *Physical abuse*: may involve hitting, shaking, throwing, poisoning, burning or scalding, drowning, suffocating or otherwise causing physical harm to a child. Also known as non-accidental injury (NAI).
2. *Neglect*: persistent failure to meet a child's basic physical and/or psychological needs, likely to result in the serious impairment of the child's health and development.
3. *Emotional abuse*: persistent emotional maltreatment such as conveying to children that they are worthless or unloved, inadequate or valued only insofar as they meet the needs of another person such as to cause severe and persistent adverse effects on the child's emotional development.
4. *Sexual abuse*: involves forcing or enticing a child to take part in sexual physical contact (penetrative or non-penetrative) or non-contact activities (looking at/producing sexual online images, or encouraging sexually inappropriate behaviour).
5. *Fabricated and induced illness (also known as Munchausen syndrome by proxy)*: a parent or carer fabricates the symptoms of or deliberately induces illness in a child (part of physical abuse).

AETIOLOGY
Carer inflicted: Family/household members, babysitter.

ASSOCIATIONS/RELATED   Drug abuse, lack of social support, mental illness, learning difficulties, unemployment, high number of siblings, domestic violence.

EPIDEMIOLOGY   Rising incidence may be due to changing definitions, ↑ recognition and documentation. Mean age of death from physical abuse/neglect is 20 months.
NSPCC data:

- 7% of children experienced serious physical abuse
- 6% of children experienced serious absence of care at home
- 6% of children experienced frequent and severe emotional maltreatment
- 11% of boys and 21% of girls <16 years have experienced sexual abuse.

HISTORY AND EXAMINATION   Careful documentation of social history, other adults and children in the home, previous involvement with social care.
General: All may present with failure to thrive or developmental delay.
Neglect: Poor school/health surveillance attendance, unkempt appearance, poor dental hygiene.
Emotional: Withdrawn child, lack of eye contact, lack of interaction.
Physical: History is inconsistent with injury, is delayed, elusive or vague. Recurrent or characteristic injuries:

1. Bruises at unusual sites: angle of jaw, fingertip marks on trunk/inner thigh/upper arms from gripping; bruising with outlines of objects used (e.g. belt), slap marks over face or buttocks
2. Head injury/skull fractures in a non-ambulant child, retinal haemorrhages (shaking)
3. Burns and scalds (symmetrical, affecting the back, cigarette burns)

4. Spiral fractures of the long bones, metaphyseal (ends of long bone) fractures, and multiple rib fractures at different stages of healing
5. Hair avulsion, torn frenulum
6. Adult bites.

Sexual: Inappropriate sexual behaviour, bruising, tear or abrasions around or on genitalia, gaping anus, sexually transmitted infection (especially anogenital warts), teenage pregnancy.

PATHOPHYSIOLOGY   10% of abusers have been abused, 90% (the majority) have not.

INVESTIGATIONS
Measure: Height, weight, and head circumference.
Photographs of injury sustained: Consent from parent is not always required.
Bloods: FBC and clotting screen to exclude bleeding disorders.
X-ray: All suspected fractures.
Skeletal survey: All children ≤2 years with suspected abuse to assess previous fractures or underlying medical condition (e.g. osteogenesis imperfecta).
Ophthalmology: All children ≤2 years with suspected abuse to assess retinal haemorrhage.
Psychiatric consultation: If appropriate for the child or carer.

MANAGEMENT
'Child in need' proceedings:

1. Complete Common Assessment Framework form (parental consent required)
2. 'Child in need' referral to Social Services (parental consent required)
3. Inform GP.

'Child at risk of significant harm' proceeding:
Immediate action (parental consent not required):

1. Inform senior paediatrician and child health protection team
2. Referral to Social Services and/or police child protection team
3. Child may require admission for immediate protection (emergency protection order).

Subsequent action:

1. Convene a child protection strategy meeting or case conference involving parent (where appropriate), paediatrician, GP, social worker +/− NSPCC, police, teacher
2. Child may require a 'child protection plan' (previously known as being put on the Child Protection Register)
3. Legal enforcement may be required and the child may require emergency foster placement (or with extended family) if they are not safe to go back home.

COMPLICATIONS   Poor school performance, truancy, sleep disorders, precocious sexual activity, phobias, mental health problems and failure to thrive.

PROGNOSIS   Abused children often develop low self-esteem, aggressive behaviour and substance abuse, and have difficulties establishing relationships in later life.

DEFINITION   Eruptive skin reaction caused by a parasitic infestation.

AETIOLOGY
Infestation by arthropod *Sarcoptes scabiei*: The adult female mite is 0.3–0.5 mm long and has 4 pairs of legs. The average patient is infected with 10–15 live adult female mites at any given time.
Mechanism of spread: Via prolonged direct human contact (>20 min) such as holding hands or playing contact games. Scabies is often incorrectly viewed as a sexually transmitted disease (STD) as may be transmitted by being in the same bed as an infected person. Fomite transmission is possible from towels, underclothing and toilet seats.

ASSOCIATIONS/RELATED   Urban areas, increased in children and women, peak during winter.

EPIDEMIOLOGY   100/100,000 UK patients consult their GP with scabies each month.

HISTORY
Itch: Occurs 2–6 weeks after infestation, worse at night and in warm conditions; may remain for many weeks after the mites are killed as irritants remain in the skin until that part of the skin is shed.
In young infants: Irritability, especially during sleep, may be the only symptom.

EXAMINATION
Burrows: Tortuous erythematous tracts, with the mite (occasionally visible) in a vesicle at one end, are pathognomic but hard to identify in the presence of 2° infection due to excoriations, papules, vesicles and pustules.
Rash: Itchy, ill-defined urticarial hypersensitivity reaction. May be confused with eczema.

Distribution
Neonates: Head, neck and face can be involved.
Infants and younger children: Palms, soles and trunk.
Older children: Webs between fingers and toes, axillae, wrists (flexor aspects), abdomen (waistband area), around nipples, penis and buttocks.

PATHOPHYSIOLOGY   Lesions are caused by the gravid female mite burrowing beneath the stratum corneum. The mite leaves behind a trail of debris, eggs and faeces, which induces a hypersensitivity response.

INVESTIGATIONS
Scabies is mainly a clinical diagnosis: Mites, eggs and faeces may be seen in skin scrapings from lesions under microscopic examination.

MANAGEMENT
Treat child and all close/family contacts. Provide written action plan.

1. Permethrin 5% dermal cream is the most effective treatment; apply to all areas below the neck overnight. Do not use 1% cream rinse (licensed for head lice).
2. Second-line treatment (e.g. if allergic to permethrin) is malathion 0.5% aqueous liquid.
3. Benzyl benzoate 25% is less effective than permethrin or malathion, it smells bad and is an irritant.
4. Mittens in children <2 years to prevent excoriation and 2° infection.
5. Rash and itch may take a few weeks to settle; treat with topical crotamiton. Topical steroids should only be used if the diagnosis is certain. Sedating antihistamines may be helpful.
6. Wash towels and linen at ≥50 °C on the same day as commencing treatment.

COMPLICATIONS
2° bacterial infection: Impetigo requires treatment with topical mupirocin or oral flucloxacillin if not responding to topical treatment.
Psychosocial impact: 2° to stigma associated with infestation.

PROGNOSIS   Good with appropriate treatment, environmental eradication and treatment of contacts.

DEFINITION Significant child-motivated refusal to attend school and/or difficulties remaining in class for a whole day.

AETIOLOGY

Separation anxiety disorder: Separation anxiety is part of normal development until the age of 3–4 years after which it may have adverse effects on development and social interactions and may → school refusal and other behavioural problems.

Environmental: Distress associated with an issue related to school attendance: peer group interactions; bullying (physical, psychological) and academic performance related (examinations, presentations).

ASSOCIATIONS/RELATED

Parental separation anxiety disorder: Associated with overprotective, needy or depressed parent.

Adverse life events: Death in family, parental separation. Lack of structure and discipline and disorganisation of family.

DD: Truancy is the willful avoidance of school without parental knowledge.

EPIDEMIOLOGY Peaks at the age of entry into new schools, e.g. 5 years and 11 years, as well as during adolescence 14–15 years. Overall prevalence rate 2–5%. Slightly more prevalent in lower socio-economic group families.

HISTORY AND EXAMINATION Use structured diagnostic interview to elicit the reasons behind refusal.

Range of presentation: Entirely absent from school, leaving before end of school day, crying, clinging, tantrums or other intense behaviour prior to going to school, exhibiting unusual distress during school days that → pleas for future absenteeism.

Can be grouped into 2 types of problematic behaviour:

1. *Internalisation*: generalised worrying, fatigue, somatisation (stomach aches, nausea and headaches), social anxiety and isolation
2. *Externalisation:* tantrums, aggressive behaviour (verbal and physical)

Screen for depression: Low mood, anhedonia, feelings of worthlessness.

Screen for other behavioural problems: Sleep disorders, eating disorders, conduct disorder, substance abuse.

Screen for symptoms and signs of organic cause: Lethargy, failure to thrive, pallor, polyuria and polydipsia, focal neurological signs.

PATHOPHYSIOLOGY

Reinforcement of behaviour patterns:

- *Negative reinforcement*: tantrums allow children to avoid distressing situations
- *Positive reinforcement*: obtaining more enjoyment, e.g. playing computer games at home instead of working at school.

INVESTIGATIONS No investigations are done by most community paediatricians

If organic cause suspected: FBC, TFTs, urine dipstick for glycosuria.

Urine toxicology (if indicated): For drugs of abuse.

MRI/CT: If suggestive of neurological cause.

Assessment of hearing or vision if concern.

MANAGEMENT Early stepwise return to school, which is tolerable to the child. Close liaison with the school.

CBT: Encourages more assertive and adapting approaches to school attendance, toleration of separation, using modelling, role playing and relaxation techniques.

Medical: SSRIs (e.g. fluoxetine) may be appropriate in certain children who show signs of depression.

COMPLICATIONS   Deteriorating school performance, social isolation, family tension/ conflict, reduced probability of attending higher education. Substance abuse, anxiety and depression in adulthood.

PROGNOSIS   Related to duration of refusal before treatment onset. Complications are more likely to develop the longer the delay in dealing with the problem.

DEFINITION
Bacteraemia: Proliferation of bacteria in the circulation.
Septicaemia: Systemic response to infection; tachypnoea, tachycardia and fever or hypothermia.
Sepsis syndrome/systemic inflammatory response syndrome (SIRS): Evidence of reduced end-organ perfusion (oliguria/altered GCS) with elevated lactate levels.
Septic shock: Sepsis syndrome plus hypotension that does not respond to fluid therapy.

AETIOLOGY
Early-onset neonatal sepsis: Usually multiorgan system disease with respiratory failure, meningitis, circulatory shock and ATN due to GBS or *E. coli*.
Late-onset neonatal sepsis: Usually occurs due to *Neisseria meningitidis*, *Streptococcus pneumoniae*, Hib, HSV, CMV or enterovirus.
Hospital acquired: Occurs predominantly among preterm infants in NICU due to *Staphylococcus aureus*, *Staph. epidermidis* or gram-negative organisms.
Immunocompromised septicaemia: Infected by broader spectrum of pathogens including fungi.
Older children: Usually caused by *Neisseria meningitides* or *Strep. pneumoniae*.

ASSOCIATIONS/RELATED
Neonatal early onset: Vaginal colonisation with GBS, PROM (>24 h term, >18 h preterm infants), preterm delivery.
Medical instrumentation: In-dwelling central venous lines and ET tubes, peritoneal dialysis, surgery and prosthetic heart valves.
Epidemiology: Most common cause of bacteraemia is pneumococcus. Most common cause of septic shock is meningococcal septicaemia.

HISTORY AND EXAMINATION
Determine immunisation status.
Presentation depends on the 1° system affected:

- *CNS*: infant: bulging fontanelle (neonates), lethargy, irritability, poor feeding. Child: headache, photophobia, neck stiffness, seizures, ↓GCS.
- *Respiratory*: tachypneoa, apnoea, grunting, cyanosis.
- *Cardiovascular*: tachycardia, hypotension.
- *GI*: poor feeding, abdominal pain, vomiting, diarrhoea.
- *General*: lethargy, fever, hypothermia, purpuric rash.

PATHOPHYSIOLOGY
Septic shock results from the following components:

1. Gram-positive bacteria peptidoglycans
2. Gram-negative bacteria lipopolysaccharides
3. *Host response*: release of inflammatory cytokines, coagulation cascade, prostaglandins and NO → vasodilation, ↑capillary permeability and shift in intravascular compartment, resulting in hypotension.

Toxic shock syndrome (TSS): *Staph. aureus* and *Strep. pyogenes* may act as 'superantigens' that activate entire classes of T cells and initiate a particularly severe form of SIRS.

INVESTIGATIONS
Bloods: ↑/↓WCC (neutropenia/neutrophilia), ↑CRP, U&E, blood glucose, clotting, ABG (hypoxia, metabolic acidosis).
Radiology: CXR, USS abdomen if intra-abdominal sepsis is suspected.

MC&S: MSU, blood culture CSF (LP if vital signs are stable enough to tolerate procedure). LP is contraindicated if there are signs of raised ICP, purpura or deranged clotting (DIC).

MANAGEMENT

Transfer to NICU/PICU.

Supportive: Fluid resuscitation $+/-$ inotropes to maintain BP and perfusion, adequate oxygenation by non-invasive or ventilatory means.

Empirical antimicrobial therapy: Follow local hospital guidelines.

Neonatal septicaemia:

* < *48 hours*: benzylpenicillin + gentamicin. If meningitis, cefotaxime + amoxicillin.
* > 48 hours: third-generation cephalosporin (cefotaxime).

Hospital-acquired infections: Vancomycin + gentamicin.

Immunocompromised patients: Wider cover usually required.

Prevention: Immunisation (includes pneumococcus). Intrapartum IV penicillin in mothers colonised with GBS or PROM, previous GBS infant.

COMPLICATIONS　Multiorgan failure, DIC, residual neurological deficit.

PROGNOSIS

Mortality: Septic shock 40–70%; multiorgan failure 90–100%.

DEFINITION   Height below the second centile (>2 SD below the mean) for gender and sex.

AETIOLOGY

Familial: Compare child's height to mid-parental height, not the normal population. Bone age is appropriate for chronological age and a normal growth velocity. Exclude inherited growth disorder affecting parents and child.

IUGR: 33% of infants with severe IUGR/extremely premature infants remain short.

Constitutional delay of growth and puberty: See delayed puberty chapter; may be induced by dieting or excessive exercise.

Endocrine: ↓d linear growth > weight loss and bone age delay. 2° to hypothyroidism (congenital/autoimmune thyroiditis), growth hormone deficiency (possibly 2° to craniopharyngioma affecting pituitary), corticosteroid excess (usually iatrogenic).

Nutritional/chronic illness: Relatively common cause; children short and underweight 2° to malnutrition from insufficient food intake, unbalanced diets or anorexia associated with a underlying chronic disease (coeliac disease, Crohn's disease, chronic renal failure, cystic fibrosis, congestive cardiac failure and chronic hypoxia).

Psychological: Emotional deprivation/neglect.

Chromosomal disorders: Trisomy 21, Turner syndrome (45XO).

Disproportion: Short-limbed dysplasia, achondroplasia, mucopolysaccharidoses.

ASSOCIATIONS/RELATED   See Aetiology.

EPIDEMIOLOGY   By definition, 2% of the paediatric population has short stature. Ethnic variations. M > F in presentation rates.

HISTORY
General:

- Original birth records to confirm length, weight and frontal occipital circumference
- Parental height/weight and pubertal timing in first-degree relatives
- Target height for a girl = [mother's height in cm × (father's height in cm − 13)/2
- Target height for a boy = [(mother's height in cm + 13) × father's height in cm]/2.

Specific:

- *Systemic review:* possible indication of underlying disease
- *Detailed SHx:* sports history and social situation.

EXAMINATION

Measure: Height (measured whilst standing in triplicate using a calibrated wall-mounted stadiometer), weight, with frontal-occipital circumference in infants.

Long bone growth: In children who can't stand or recline completely (spina bifida, contractures), arm span provides a reliable alternative for longitudinal assessment of long bone growth.

Growth velocity: Can be calculated as the change in standing height over at least 6/12 for children or change in length over 4/12 for infants.

Specific: Height of sitting body (short-limbed dwarfism), thyroid examination, shortened fourth metacarpals (Turner syndrome), ulcerative stomatitis (Crohn's disease).

PATHOPHYSIOLOGY   See Aetiology.

INVESTIGATIONS

Bloods: ↓Hb (coeliac/Crohn's disease), U&Es (CRF), ESR/CRP (Crohn's disease), TFTs (hypothyroidism), serum transferrin and prealbumin concentrations (malnutrition), insulin-like growth factor-binding protein-3 (IGFBP-3) for GH deficiency.

Karyotype: Genetic conditions.

Sweat test: Cystic fibrosis.

Immunoglobulin assays: Endomysial gliadin antibodies (coeliac disease).

X-ray: Hand and wrist to assess bone age.

MRI: If neurological symptoms/signs for craniopharyngioma or intracranial tumour.

MANAGEMENT   Optimisation of diet, recombinant human growth hormone (rhGH) or thyroid hormone in deficient states, treatment of chronic disease, removal of pituitary tumours if causative. Skeletal lengthening is not recommended.

COMPLICATIONS   Depends on underlying condition, suggested ↑d risk of osteoporosis.

PROGNOSIS

Familial/constitutional short stature: Persists into adulthood; has no effects on life expectancy but may have psychological implications.

Growth hormone/thyroid hormone deficiency: Can expect to attain height consistent with genetic potential if hormone therapy is started 5 years before puberty.

Chronic disease: Final height depends on when treatment of the underlying condition is initiated.

DEFINITION   Genetic condition with abnormal sickle-shaped red blood cells 2° to haemoglobin S (Hb S) production instead of haemoglobin A.

AETIOLOGY   Autosomal recessive inherited point mutation in the β-globin gene resulting in a substitution of valine for glutamic acid on position 6, producing the abnormal protein, haemoglobin S.
Disease depends on the karyotype: homozygous Hb S (sickle cell anaemia), heterozygous HbS (sickle cell trait), heterozygous Hb S and Hb C, Hb S, β-thalassaemia (sickle cell disease).

ASSOCIATIONS/RELATED   Malaria-prevalent countries.

EPIDEMIOLOGY   1/1000 (UK). Manifests >6/12 old (Hb-F in <6/12). Common (5–12%) in African, Caribbean and Middle Eastern areas.

HISTORY AND EXAMINATION
Predisposing factors for a crisis: Infection, temperature change, dehydration.
Thrombotic crisis: Severe abdominal pain (mimics acute abdomen), acute chest syndrome (SOB, cough, pain, pyrexia), severe bony tenderness and swelling especially of the small bones in hands and feet (avascular necrosis may follow), priapism.
Aplastic crises: 2° to parvovirus B19 infection of RBC progenitors causing temporary cessation of erythropoiesis and RBC lifespan shorten to 10–20/7. Characterised by sudden lethargy and pallor 2° to sudden ↓Hb.
Splenic sequestration crisis: Sickled RBC pools in spleen, leading to sudden rapid enlargement, repeated splenic infarction, impaired splenic function (immunodeficiency) Repeated events cause splenic fibrosis and hypoplasia (autosplenectomy).

PATHOPHYSIOLOGY   With deoxygenation, Hb S has ↓↓ solubility, ↑d viscosity and polymer formation at concentrations exceeding 30 g/dl. ↓d RBC survival (20/7; normal 120/7) 2° to sequestration and destruction.

INVESTIGATIONS
Bloods: ↓Hb, ↑ reticulocytes in haemolytic crisis, ↓ reticulocytes in aplastic crisis, U&Es.
Blood film: Sickle cells, anisocytosis, features of hyposplenism (target cells, Howell-Jolly bodies).
Haemoglobin electrophoresis: Hb S, absence of Hb A (in Hb SS) and ↑d levels of Hb F.

MANAGEMENT
Acute crisis: O_2, IV fluids with fluid resuscitation, opiate analgesia, antibiotics.
Infection prophylaxis: Penicillin V OD, pneumococcal, meningococcal, Hib vaccination.
Folic acid: For ↑d cell turnover.
Hydroxurea: Inhibitor of deoxynucleotide synthesis; ↑s Hb F levels and ↓s frequency and duration crisis.
RBC transfusion: Maintain Hb S level to <30%. Iron chelators are required for those who have frequent transfusions.
Exchange transfusion: In sequestration crisis and before surgery.
Advice: Nutrition, genetic counselling, prenatal diagnosis.
Bone marrow transplantation: Allogenic BMT can effect cure (dependent on suitable donor and risk:benefit ratio)/cord blood stem cell transplantation.
Surgery: Limited to disease complications treatment (AVN-joint replacements, skin graft for chronic leg ulcers, laparoscopic cholecystectomy).

COMPLICATIONS   ↑d risk of infections with encapsulated organisms (*Streptococcus pneumoniae*, *Haemophilus influenzae*, meningococcus, *Salmonella*) 2° to autosplenectomy. Gallstones, renal papillary necrosis, leg ulcers, cardiomyopathy and cerebral infarction.

PROGNOSIS   Major mortality in children is usually the result of infection. Lifespan generally good dependent on complications.

DEFINITION
Night terrors: Disturbance of the structure of sleep.
Nightmares: Repeated episodes of frightening dreams.
Difficulty settling to sleep: Child is unable to sleep without parent present.

AETIOLOGY
Night terrors: Fevers, stress, lack of sleep, medication.
Nightmares: Stressful life event, drugs, fever, family history.
Difficulty settling to sleep: Separation anxiety.

ASSOCIATIONS/RELATED   Learning disability, depression, PTSD, ASD, ADHD.

EPIDEMIOLOGY   1/3 of children affected. M = F.
Night terrors: Onset usually at ages 4–12 years.
Nightmares: Mainly affect ages 3–6 years.
Difficulty settling to sleep: Common in toddlers.

HISTORY
Night terrors: Recurrent episodes of intense crying and fear about 1 h 30 min after falling asleep, lasting ~2 min. Following night terror, child is difficult to rouse and is disorientated for up to 30 min. During night terror child becomes tachypnoeic, tachycardic and sweats profusely. There is no recollection of the episode in the morning.
Nightmares: Usually occur in the middle of the night. Usually involve a threat to the child, loss of control or fear of injury. The child is highly alert on waking. May cause stress and discomfort throughout the day.

EXAMINATION   Usually unremarkable.

PATHOPHYSIOLOGY
Night terrors: Occur during the transition from non-REM sleep to REM sleep with sudden autonomic activation.
Nightmares: Occur during REM sleep.

INVESTIGATIONS   None are usually required.
EEG: If associated nocturnal seizures.

MANAGEMENT   Parental reassurance.

Methods to facilitate better sleeping patterns
Night terrors:

1. Ensure the child's sleeping environment is safe
2. Regular bedtimes, and remove any possible triggers that could stop the child sleeping
3. Keep a record of the times when they occur and wake child shortly before expected night terrors.

Nightmares:

1. Encourage parents to spend periods of time relaxing with the child
2. Psychiatric consultations may be required if there is an underlying stressful event leading to PTSD.

Difficulty settling to sleep:

1. Routines for sleeping
2. In extreme cases sedation for a couple of nights followed by increasing lengths of time between leaving the bedroom and returning, until the child falls asleep in the time that the parent is away.

COMPLICATIONS   Parental distress and daytime somnolence/anxiety in the child.

PROGNOSIS   Night terrors usually occur over a few weeks at a time. Children usually outgrow all sleep disorders.

DEFINITION Congenital malformation of the gastrointestinal tract (duodenum, jejunum and ileum) resulting in absence or complete closure of a portion of its lumen.

AETIOLOGY
Duodenal atresia: The duodenum ends in a blind pouch either distally to the ampulla of Vater (75%) or proximally (25%). Type I (duodenal web or 'windsock'), type II (complete obstruction with fibrous cord between proximal and distal pouches) and type III (complete gap between pouches).
Jejunal and ileal atresia: Type I (membranous obstruction), type II (intact mesentery and fibrous cord between pouches), type III (mesenteric defect with gap between pouches), type IIIb (apple-peel deformity), type IV (multiple jejunoileal atresias). Commonest: 30% proximal jejunum, 35% distal ileum.
General: Exact causes unknown. Possible failure of recanalisation of the duodenum during the embryonic solid core stage or *in utero* mesenteric vascular accident.

ASSOCIATIONS/RELATED
Duodenal: Maternal polyhydramnios (60%), Down syndrome, congenital cardiac abnormalities, malrotation, early intrauterine intussusception, gastroschisis.
Jejunoileal: Prematurity, LBW, consanguineous, maternal infections.

EPIDEMIOLOGY
Duodenal: 1/5000.
Jejunoileal: 2/5000.

HISTORY AND EXAMINATION Depends on the level of the atresia. Often diagnosed antenatal by ultrasound (>20/40); NNU admission, initial abdominal radiograph and transfer to paediatric surgical centre postnatally. If no diagnosis, will present with a history of obstruction. More distal atresias will present later than proximal ones (vomiting/abdominal distension occur later). Vomiting commonly bile-stained, although may be non-bilious depending on site of duodenal atresia.

PATHOPHYSIOLOGY See Aetiology.

INVESTIGATIONS
Duodenal: AXR shows dilated proximal bowel, i.e. 'double bubble', and absent or reduced gas beyond the obstruction. Fluid levels are common. Constrast studies may aid the diagnosis (Accuracy ↑d with injection of 30-40mls of air via NGI).
Jejunoileal: Dilated loops of bowel.

MANAGEMENT
General: Stabilisation of the neonate with NGI decompression, NBM and thorough examination for other associated anomalies and ECHO for ?cardiac defects prior to anaesthesia.
Surgical: Transverse supraumbilical incision, examination for malrotation, mobilisation of the distal and proximal pouches. Primary anastomosis is achieved in the majority of cases (end-to-oblique enteroenterostomy). Ladd procedure if malrotation is present (40%) and also intra-operative examination of the total small bowel to exclude multiple atretic segments.

COMPLICATIONS Pulmonary aspiration, anastomotic complications (stenosis/leak), proximal bowel may have abnormal peristalsis so there may be a prolonged postoperative course of parenteral nutrition. May result in short bowel syndrome depending on length present.

PROGNOSIS Mortality directly related to the severity of the associated anomalies and to the degree of prematurity.

DEFINITION   Mucoid/purulent discharge from the eye.

AETIOLOGY
Newborn: blocked lacrimal duct.
Infectious cause:

1. *Staphylococcus aureus/epidermidis, Streptococcus pneumoniae, Strep. viridans*
2. *Chlamydia trachomatis*; vertical transmission most common
3. *Neisseria gonorrhoeae*; ophthalmia neonatorum
4. *Viral*: adenovirus; exclude herpes simplex conjunctivitis (HSV).

Allergic cause: Vernal keratoconjunctivitis (VKC): chronic allergic inflammation.

ASSOCIATIONS/RELATED
Infectious cause: Maternal genital chlamydia or gonococcal infection.
Allergic cause: Atopy. Family history of allergy.

EPIDEMIOLOGY
Sticky eye in the newborn: 1% live births.
VKC: rare.

HISTORY AND EXAMINATION
Newborn: Present within the first week of life; mild mucoid discharge with no overt
conjunctival inflammation. Non-canalised lacrimal duct may persist until 1 year.

Infectious (conjunctivitis)
Staphylococcal/streptococcal organisms: Mild presentation; may present with lid
oedema, conjunctival injection, chemosis (swelling/oedema of the conjunctiva) and/or
discharge.
Gonococcal: Usually presents on day 1, bilateral purulent conjunctivitis, associated with
marked lid oedema and chemosis. May also present with rhinitis, stomatitis, arthritis or
meningitis.
Chlamydial: Incubation period is 5–14 days. Presentation ranges from mild hyperaemia with
scant mucoid discharge to lid swelling chemosis and pseudomembrane formation. May
present with pneumonitis, pharyngitis, otitis media.
Viral: Usually presents as a unilateral red watery eye. May become purulent.
VKC: Classically presents with stringy white discharge in spring (tree-pollen sensitivity)
but may be perennial. Itchy +++. Giant papillae are classically visualised in the upper
tarsal conjunctiva.

PATHOPHYSIOLOGY   The conjunctiva is a mucous membrane that forms the outermost
layer of the eye. Any type of irritation to the eye causes vasodilation of the conjunctival blood
vessels, giving the typical red appearance as well as chemosis and excessive secretions. The
reaction is more severe in the neonate because of lack of immunity, absence of lymphoid
tissue and absence of tears at birth.

INVESTIGATIONS   Not usually required for sticky eye of the newborn. If needs cleaning
>4 hours need to screen for infection. In older child check visual acuity.
Microsopy, culture and sensitivity: Swab any discharge.
Chlamydial culture: If treatment is contemplated prior to results, chlamydial swab should
also be taken and sent in virus transport medium.
Viral swab: PCR/culture for HSV if clinical suspicion.
Skin prick test/specific IgE: If VKC is suspected.
Intraocular pressure measurement: In long-term topical steroid use for VKC.

MANAGEMENT
Sticky eye of the newborn: Regular saline cleaning.

Empirical treatment; Chloramphenicol eye drops/ointment 4 hourly.
1. *Staphylococcus/Streptococcus*: chloramphenicol eye drops/ointment.
2. *N. gonorrhoeae*: IV benzylpenicillin.
3. *Chlamydia*: oral erythromycin.
4. *HSV*: topical antiviral and IV aciclovir.

Prevention: Antenatal treatment of maternal and paternal STDs.
Notification: Ophthalmia neonatorum is a notifiable disease.
VKC: Topical mast cell stabilisers, antihistamines and steroids.

COMPLICATIONS
HSV: Corneal ulceration.
Gonococcal: Corneal ulceration, abscess, perforation.
Chlamydia: Inversion of the eyelids, irritation, corneal infections and scarring.
All can lead to blindness.

PROGNOSIS   Good with prompt investigation and treatment.

DEFINITION The sudden death of an infant <1 year that remains unexplained after a thorough case investigation, including performance of a complete postmortem, examination of the death scene and a review of the clinical history (National Institute of Child Health and Development).

AETIOLOGY Many factors have been implicated but none has been proven.
Prolonged QT interval: Is a marker of reduced cardiac electrical stability and is strongly associated with SIDS. ↑ Sympathetic activity in these infants may be sufficient to cause fatal arrhythmias such as torsades de pointes.
Upper airways obstruction:

1. Infants have sites of anatomical and physiological vulnerability such as a shallow hypopharynx and position of the tongue and epiglottis
2. Infants are obligate nasal breathers for the first few months of life and so prone positioning may compress their only airway.

Central apnoea: Infants can have reflex-like apnoeic responses to a number of conditions such as hypoxia, hypoglycaemia, infection and stimulation of the upper larynx (e.g. GOR). Such apnoeic responses are probably due to incomplete development of the CNS, ↑ vagal tone and ↓ respiratory muscle reserve.
Thermoregulatory dysfunction: Minor changes in temperature (hot or cold) can induce autonomic dysfunction in infants.
Brainstem dysfunction: Cardiorespiratory function, autonomic mechanisms, chemoreceptor sensitivity and thermoregulation are all controlled by the medullary and related structures of the brain. Autopsy examinations of the brainstems of infants with a diagnosis of SIDS have demonstrated hypoplasia or ↓ neurotransmitter binding of the arcuate nucleus (medulla).

ASSOCIATIONS/RELATED
Acute life-threatening events (ALTE): Characterised by some combination of apnoea (central, occasionally obstructive), colour change (usually cyanotic or pallid), hypotonia, choking or gagging. Survivors of an ALTE share many risk factors for SIDS and are at a significantly ↑ risk.
Risk factors: Prematurity, low birth-weight, environmental (see prevention below), low socio-economic status, bottle- rather than breastfed infants, young maternal age.

EPIDEMIOLOGY SIDS is the most common cause of death in infants aged 1 month to 1 year.
Peak incidence: 1–4 months.
UK incidence: 300 cases/year. M > F.
Prevalence: 1.7 cases/1000 live births.
Seasonal variation: More common during winter.

HISTORY SIDS is a diagnosis of exclusion so a thorough history describing the details surrounding the event and examination are required to look for possible medical conditions leading to demise. History should include developmental stage of child, family and social history (including parents' and siblings' full names, dates of birth and whereabouts).
Classic presentation:

1. Usually occurs during hours of extended sleep (10pm–10am)
2. Child is found dead usually in the position the child was put to bed
3. Checks whilst the child was asleep usually revealed no problems
4. Parent may report that the child 'was not himself or herself' before going to sleep
5. May report GI or respiratory infection in the weeks preceding death.

Alerts for child abuse: Unclear, inconsistent history, unwanted child, poor antenatal/postnatal care, age >6 months.

EXAMINATION   Fully undress the child and note:

1. General condition of child (hygiene, nutrition, growth parameters)
2. Signs of illness (vomit, hydration, nasal discharge, rash)
3. Signs of trauma, abuse (see Safeguarding Children chapter) or evidence of bleeding
4. Clothing (do not discard – should stay with the child).

PATHOPHYSIOLOGY   See Aetiology.

INVESTIGATIONS   Blood culture should be obtained in all cases. Depending on history and examination, further microbiological samples may be taken (swabs, SPA, LP) or metabolic samples (blood, urine, CSF) may be required. Postmortem examination.

MANAGEMENT
Resuscitation: Should always be initiated by paramedic and emergency staff unless clearly inappropriate. Resuscitation should only be discontinued when the most senior paediatrician is present. If there is no detectable cardiac output or sign of cerebral activity for 20 minutes, it is reasonable to withdraw.
Following unsuccessful resuscitation:

1. Provide support and a calm environment for the family
2. Allow both parents to spend time with the child, allow photographs if desired
3. Avoid mention of risk factors which attribute blame
4. Put in touch with SIDS support groups.

Information cascade: Parents must be told of the legal requirement to inform the coroner and that the police will wish to visit the place of death and take a statement.

1. *Immediate*: inform attending consultant paediatrician, coroner, police (if unexpected), duty social worker and police child protection team (if relevant)
2. *Within 24 hours*: GP, paediatric clinical director, emergency consultant, designated doctor and nurse who will cascade to further relevant parties.

Prevention

1. Avoid smoking during pregnancy and by family members following birth.
2. Avoid overheating the baby, e.g. with duvets. Room temperature should be 16–20 °C
3. Use thin flat sheets that are firmly fastened and will not cover the baby's head.
4. Place the baby on their back to sleep with their feet touching the foot of the cot.
5. Use firm flat bedding, infants are more likely to sleep face down with soft bedding.
6. Avoid bed-sharing with parents, especially if parent has drunk alcohol, been smoking or taken medication that makes them drowsy.
7. Dummies have been shown to decrease the risk of SIDS. In breastfed child, should only be used >1 month to avoid confusion.

COMPLICATIONS   Psychological distress in family members. Plagiocephaly may occur due to 'back to sleep', but this can be improved by putting child on their front for 'tummy time' when they are awake.

PROGNOSIS   Future siblings of children who have died from SIDS have a slightly increased risk of SIDS. The Care Of Next Infant (CONI) programme provides increased support for parents and future siblings.

DEFINITION   Narrow complex tachycardia 2° to an abnormal mechanism originating proximally to the bifurcation of the bundle of His.

AETIOLOGY
General: 15% of infants (<4/12) and 93% of children (>9/12) have predisposing factors (congenital heart disease/drug administration/illness/pyrexia).
Four major categories:

1. 1° Atrial tachycardia
2. SVT using an accessory pathway such as Wolff–Parkinson–White syndrome (WPW) or concealed accessory connection. Most common form.
3. Re-entrant tachycardia without an accessory pathway such as atrioventricular node re-entry tachycardia or atrial flutter. Functional additional connection without visible histology.
4. Junctional ectopic tachycardia.

Often recurrent episodes are life altering, not threatening.

ASSOCIATIONS/RELATED   Electrolyte, acid/base disturbances, cardiac surgery.

EPIDEMIOLOGY   1–4/1000. Peak presentation <1 year old.

HISTORY AND EXAMINATION
General: Characterised by sudden onset and resolution. Usually occurs at rest.
Children: HR = 180–300 beats/min. Palpitations may be the only complaint. Episodes generally tolerated very well; only exceptionally rapid rates or prolonged attacks progress to heart failure.
Young infants: More obscure diagnosis as HR is normally rapid and difficult symptom communication. Rate ranges from 200 to 300 beats/min. Usual presentation is with heart failure. May become acutely ill in attacks lasting >6 hours with ashen complexion and irritability.
Neonates: Differentiation from sinus tachycardia is difficult, but if the HR is invariable, an abnormal P wave axis is present and rate >230 beats/min, SVT should be suspected.

PATHOPHYSIOLOGY   Re-entrant tachycardia using an accessory pathway: Premature atrial beat → conducted to the ventricle through the normal AV nodal pathway → ventricular response finds the AV nodal pathway refractory, but the bypass tract readily conducts in a retrograde fashion → returns to the atrium as an echo beat → echo beat then is transmitted to the ventricle → cycle repeats itself.

INVESTIGATIONS
ECG (MA Tipple criteria): Narrow complex tachycardia of 250–300 beats/min. With severe heart failure there may be myocardial ischaemic changes (T wave inversion in the lateral precordial leads).
WPW syndrome: Characteristic features are usually seen when the patient is not experiencing tachycardia; short PR interval and slow upstroke of the QRS (delta wave).

MANAGEMENT
Medical conversion to sinus rhythm:

1. *Vagotonic manoeuvres:* Valsalva manoeuvres, submersion of the face in iced saline (diving reflex), breath-holding or carotid sinus massage.
2. IV/IO adenosine is the treatment of choice in the acute situation and induces AV block, hence terminating the re-entry circuit (12–25 s).
3. Synchronised DC cardioversion may be used if treatment with adenosine fails or if the child is haemodynamically compromised.

Recurrent SVTs: Accessory pathways are usually identified and ablated.

COMPLICATIONS Hydrops fetalis, severe heart failure, myocardial dysfunction, tachycardia-induced cardiomyopathy.

PROGNOSIS Symptomatic WPW syndrome patients have a small risk of sudden death. Excellent prognosis with a structurally normal heart.

DEFINITION   Rotation of testicle around its vascular pedicle resulting in testicular ischaemia.

AETIOLOGY

Intravaginal torsion: The typical testicle is covered by the tunica vaginalis, which attaches to the posterolateral surface of the testicle and allows for little mobility. Torsion may be idiopathic or 2° to the congenital bell clapper deformity (12% of cases and 80% are bilateral). In this condition patients have a narrow attachment of the tunica to the cord 2° to its high insertion onto the cord. This enables free rotation of the testicle on the cord and therefore torsion within the tunica.

Extravaginal torsion (5%): Occurs in the prenatal or neonatal period. Poor prognosis for testicular salvage. Prenatally occurs at 32/40. Neonatal torsion is difficult to differentiate from scrotal haematomas.

ASSOCIATIONS/RELATED

Differential diagnosis: Torsion of testicular appendage (hydatid cyst of Morgagni), epididymitis, orchitis, epididymo-orchitis, idiopathic scrotal oedema or acute appendicitis.

EPIDEMIOLOGY   1/4000 boys. L > R. Age distribution is bimodal with two peaks: neonatal period and 13 years old.

HISTORY AND EXAMINATION

Extravaginal torsion: Manifests as a firm, hard, scrotal mass. Scrotal skin characteristically fixes to the necrotic testis.

Intravaginal torsion: Variable presentation with hemi-scrotal pain. May either be of sudden onset or with an intermittent severe pain history. Torted testicle has a high scrotal position, a transverse lie, is hard to palpation and there is ipsilateral loss of the cremesteric reflex (although absence of these signs doesn't exclude torsion).

PATHOPHYSIOLOGY   Twisting of the testicle on the spermatic cord leads to venous occlusion and engorgement, with subsequent arterial ischaemia causing infarction of the testicle.

INVESTIGATIONS   Diagnosis is clinical. Urine dipstick/Doppler USS can aid diagnosis but should not delay scrotal surgical exploration. USS findings include ↓d blood flow, ↑d testicular volume and testicular heterogeneous appearance with torsion, ↑d blood flow with thickened epididymis (epididymo-orchitis). Sensitivity 89% (therefore not routinely used).

MANAGEMENT   "Testicular pain - don't engage brain" (always explore if any doubt). Surgical emergency as testicle must be untorted in <6 hours for good testicular salvage rates. If the testicle is viable at exploration a three-point fixation is performed +/− the formation of a Dartos pouch. The testicle should be wrapped in warm saline-soaked gauze for several minutes. The testicle is removed if not viable (orchidectomy). Contralateral testicular three-point fixation is normally undertaken with true torsion regardless of testicular viability.

COMPLICATIONS   Delayed diagnosis +/− surgical exploration leads to decreased testicular salvage rates. Antisperm antibody formation possibility with reaction to any suture material used in testicular fixation.

PROGNOSIS   Excellent with prompt surgical intervention.

DEFINITION   Cyanotic congenital heart disease consisting of four structural defects:

1. Large ventricular septal defect (VSD)
2. Infundibular and valvular pulmonary stenosis
3. Right ventricular hypertrophy (RVH)
4. Over-riding of the aorta relative to the ventricular septum (aorta superior to VSD).

AETIOLOGY   Complex of anatomical abnormalities arising from the abnormal development of the right ventricular infundibulum.

ASSOCIATIONS/RELATED   Fetal: hydantoin, carbamazepine and alcohol syndrome. CATCH 22, DiGeorge syndrome, trisomy 21.

EPIDEMIOLOGY   5/10,000, M > F.

HISTORY AND EXAMINATION
Neonatal: Severe cyanosis with ductus arteriosus closure if pulmonary atresia present. Low birthweight.
Infants:

- Hypoxic 'spells' give rise to pallor or cyanosis with respiratory distress
- Harsh ejection systolic murmur at left sternal edge/pulmonary area which radiates to the back
- Loud single second heart sound due to loss of the pulmonary valve
- Parasternal thrust in RVH.

Older children:

- Often adopt a squatting position with 'spells' Squatting ↑s systemic vascular resistance and ↑s systemic venous return → ↓d R-L shunt, ↑d pulmonary blood flow, ↑d blood oxygenation
- Signs of congestive cardiac failure
- Delayed development and puberty.

PATHOPHYSIOLOGY
Severity of disease is determined by degree of pulmonary outflow tract obstruction: ↓d blood flow into lungs → ↑d right ventricular pressure = RVH → ↑d resistance to ejection into the pulmonary circulation → R-L shunting and deoxygenated blood flow into the systemic circulation.
Hypoxic spells: ↑d R-L shunting = ↓d pulmonary flow.

INVESTIGATIONS
CXR: Normal/small heart with uptilted apex 2° to RVH and concave pulmonary segment – coeur en sabot ('boot-shaped') heart. ↓d lung markings as ↓d lung vascularity reflecting ↓d pulmonary flow.
ECG: Right axis deviation, RAH, RVH, partial or complete RBBB.
Bloods: ↑ Hb (polycythaemia 2° to hypoxia).
Echo: Confirms diagnosis.

MANAGEMENT
Treatment of cyanotic spells: Soothe the distressed infant to try and induce sleep. Knee–chest position (calms/↑d SVR/↓d systemic venous return). If prolonged (>15 mins): IV sedation (morphine sulphate)/IV phenylephrine (↑d SVR)/IV propranolol.
Corrective surgical intervention: VSD patch closure with ventricular outflow obstruction relief. Associated anomalies also repaired (ASD/patent foramen ovale). Repair at <1 year old. Cyanotic infants are stabilised preoperatively with prostaglandin use (PDA).

COMPLICATIONS   Hypoxic attacks (myocardial infarction, cerebrovascular accidents and death), 2° polycythaemia (cerebral thromboembolic events), infective endocarditis, cerebral abscess, delayed growth and development.

PROGNOSIS   Pre-surgery 30% mortality in the first year of life and 75% by 10 years. With surgery now 90% survive to adult life and 90% of these have a normal lifestyle.

DEFINITION   Inherited disorders of haemoglobin synthesis affecting α- and β-chain genes.

AETIOLOGY
General: Hb composed of 2α and 2β chains. Four genes code for α-chains (2 on each chromosome 16) and 2 for β-chains (1 on each chromosome 11). Clinical manifestation depends on the amount of genes affected. α-Thalassaemia results from major deletions, β-thalassaemia from single base changes, small deletions of insertional mutations. Lack of major deletions with β-thalassaemia = variable degrees of ↓d β-chain production.

Classification (α-thalassaemia)
Silent carrier state: 1-gene deletion, slight ↓d α-chain production but haematologically normal.
Mild α-thalassaemia: 2-gene deletions, small RBCs, mild anaemia, usually asymptomatic.
Haemoglobin H disease: 3-gene deletion causes severe anaemia, small abnormal RBCs and red cell fragments, splenic and bone changes. Haemoglobin-H formed from normal β-chain tetramers; has impaired O_2 transport and leads to ↑d cell breakdown 2° to membrane instability. Regular blood transfusions required.
Hydrops fetalis (α-thalassaemia major): 4 gene deletion, incompatible with life → *in utero* death. Antenatally produced η-chains associate to form Hb-Barts.

Classification (β-thalassaemia)
Thalassaemia minor (trait): 1-gene β-thalassaemia; 1 normal gene and 1 affected gene (varied production of β-globin).
Thalassaemia intermedia: 2-gene β-thalassaemia (compound heterozygous state) dependent on residual β-globin production in the affected genes. Significant anaemia present but transfusions not required.
Thalassaemia major (Cooley anaemia): As intermedia but requires transfusions.

ASSOCIATIONS/RELATED   Malaria regions.

EPIDEMIOLOGY
α-Thalassaemia: 5–10% (Mediterranean), 20–30% (West Africa), 68% (South Pacific), <1% North Europe.
β-Thalassaemia: >1% (Mediterranean/India/South East Asia/North Africa/Indonesia), uncommon in other areas. M = F.

HISTORY AND EXAMINATION
Minor thalassaemia: Normal examination, usually asymptomatic.
Major thalassaemia: Variable presentation but may include severe pallor, slight to moderately severe jaundice, marked hepatosplenomegaly, growth retardation, bony abnormalities (frontal bossing, prominent facial bones and dental malocclusion), complications of severe anaemia (exercise intolerance/cardiac murmur/CCF), signs of endocrinopathy caused by iron deposits (2° iron overload). Diabetes and thyroid or adrenal disorders.

PATHOPHYSIOLOGY   See above.

INVESTIGATIONS
Bloods: ↓Hb, ↓MCV/MCH, ↑WBCs, left shift, normal platelets, ↑ serum Fe^{2+}/ferritin level.
Peripheral blood film: Marked hypochromasia and microcytosis, hypochromic macrocytes (polychromatophilic cells), nucleated RBCs, basophilic stippling and occasional immature leucocytes.
Hb electrophoresis: ↑Hb-F +/− Hb-H/Hb-Barts.
Imaging: Bone surveys, AUSS.

MANAGEMENT

Medical: Genetic counselling (mild/trait). Blood transfusion with chelation therapy may be required. Deferasirox (PO chelation agent) minimises Fe^{2+} accumulation and hence overload. Parenteral desferrioxamine (DFO) may also be used in combination with PO therapy. Haematopoietic stem cell transplantation for selected patients.

Surgical: Splenectomy may be necessary via the open approach if massive splenomegaly present. Placement of a CVC/Portacath for venous access for transfusions.

COMPLICATIONS Fe^{2+} overload, ↓ growth, sexual development, ↓ fertility, osteoporosis, osteopenia, diabetes mellitus, hypothyroidism, hypoparathyroidism, hypoadrenalism.

PROGNOSIS Dependent on thalassaemia severity/Fe^{2+} overload/age at diagnosis.

DEFINITION

Tics: Stereotyped movements of muscle groups that have no useful function.

Tourette syndrome: Chronic idiopathic syndrome with both motor and vocal tics beginning before adulthood.

AETIOLOGY

Genetic: Suggested by significantly higher concordance in monozygotic twins compared to dizygotic twins, and significantly higher incidence in first-degree relatives of sufferers.

Acquired: There is a possible subgroup that have antibodies to β-haemolytic streptococci that cross-react with neurons.

ASSOCIATIONS/RELATED   ADHD in >30%, OCD in >20%.

EPIDEMIOLOGY

Tic disorders: 3–15% of children according to different studies, declining to 2–3% by adolescence. Usual onset 7–9 years.

Tourette syndrome: 0.5–1%. M : F = 2 : 1.

HISTORY AND EXAMINATION

Simple tics: Brief movements involving few muscle groups, e.g. eye blinking, shoulder shrugging, clearing the throat, humming. May be transient (>4 weeks but <1 year) or chronic (>1 year).

Complex tics: Co-ordinated patterns of successive movements involving several muscle groups e.g. jumping, touching the nose, echolalia (repeating another's speech) and coprolalia (outbursts of obscenities). Tics are worsened by stress and reduced by absorbing activities, markedly reduced during sleep and suppressible for brief periods of time.

Tourette syndrome: Multiple motor and vocal tics occur (not necessarily concurrently). Tics occur many times a day, nearly every day for more than 1 year and frequently vary in nature, severity and location. *Rage attacks* consist of explosive, unpredictable outbursts out of proportion to stimuli, threatening destruction and self injury, followed by immediate remorse.

PATHOPHYSIOLOGY Unknown. Theories include a reduction in the basal ganglia's inhibition of undesired motor programmes.

INVESTIGATIONS

Usually none required. In specific cases investigations may be appropriate to exclude organic cause.

1. Antistreptolysin titre (ASOT), especially if there was sudden onset of tics post impetigo, pharyngitis or otitis media.
2. TFTs to exclude hyperthyroidism.
3. Serum caeruloplasmin to exclude Wilson disease.
4. EEG to assess for absence seizures.

To assess for co-morbid mental health problems: ADHD and OCD.

MANAGEMENT

Multidisciplinary team approach.

- *Supportive*: parental education and notify school of diagnosis.
- *Behavioural/psychotherapy*: reversal of habit.
- *Medical treatment*: only required if there is significant impairment of school and daily activities and distress. Treatment options include neuroleptic drugs (lower dose than for psychosis) and dopamine agonists.

Treatment of co-morbid psychiatric disease:

1. *OCD*: SSRIs.
2. *ADHD*: psychostimulants such as methylphenidate used in treating ADHD can cause/ exacerbate tics. Recent studies have shown that children with co-morbid ADHD and tics may show improvement of both disorders with atomoxetine (selective noradrenaline reuptake inhibitor).

COMPLICATIONS   Stigma associated with outbursts may → social withdrawal. Interruption in thought and conversation affects education. Self-injurious behaviour may arise from depression.

PROGNOSIS   Tics may progressively worsen in childhood but abate or diminish markedly by the age of 18 in 90% of cases. There is significant morbidity associated with co-morbid psychiatric disease.

DEFINITION Acute, self-limiting tachypnoea in the absence of other cause such as metabolic acidosis, respiratory distress syndrome or infection.

AETIOLOGY 2° to delayed resorption of fetal lung fluid causing ↓d pulmonary compliance and ↓d tidal volume with ↑d dead space.

ASSOCIATIONS/RELATED Elective caesarean section and precipitate deliveries (neonate has not experienced all stages of labour), maternal asthma.

EPIDEMIOLOGY Most common cause of respiratory distress in full-term infants. 1–2% of neonates have respiratory distress; of these, 33–50% have TTN. M = F. Nil ethnic variation. Term neonates.

HISTORY Usually occurs in the first 1–3 hours following an uneventful normal preterm, term vaginal or elective caesarean section delivery. Most cases resolve <72 hours.

EXAMINATION Early onset of tachypnoea in the neonate +/− signs of respiratory distress; recession (intercostal/subcostal/sternal), expiratory grunting, nasal flaring and cyanosis (severe cases).

PATHOPHYSIOLOGY *In utero* lung epithelium secretes Cl^- and fluid but doesn't have the ability to actively reabsorb Na^+ (occurs late gestation). Postdelivery switch to Na^+ resorption 2° to circulating catecholamines. Changes in O_2 tension, also ↑Na^+ resorption ability and ↑ amount of epithelial Na^+ channels (↑ gene expression). With a shorter delivery/lack of some stages of labour (caesarean section) then Na^+ resorption does not occur, leading to TTN

INVESTIGATIONS
CXR: Prominent perihilar streaking (distended pulmonary veins and lymphatics), patchy infiltrates, fluid in the horizontal fissure, flat diaphragms and occasional pleural fluid.
ABG: Degree of ↓pO_2 depends on the amount of fluid on the lungs.
Blood cultures: To exclude infectious cause of respiratory distress.

MANAGEMENT

- Exclusion of other causes of neonatal respiratory distress; pneumonia (e.g. group B haemolytic streptococcus), meconium aspiration, pulmonary haemorrhage or cerebral hyperventilation that follows birth asphyxia.
- Ventilatory support as required including supplemental oxygen and occasionally continuous positive airways pressure (CPAP).
- Maintenance hydration and intravenous fluids.
- NBM until respiratory rate <60/min to ↓ aspiration incidence.
- Prophylactic antibiotics, discontinued once exclusion of infectious causes (−ve BC).
- Diuretics (frusemide) do not improve outcome (Cochrane database review evidence).

COMPLICATIONS Usually no complications if managed with good supportive measures.

PROGNOSIS Excellent as self-limiting disorder. Possible link with development of wheezing syndromes in childhood.

DEFINITION   Cyanotic congenital cardiac malformation characterised by transposition of the aorta and the pulmonary arteries.

AETIOLOGY   Unknown. Embryologically likely to involve abnormal persistence of the subaortic conus with resorption or underdevelopment of the subpulmonary conus (infundibulum). This abnormality aligns the aorta anterior and superior to the right ventricle during development and is characterised by atrioventricular concordance and ventriculoarterial discordance. Classification is anatomical and depends on the relationship of the great vessels to each other $+/-$ the infundibular morphology. Isolated malformation (50%). Associated non-cardiac malformations (10%).

ASSOCIATIONS/RELATED   Maternal factors: rubella, poor prenatal nutrition, fetal alcohol syndrome, exposure to rodenticides/herbicides, age >40 and diabetes. Several genetic mutations have been identified.

EPIDEMIOLOGY   2–3/10,000. M:F $= 3:2$.

HISTORY AND EXAMINATION   Depends on the extent of intercirculatory mixing and presence of associated anatomical lesions.
TGA with intact ventricular septum: Prominent and progressive cyanosis within <24 hours.
TGA with large ventricular septal defect: May be asymptomatic initially or may exhibit mild cyanosis when crying. Parasternal heave $2°$ to RVH. $<3–6$ weeks may exhibit signs of CCF as pulmonary blood flow ↑s.
TGA with ventricular septal defect and left ventricular (pulmonary) outflow tract obstruction: Similar to tetralogy of Fallot neonates.
TGA with ventricular septal defect and pulmonary vascular obstructive disease: Progressive cyanosis, despite early balloon atrial septostomy.

PATHOPHYSIOLOGY   Circulations are in parallel instead of in series. Two closed circuits of flow: oxygenated blood through a closed circuit of the pulmonary circulation and left cardiac chambers, deoxygenated through the right cardiac chambers. Survival is reliant on transfer of blood across from each circuit into the other via a patent foramen ovale, PDA or atrio-/ventriculoseptal defect.

INVESTIGATIONS
CXR: Narrow mediastinum ($2°$ to great vessels anteroposterior relationship, ↑d pulmonary vascular markings due to ↑d pulmonary flow. 'Egg-shaped' heart $2°$ to RVH (severe cases).
Echocardiogram: Diagnostic.

MANAGEMENT
Medical: Preoperative correction of electrolyte abnormalities and prostaglandin infusion to maintain PDA/↑left atrial pressure/promote atrial intercirculatory mixing.
Interventional: Balloon atrial septostomy; catheter with expandable balloon passed into left atrium via the right atrium and foramen ovale. Balloon is inflated and pulled through the atrial septum, tearing the atrial septum and thus allowing atrial intercirculatory mixing.
Surgical: 'Arterial switch procedure' $+/-$ correction of associated anomalies $<4/52$ of age. Pulmonary artery and aorta are transected above the arterial valves and switched over. Coronary arteries are also transferred across to the new aorta.

COMPLICATIONS   CCF, heart arrhythmias, progressive PHT, polycythaemia ($2°$ to prolonged hypoxia), Eisenmenger syndrome.

PROGNOSIS   Untreated, the mortality rate is 90% by the end of the first year. Survival rate post-arterial switch operation is 90%.

DEFINITION   Genetic defect, in females, resulting from the complete or partial absence of an X chromosome.

AETIOLOGY
Classic TS: 45XO. **Mosaic TS**: 45X0/46XX and rarely 45X0/46XY. Two-thirds of classic TS lack paternal X chromosome. Not all the genes have been identified but loss of one copy of the SHOX gene leads to similar phenotype of short stature and skeletal abnormalities (Leri–Weill dyschondrosteosis).

ASSOCIATIONS/RELATED   Crohn's disease, ulcerative colitis.

EPIDEMIOLOGY   1/2500 females. No race/ethnic trends.

HISTORY   ↑d incidence of spontaneous abortions with TS. Possible swollen hands and feet at birth. May present with signs of ovarian failure (1° or 2° amenorrhoea, infertility, failure of breast development) although there is normal pubic hair development. Short stature presentation common.

EXAMINATION
General: 95% have short stature (normal until 4 years when ovaries involute) and ovarian failure. Normal intelligence.
Congenital malformations: Congenital heart defects (20%): coarctation of the aorta (obstructed lymphatic system compression of developing aorta), hypoplastic left heart syndrome, horseshoe kidneys (40%) and ovarian dysgenesis (95%).
Physical signs: Neonatal lymphoedema of the hands and feet and cutis laxa (loose folds of skin, especially at the neck), neck webbing (2° to lymphoedema *in utero*), wide carrying angle (cubitus valgus), broad chest with widely spaced nipples (shield chest), high pigmented naevi, hypoplastic or hyperconvex nails, ptosis, strabismus, amblyopia and short fourth metacarpal.

PATHOPHYSIOLOGY
Classic TS: Nondysjunction in oogenesis.

INVESTIGATIONS
Antenatal: Amniocentesis or chorionic villious sampling and karyotype analysis if diagnosis suspected (nuchal cystic hygroma/horseshoe kidney/left-sided cardiac anomalies, non-immune fetal hydrops).
Chromosomal studies: Karotype confirmation, confirmation of presence of possible Y chromosomal material (Y-centromeric probe). Differentiation from Noonan syndrome (phenotypically very similar).
Bloods: ↑d LH and FSH confirm ovarian failure.

MANAGEMENT
Surgical treatment: ↑d risk of keloid formation. Specific surgical interventions: congenital heart defect correction, grommets (significant secretory otitis media), plastic surgery (neck webbing), remove of gonads if present (50% malignant change).
Hormonal treatment: Growth hormone therapy from mid-childhood ↑s final height. Oestrogen replacement therapy (12–15 years) promotes the development of 2° sexual characteristics.

COMPLICATIONS   Infertility. Y chromosome presence; malignant gonadoblastomas, testicular tissue. Aortic dissection. Conductive hearing loss (secretory otitis media). Hypothyroidism (50% have antithyroid antibodies). ↑d HT/DM/osteoporosis.

PROGNOSIS   Excellent although suggested 10 years ↓d life expectancy.

DEFINITION   A number of different conditions such as the common cold (coryza), sore throat (pharyngitis and tonsillitis), and middle ear infection (otitis media).

AETIOLOGY   Viruses cause >90% of URTIs.
Coryza: Rhinovirus, coronavirus, RSV.
Pharyngitis: Adenovirus, enterovirus, rhinovirus, group A β-haemolytic streptococcus in older children.
Tonsillitis: EBV (infectious mononucleosis), group A β-haemolytic streptococcus.
Otitis media: Influenza, parainfluenza, enteroviruses and adenovirus, *Streptococcus pneumoniae*, non-typeable *Haemophilus influenzae* (i.e. not Hib), *Moraxella catarrhalis*.
Non-immunised child: *Corynebacterium diphtheriae* is a severe, life-threatening cause of pharyngitis and tonsillitis.

ASSOCIATIONS/RELATED   M > F. Immunodeficiency. URTIs are universally prevalent and are not associated with factors associated with low socio-economic class (e.g. household smoking), as are LRTIs.

EPIDEMIOLOGY   Very common. Two peaks: starting nursery (2–3 years) and primary school (4–5 years).

HISTORY
General: Lethargy, poor feeding.
Coryza: Sneezing, sore throat, fever is variable.
Pharyngitis/tonsillitis: Fever, sore throat, cough, abdominal pain; mesenteric adenitis is often preceded by a URTI with subsequent enlargement of the mesenteric lymph nodes.
Infectious mononucleosis: Prolonged lethargy, malaise, sore throat.
Otitis media: Ear pain; infant may scream and pull at ear, conductive hearing loss in chronic secretory otitis media.

EXAMINATION
General: Pyrexia, tachycardia, cervical lymphadenopathy.
Coryza: Nasal discharge.
Pharyngitis: The pharynx, soft palate and tonsillar fauces are inflamed and swollen.
Tonsillitis: Red, swollen tonsils with or without white exudates. Follicular tonsillitis with white exudates may be due to adenovirus, EBV or group A β-haemolytic streptococcus.
Otitis media: Tympanic membranes bright red and bulging on otoscopy with loss of normal light reflex. May see pus in the middle ear.

PATHOPHYSIOLOGY
Macro: Reactive inflammation of the URT to infectious agent with production of serous discharge (coryza) and swelling of mucosal lining.

INVESTIGATIONS
Throat swab: May grow group A β-haemolytic streptococcus. Use in non-immunised child/ complicated tonsillitis/pharyngitis to rule out diphtheria.
Bloods: ASOT, monospot test (EBV).

MANAGEMENT
Symptomatic pyrexia: Explain to parents that the aim of controlling fever is to ease symptoms and prevent dehydration. Tepid sponging and fanning are not recommended. Regular paracetamol or ibuprofen may be used if the child is distressed by the fever. Reducing fever will not prevent febrile seizures (see chapter). Do not use aspirin as may precipitate Reye syndrome (severe liver disease).
Active treatment: Oral antibiotics such as penicillin or erythromycin (if penicillin allergic) for 10 days to prevent rheumatic fever are indicated if group A β-haemolytic streptococcus grows on throat swab.

Surgical intervention: Tonsillectomy is rarely indicated, only when recurrent tonsillitis is causing significant loss of schooling or upper airways obstruction and sleep apnoea.

COMPLICATIONS

1. Recurrent acute tonsillitis/tonsillar hypertrophy.
2. Peritonsillar abscess: quinsy.
3. Post-streptococcal immunological response, e.g. acute GN, rheumatic fever.

PROGNOSIS   Excellent; duration of illness 1–2 weeks. 'Treat a cold, it lasts a week, don't treat and it lasts 7 days.'

DEFINITION   Congenital structural abnormalities of the kidneys, bladder or urethra.

AETIOLOGY
General: Also known as CAKUT (congenital anomalies of the kidney and urinary tract), associated with severe different chromosomal loci abnormalities and PAX2 gene mutation.
Renal abnormalities:

- *Multicystic dysplastic kidneys (MCDK)*: multiple renal cortex and medulla cysts +/− hepatic cysts. 2° to early ureteric obstruction
- *Medullary sponge kidney*: congenital cystic dilation of the collecting ducts allowing calculi formation
- *Nephronophthisis*: multiple cyst formation at the corticomedullary junction with progressive glomerular sclerosis
- *Unilateral renal agenesis*: congenital absence of a kidney 2° to lack of induction of the metanephric blastema by the ureteral bud
- *Ectopic/horseshoe kidney*: fusion of the lower poles (>90% cases) resulting in either symmetrical or asymmetrical horseshoe.

Non-renal abnormalities:

- *Pelviureteric junction (PUJ) obstruction*: 2° to stenosis or atresia of the proximal ureter
- *Vesicoureteral reflux (VUR)*: with associated hydronephrosis (VUR Grades I → V).
- *Non-obstructed non-refluxing 1° megaureter*: aperistaltic and narrowed prevesical portion of the ureter
- *Bladder outlet obstruction*: 2° to posterior urethral valves (PUV); congenital lesions causing variable degrees of obstruction (may present with severe renal failure).
- *Ureterocoele*: presence of an intrabladder hernia or cystic ballooning at the lower end of a ureter
- *Hypospadias/epispadias*: abnormal ectopic urethral opening along the ventral (hypospadias) or dorsal surface (epispadias) to variable degrees.

ASSOCIATIONS/RELATED   Other congenital malformations (cardiac, pulmonary, cleft palate, CNS).

EPIDEMIOLOGY   3–6/1000.

HISTORY AND EXAMINATION
Antenatal: Commonly with oligohydramnios 2° to ↓d fetal urine output. Pulmonary hypoplasia in severe cases. Antenatally diagnosed hydronephrosis is common.
Postnatal: Intra-abdominal masses, UTI, pain (associated with ↑d fluid intake), haematuria, renal calculi, renal failure, hypertension, hepatosplenomegaly, liver fibrosis complications (oesophageal varices, haemorrhage) urinary voiding dysfunction, depending on underlying cause and age at presentation.

PATHOPHYSIOLOGY   See Aetiology.

INVESTIGATIONS
Ultrasound: Non-invasive, operator dependent, diagnostic in majority of congenital malformations.
Intravenous urogram (IVU): Visualisation of majority of anomalies including VUR/PUV that are not visualised that well by USS.
Nuclear renal imaging: DMSA and MAG3 for assessment of kidney function and perfusion. May overestimate function in an obstructed system, however.

MANAGEMENT

General: Antenatal counselling with screening for associated anomalies or karyotyping as appropriate.

Medical: Symptom control (hypertension), Ca^{2+} supplements, PO_4^{2-} binders, 1,25-dihydroxyvitamin D3 for PTH suppression (renal osteodystrophy), antibiotics (UTI/prophylaxis), dialysis (renal failure).

Surgical: Treatment of cause, e.g. nephrectomy (MCDK/non-functioning kidney), hypospadias correction (e.g. Snodgrass procedure), open/laparoscopic pyeloplasty (PUJ obstruction), PUV or ureterocoele puncturing (endoscopic procedures) nephrostomy placement (obstructed system), suprapubic catheter placement.

COMPLICATIONS   Hypertension, renal osteodystrophy, urinary tract infections and calculi.

PROGNOSIS   Most renal anomalies may lead to end-stage renal failure and its associated complications. Prognosis is good with non-renal anomalies if adequately treated.

DEFINITION

Symptomatic bacteriuria: Presence of urine bacteria which is not a contaminant of urethral flora with concomitant pyuria. Broad clinical categories: upper UTI (acute pyelonephritis) and lower UTI (cystitis, urethritis).

Asymptomatic bacteriuria: Detection of incidental bacteriuria in an asymptomatic child.

AETIOLOGY

General: Proliferation of bacteria in the urinary tract, ascending infections 2° to bacteria in the periurethral flora and distal urethra. F > M as short urethra and closer proximity of perianal colonic organisms.

Neonates: 70% ascending infection, 30% are of haematogenous origin.

Infants, children, adolescents: Majority are ascending infections.

Organisms:

- *Gram-negative bacteria*: *Escherichia coli (90%)*, *Streptococcus faecalis* and *Klebsiella* species from the child's faecal flora
- *Proteus* (males; present under the prepuce)
- *Staphylococcus saprophyticus* (common in adolescent girls)
- *Pseudomonas* (usually in children with congenital urinary tract anomalies (see chapter) or acquired renal problems, e.g. stones)
- *Adenovirus* 11 and 12 in haemorrhagic cystitis.

Atypical UTI: Seriously ill child, poor urine flow, abdominal/bladder mass, ↑d creatinine, septicaemia, failure to respond to treatment <48°, non-*E. coli* infections.

Recurrent UTIs: 2 + acute pyelonephritis/upper UTIs, 1 upper with 1 + lower UTI episodes, 3 + lower UTI episodes.

ASSOCIATIONS/RELATED   Congenital GU malformations and urinary obstruction (posterior urethral valves, PUJ obstruction). Vesicoureteric reflux. Chronic constipation. Voiding dysfunction. Neuropathic bladder.

EPIDEMIOLOGY

General: F > M (F 3–8%, M 0.5–1%).

Specific: ↑d upper UTIs <1 year (M > F), ↑d lower UTI >2 years (F > M).

HISTORY AND EXAMINATION

NICE Guidelines

Upper UTI: Bacteriuria and pyrexia >38° or loin pain with pyrexia <38°.

Lower UTI: Bacteriuria with no systemic symptoms.

		Common	→	**Least common**
Infants <3/12		Pyrexia	Poor feeding	Abdominal pain
		Vomiting	Failure to thrive	Jaundice
		Lethargy		Haematuria
		Irritability		Offensive urine
Infants/children >3/12	**Preverbal**	Pyrexia	Abdominal pain	Lethargy
			Loin tenderness	Irritability
			Vomiting	Haematuria
			Poor feeding	Offensive urine
				Failure to thrive
Infants/children >3/12	**Verbal**	Frequency	Dysfunctional voiding	Pyrexia
		Dysuria	Continence changes	Malaise
			Abdominal pain	Vomiting
			Loin tenderness	Haematuria
				Offensive urine
				Cloudy urine

PATHOPHYSIOLOGY

Acute pyelonephritis: Renal parenchymal infection with neutrophil infiltration 2° to ascending ureteric infection or haematogenous spread (bacteraemia).

Chronic pyelonephritis: Reflux nephropathy shows cortical scarring and clubbing of calyces.

INVESTIGATIONS

Urine collection: All infants and children presenting with an unexplained pyrexia >38° should have a urine sample tested <24 hours. 'Clean-catch' sample/urine collection pads/ suprapubic aspiration/mid-stream urine sample (MSU) dependent on age. Adhesive plastic bags/cotton wool balls may be contaminated with faecal +/− genital flora and are therefore not used.

Urine dipstick: May be diagnostic; Leucocyte esterase + ve/nitrite + ve (UTI). Leucocyte esterase −ve/nitrite + ve (suspected – treat as UTI). Leucocyte esterase + ve/nitrite −ve (suspected – await MC&S unless clinically apparent). Leucocyte esterase −ve/nitrite −ve (no UTI).

Urine MC&S: Pyuria + ve/bacteriuria + ve (UTI). Pyuria + ve/bacteriuria −ve and pyuria −ve/ bacteriuria + ve (suspected – treat as UTI). Pyuria −ve/bacteriuria −ve (no UTI).

Bloods: Possible ↑WCC, ↑CRP, U&Es.

Radiological investigation:

- *<6/12*: atypical/recurrent UTIs should have immediate USS and follow-up DMSA (4–6/12) and MCUG. Follow-up USS only, within 6/52, if response to therapy is <48°
- *6/12–3 years*: atypical UTIs should have immediate USS and follow-up DMSA. Recurrent UTIs have USS within 6/52 and DMSA at 4–6/12
- *>3 years*: atypical UTIs should have immediate USS. Recurrent UTIs have USS within 6/52 and DMSA at 4–6/12. MCUG not indicated and no investigations if responds <48°.

USS: Quick, non-invasive and no radiation. Identifies structural anomalies, scars or hydro-nephrosis, low sensitivity for detecting VUR.

Radio-isotope scanning (DMSA): IV radio-labelled DMSA taken up and binds to the cortical tubular cells, allows visualisation of the renal parenchyma, independent of activity in the pelvicalyceal system. Distinguishes areas of acute inflammation from normal renal parenchyma and degree of renal involvement.

MCUG: Bladder filled with contrast via urethral catheter. Voiding XRs. Significant radiation but is very sensitive/specific for detecting VUR. Performed once the urine is sterile so as not to precipitate septicaemia. May be an unpleasant and traumatic investigation. 3/7 prophylactic antibiotics with procedure.

MAG 3 indirect cystogram: IV MAG3 which has renal excretion. Once all the tracer is visualised in the bladder on screening, the child voids detecting VUR.

MANAGEMENT   Prompt treatment is important as risk of irreversible renal damage is high, especially in infants.

Treatment: PO cephalosporin or co-amoxiclav. In infants and severely ill children IV cefotaxime or gentamicin may be required. Ensure good oral intake.

Prevention: Regular and complete voiding, good hygiene, avoidance of constipation and long-term low-dose antibiotic prophylaxis (trimethoprim) for children with recurrent UTIs, reflux, scarring and whilst awaiting investigations.

COMPLICATIONS   Chronic pyelonephritis, chronic renal failure (CRF) and hypertension (3%). VUR accounts for CRF in 20% of children and 5–10% in adults.

PROGNOSIS   Infants who present with first symptomatic UTI aged <1 year are significantly more at risk of having recurrence (30% risk). Preschool presentation of a UTI has a recurrence of 12%.

DEFINITION Contagious infectious disease caused by the DNA herpes virus varicella zoster.

AETIOLOGY
Antenatal: Varicella embryopathy (VE) is caused by transplacental transmission during maternal infection in 2.2% of fetuses if <20 weeks' gestation.
Perinatal: Varicella of the newborn (VON); severity depends on the time of maternal infection:

- *21–5 days before delivery*: VON appears in first 4 days and there is a good prognosis
- *5 days before delivery or 2 days after delivery*: VON presents day 6–26; may be mild or severe (30% mortality).

Postnatal: Transmission via the respiratory route; preterm infants are at higher risk due to lack of placental varicella IgG transfer in the third trimester.
Childhood: Virus enters the respiratory tract and undergoes replication in the regional lymph nodes. At 4–6 days a 1° viraemia spreads the virus to the reticuloendothelial cells primarily in the spleen and liver. At 11–24 days there is a 2° viraemia to the viscera and skin, which elicits typical skin lesions.

ASSOCIATIONS/RELATED Maternal, family contact and school contact with infected individuals.

EPIDEMIOLOGY 15% of pregnant women are susceptible to varicella infection. Incidence of varicella during pregnancy is 3/1000 in the UK. Household transmission rates are 80–90%.

HISTORY AND EXAMINATION
VE manifestations:

1. *CNS*: microcephaly, paralysis, developmental delay, seizures
2. *Ocular*: cataracts, chorioretinitis, microphthalmia, nystagmus
3. *Musculoskeletal* : cicatricial dermatomal skin lesions and scarring, unilateral atrophy of a limb with scarring and paresis, rudimentary digits.

VON manifestations:

1. *Prodrome*: poor feeding, mild pyrexia and malaise
2. *Rash*: morbilliform rash in the prodrome develops into a generalised pruritic vesicular rash.

Childhood manifestations:

1. *Prodrome*: mild pyrexia precedes skin manifestation by 1–2 days
2. *Rash*: appears in crops at different stages (papule, vesicle, pustule and crust). Varicella's hallmark is the simultaneous presence of different stages of skin lesions and intense pruritus
3. *Systemic*: abdominal pain, headache, malaise, anorexia, cough, coryza, sore throat.

PATHOPHYSIOLOGY See Aetiology.

INVESTIGATIONS Varicella infection is usually a clinical diagnosis.
Specific tests: Serology (varicella-specific IgM) in fetal blood, detection of varicella antigens by ELISA, virology from vesicular fluid.

MANAGEMENT
Conservative: Cool compresses, calamine lotion, regular bathing to manage pruritus, discourage scratching to prevent scarring (mittens may be necessary).
Medical: Sedating antihistamines for pruritus, aciclovir is indicated for moderate to severe disease.

VZ Ig indicated in:

1. Infants born to mothers with infection 5 days before delivery or 2 days after
2. At-risk infants (<28 weeks or <1000 g)
3. Exposed seronegative pregnant women.

Prevention: Routine VZ immunisation is available in some countries (USA, Canada, Germany, Australia, Uruguay).

COMPLICATIONS   In childhood varicella 1/50 cases are associated with complications.
Neurological: Meningoencephailitis, encephalitis, acute cerebellar ataxia, Reye syndrome.
Skin: Impetigo (most common complication), scarring, necrotising fasciitis.
Other: Pneumonia, GN, myocarditis, pancreatitis, HSP.

PROGNOSIS   In otherwise healthy children aged 1–14 years, mortality rate is 2/100,000 cases. Patients with previous VE have a higher incidence of VZ in the first 10 years of life.

DEFINITION   Insertion of a central venous catheter (CVC) as a method of accessing a vein.

AETIOLOGY   Various types of devices used. Ideally placed at the superior vena cava and right atrial junction for the administration of parenteral nutrition.

Indications: TPN, medications (chemotherapy/antibiotics), repeated phlebotomy, failure of peripheral cannula insertion (by senior clinician), repeated transfusions.

Long line: Single-lumen line inserted into a peripheral vein and advanced to the SVC/RA junction. Used in neonates and infants. Neonatal scalp veins are often used.

PICC: Peripherally inserted central catheter; depending on the age of the patient, may be single/double lumen. Used for access for a short period of time (antibiotic treatment for osteomyelitis/intra-abdominal abscess).

Non-tunnelled CVC: Inserted into the internal jugular/subclavian/femoral veins. Surgeon/anaesthetist insertion. Double/triple lumen.

Tunnelled CVC (Hickman and Broviac): Surgically inserted into right/left internal jugular vein via open or percutaneous techniques. Cuff causes fibrosis and hence partially secures line, tunnelled under the skin prior to vein insertion. Indicated when access required for >6/52 (neonates/other children).

Portacaths: Surgically inserted, tunnelled as above but completely enclosed within the subcutaneous tissue. Disc-shaped port distally enabling phlebotomy and medication administration via hub needle. Used with older children with haematological/oncological diagnosis.

ASSOCIATIONS/RELATED   Prematurity, haematological/oncological diseases, PICU admissions.

EPIDEMIOLOGY   Very common procedure (in paediatric surgical unit). Catheter-related bloodstream infections (CRBSIs) occur in 5–40% of patients with CVCs.

HISTORY AND EXAMINATION   As above.

PATHOPHYSIOLOGY   Most common organisms causing CRBSIs are *Staphylococcus aureus*, coagulase-negative staphylococci (CONS), *Candida* spp (esp. *albicans*), *Pseudomonas aeruginosa* (very difficult to treat).

INVESTIGATIONS

Radiology: Correct position screening (image intensifier in theatre) and with possible displacement.

USS: Vein patency with run-off for repeated CVC placement.

MANAGEMENT

General: Sterile CVC access, minimal access, good dressing care, constant monitoring (prevent accidental displacement/site infection). Suture placement for securing. Non-tunnelled CVC/PICC should be only used for 7–10/7 (infection risk): femoral > internal jugular for CRBSIs incidence.

Line sepsis suspected: Stop TPN, blood cultures (peripheral/each CVC lumen), commence broad-spectrum antibiotics.

Line sepsis confirmed: Organism-targeted antibiotics, nil TPN, if repeated positive blood cultures or sepsis may require CVC removal.

Removal: Non-tunnelled removed on the ward. Portacaths need GA. Tunnelled CVC depends on time *in situ* and therefore degree of fibrosis around the cuff; usually requires GA with blunt dissection of the cuff. All types of CVC should have pressure applied to the vein >2 min on removal.

Antibiotic line locks: Gentamicin, tigecycline and daptomycin in combination with anti-coagulants as lock solutions can be used to prevent CRBSIs.

COMPLICATIONS

CVC insertion: Pneumothorax, haemothorax, haemorrhage.

CVC: Entry site cellulitis, line sepsis, CRBSIs, thrombosis or embolisation, CVC line break (may be repaired depending on position), extravasation of infused material, endocarditis/cardiac effusion.

PROGNOSIS   Dependent on underlying disease, CRBSIs can be serious but are normally resolved on CVC removal.

DEFINITION   Acyanotic congenital heart condition comprising a defect in the interventricular septum leading to an abnormal communication between the ventricular cavities.

AETIOLOGY   Can occur as 1° anomaly or be associated with other congenital heart defects (e.g. tetralogy of Fallot, TGA). Classified according to position of defect.

- *Perimembranous (infracristal)*: most common (80%), present in the LV outflow tract inferior to the aortic valve. Subclassification: perimembranous inlet/outlet/muscular.
- *Muscular (trabecular)*: common (≤20%) Present within the muscular septum, often multiple. Subclassification: central/mid-muscular/apical/marginal.
- *Supracristal*: less common (5–8%), present inferior to the pulmonary valve.

ASSOCIATIONS/RELATED   Trisomy 21, 18 and 13, maternal diabetes, phenylketonuria, alcohol intake. FHx.

EPIDEMIOLOGY   4/1000 (term) and 5–7/1000 (premature). Most common cardiac defect (30%). 95% isolated anomaly. F > M, 1.5 : 1.

HISTORY   Asymptomatic or symptomatic (size dependent). Small defects often diagnosed incidentally. Large defects include fatigue and sweating with feeds, recurrent respiratory infections (pulmonary congestion), symptoms of congestive heart failure: dyspnoea, palpitations (older children), failure to thrive. Symptoms occur earlier with premature neonates.

EXAMINATION
Small defect: Blood flowing through VSD results in a loud harsh blowing (high-pitched) pansystolic murmur, and may be associated with a parasternal thrill.
Large defect: Parasternal heave 2° to RVH, systolic murmur is considerably softer. Additional diastolic murmur may be heard due to ↑d flow through the mitral valve.

PATHOPHYSIOLOGY   Single ventricular chamber is divided into two at 4–8/40. 2° to failure of fusion of the membranous portion of the ventricular septum, the endocardial cushions and the bulbus cordis.

INVESTIGATIONS
CXR: Cardiomegaly with prominence of ventricles and PA with ↑d pulmonary vasculature.
ECG: Left and right ventricular hypertrophy.
Doppler + Echo: Diagnostic, size of defect assessment and of congestive heart failure.

MANAGEMENT
Medical: Antibiotic procedural prophylaxis, medical treatment of associated congestive heart failure.
Surgical indication: Uncontrolled CHF, large asymptomatic defects with elevated pulmonary arterial pressures, older asymptomatic defects with pulmonary: systemic flow >2 : 1, prolapse of an aortic valve cusp.
Surgical technique: Transatrial approach (perimembranous/inlet), pulmonary valve approach (outlet), left ventriculotomy with patch repair or initial pulmonary banding (multiple muscular). Minimally invasive transcatheter therapy also available in some centres (asymmetric, self-expandable, double-disc device).

COMPLICATIONS   Infective endocarditis, congestive heart failure, pulmonary hypertension leading to Eisenmenger syndrome (L → R shunt = ↑d pulmonary vasculature flow causing PHT which reverses the shunt and leads to cardiac failure).

PROGNOSIS   Spontaneous closure can occur (<2 years). Uncommon >4 years. Spontaneous closure: muscular (80%), perimembranous (40%).

Visual impairment

DEFINITION   Decreased visual acuity: <6/18 Snellen chart. Blindness: <3/60 Snellen chart.

AETIOLOGY
Developed countries: 50% genetic.
Developing countries: Mainly acquired causes.

ASSOCIATIONS/RELATED   Family history.

EPIDEMIOLOGY   10–20/10,000 UK children need special educational for visual impairment.

HISTORY   Lack of eye contact with parents, no responsive smiling by 6 weeks, impaired social bonding, visual inattention, random eye movements, squint, abnormal perceptual development, delays in mobility, other developmental delays.

EXAMINATION   May be normal if impairment is of cortical origin. However, children may lack fixation and visual tracking behaviour, or have persistent nystagmus, which is abnormal at any age. Squint and cataracts may be apparent immediately or using red reflex on ophthalmoscope.

INVESTIGATIONS   One must always assess visual acuity with a Snellen chart in children >5 years. Slit lamp exam, CT/MRI if indicated.

MANAGEMENT

- Maximise development of compensatory responses and available visual ability (e.g. correct any refractive errors).
- Advise parents on providing non-visual stimulation.
- Ensuring safe environment for child.
- Special schooling may be required for severely visually impaired children with teaching through Braille.

Strabismus (squint)

DEFINITION   Abnormal alignment of both eyes. As a result, the eyes look in different directions and do not focus simultaneously on a single point. Most commonly horizontal (convergent or divergent), but may be vertical (hypertropia – upward-looking or hypotropia – downward-looking).

AETIOLOGY   Failure to develop binocular vision.
Non-paralytic: More common and due to refractive error in one/both eyes.
Paralytic: Rare and due to paralysis of motor nerves. When onset is rapid, may be due to underlying space-occupying lesion such as a brain tumour.

ASSOCIATIONS/RELATED   Family history.

EPIDEMIOLOGY   4/100 children.

HISTORY   Neonates often give the appearance of having a squint because of overconvergence, but almost all correct in infancy. Strabismus is a persistent squint after 2–3 months of age (may be intermittent).

EXAMINATION
Corneal light reflection test: Reflection of the light simultaneously off both corneas does not appear in the same place.
Cover test: Squinting eye moves to take up fixation when normal eye is covered.
Fundoscopy and neurological examination.

INVESTIGATIONS
CT/MRI brain: If rapid onset, paralytic squint.

MANAGEMENT   Refer all children with squints after 2–3 months to orthoptist and ophthalmologist.
Principles of treatment: Develop best possible vision for each eye.

- Correct any underlying defect, e.g. cataract.
- Correct refractive error with glasses.
- Treat amblyopia with patch occlusion therapy if it occurs.

Non-paralytic strabismus can be controlled by glasses that correct for overconvergence (long-sightedness). Congenital paralytic squints require surgery as soon as possible to enable the development of good visual function.

COMPLICATIONS
Amblyopia: Interference in visual input to eye during critical period (birth to 6 years) → atrophy of retinocortical pathways, resulting in loss of visual acuity. If only one eye sees clearly, it inhibits the eye with a blur; therefore amblyopia is a neurologically active process.

PROGNOSIS   With early diagnosis and treatment, the defect can usually be corrected.

Cataracts

DEFINITION   Opacification of lens present at birth.

AETIOLOGY
Familial: Usually autosomal dominant.
Congenital infection: Rubella, CMV, toxoplasmosis, herpes simplex.
Drugs: Corticosteroids.
Metabolic: Hypocalcaemia, galactosaemia, DM.
Chromosomal: Down syndrome, Turner syndrome, trisomy 13, trisomy 18.
Idiopathic: One-third are sporadic (not associated with other disease).

EPIDEMIOLOGY   1/250 live births.

HISTORY   Congenital cataracts are present at birth but may not be identified until later in life. Some cataracts are static, but some are progressive. This explains why not all congenital cataracts are identified at birth.

EXAMINATION   Loss of red reflex, white reflex in the pupil (cataract, retinoblastoma or ROP), photophobia.

PATHOPHYSIOLOGY   Insults to developing lens fibres result in opacity.

INVESTIGATIONS   Slit lamp examination. Investigate to exclude associated conditions if suspected.

MANAGEMENT   Surgical removal of cataract, ideally before 2 months.

COMPLICATIONS   Amblyopia (if surgery is delayed), strabismus, glaucoma (post-surgery).

PROGNOSIS   Irreversibly impaired vision if untreated.

DEFINITION
'Vitamin D' encompasses ergocalciferol (vitamin D2), cholecalciferol (vitamin D3), alfacalcidol (1α-hydroxycholecalciferol) and the active form, calcitriol (1,25-dihydroxy-cholecalciferol). Vitamin D deficiency can be classified as follows.

- *Mild*: 25–50 nmol/l (10–20 ng/ml)
- *Moderate*: 12.5–25.0 nmol/l (5–10 ng/ml)
- *Severe*: <12.5 nmol/l (<5 ng/ml)

AETIOLOGY
↓ **Vitamin D intake:**

1. *Inadequate sunlight exposure* (approximately 90% of vitamin D is obtained from ultraviolet sunlight) particularly in darker skinned or modestly covered individuals
2. *Nutritional*: prolonged exclusive breastfeeding (especially if mother is vitamin D deficient), prematurity, unsupervised exclusion diet (e.g. in food allergy)
3. *Malabsorption (rare)*: coeliac disease, cystic fibrosis.

Metabolism of vitamin D:

1. Severe renal or liver disease
2. Anticonvulsant therapy (phenytoin).

ASSOCIATIONS/RELATED   Vitamin D deficiency is a risk factor for diabetes, ischaemic heart disease, tuberculosis and certain malignancies (prostate/colorectal).

EPIDEMIOLOGY   Vitamin D deficiency and rickets is increasing in the UK and is an important public health concern. Asian, Afro-Caribbean and Middle Eastern groups are particularly at risk. 85% of Asians compared to 3.3% of non-Asians had vitamin D levels <8 ng/ml (Birmingham, UK).

HISTORY AND EXAMINATION
Infant presentation: Irritability, generalised seizures 2° to hypocalcaemia.
Early childhood: Poor growth, delayed dentition, slow motor development.
Classic rickets: Bowed legs, knock-knees, thickened wrists and ankles, rachitic rosary (enlargement of the costochondral junctions), frontal bossing, pathological fractures.
Adolescent presentation: Carpopedal spasm 2° to hypocalcaemia and classic rickets.

PATHOPHYSIOLOGY   Without vitamin D, only 10–15% of dietary calcium and about 60% of phosphorus is absorbed. Low serum calcium triggers secretion of PTH to release calcium and phosphorus from bone and results in ↓ bone mineralisation.

INVESTIGATIONS
↓ **Vitamin D intake:** ↓/N calcium, ↑/↓ phosphate, ↑/N PTH, ↑ALP, ↓ vitamin D.
Radiology: Wrist X-ray; cupping and fraying of metaphysial surfaces and widened epiphyseal plate in rickets.

MANAGEMENT
Prevention: In the UK all infants should receive vitamin D daily ((280–340 IU, multivitamin or fortified infant formula) and pregnant/lactating mothers should receive 400 IU daily.
Dietary vitamin D sources: Fatty fish (herring, mackerel, sardines, tuna, salmon), egg yolk, fortified foods (infant formula, shop-bought milk, breakfast cereal, margarine).
Supplementation for vitamin D deficiency: Ergocalciferol (vitamin D2) or cholecalciferol (vitamin D3) is indicated in nutritional vitamin D deficiency. Alfacalcidol should only be used if there is severe liver or renal disease. Oral calcium supplements are usually required initially if the child is hypocalcaemic and/or dietary intake is poor. Serial bloods should be measured. Treatment usually lasts 2–4 months.

COMPLICATIONS   Rickets. Low maternal vitamin D may adversely affect the developing fetal brain and has been shown to affect postnatal head and linear growth.

PROGNOSIS   Bony abnormalities may take up to 2 years to resolve after treatment has been administered.

DEFINITION A respiratory tract infection characterised by paroxysms of coughing followed by a 'whoop' (sudden massive inspiratory effort against a narrowed glottis).

AETIOLOGY Caused by the bacterium *Bordetella pertussis*; has an incubation period of 7–10 (up to 21) days, and is communicable for 3 weeks from the start of coughing via droplet spread.

ASSOCIATIONS/RELATED Preterm infants, patients with underlying cardiac, pulmonary, neuromuscular or neurological disease are at high risk for complications of pertussis (e.g. pneumonia, seizures, encephalopathy and death).

EPIDEMIOLOGY
Incidence England and Wales: 594/year (2005). Immunisation has decreased the risk of developing whooping cough by 80–90%. Previously, epidemics occurred in the UK every 4 years.
Peak age: 3 years. In infants <6 months, it has a much higher mortality.

HISTORY AND EXAMINATION Pertussis has three stages.

1. *Catarrhal stage*: duration 1–2 weeks; indistinguishable from common URTIs with nasal congestion, rhinorrhoea, sneezing, low-grade fever and the occasional cough. At this stage pertussis is most infectious.
2. *Paroxysmal stage*: duration 1–6 weeks; consists of paroxysms of coughing, followed in the older child by a 'whoop', with associated vomiting, dyspnoea and possibly seizures. Infants <6 months do not have the characteristic whoop but may have apnoeic episodes.
3. *Convalescent stage*: duration weeks to months; chronic cough that becomes less paroxysmal.

Older children and adolescents: May not exhibit distinct stages. Symptoms in these patients include uninterrupted coughing, feelings of suffocation or strangulation, and headaches.

PATHOPHYSIOLOGY See Aetiology.

INVESTIGATIONS
Bloods: ↑WCC, absolute lymphocytosis is common, ↑CRP, U&E.
Immunocytochemistry: Direct fluorescent antibody testing of pernasal swabs.

MANAGEMENT
Immunisation is key.
Prophylaxis: Erythromycin may be used in the catarrhal phase to decrease contagiousness of an individual or prophylactically to siblings/close contacts of a case of pertussis, especially if <1 year of age and not fully immunised.
Respiratory isolation: 5 days after starting antibiotics or until 3 weeks after the onset of the coughing spasms if the person is not receiving antibiotic treatment.
Criteria for admission:

1. Age <6 months due to ↑ mortality in this age group
2. Vomiting with dehydration or weight loss
3. Respiratory distress +/− cyanosis
4. Apnoea associated with paroxysms.

Notification: Whooping cough is a notifiable disease (CCDC).

COMPLICATIONS
Paroxysmal cough: May cause petechiae and conjunctival haemorrhages. Lack of intake may cause dehydration and weight loss.

Seizures (3%): If encephalopathy follows, one-third die, one-third remain neurologically impaired, one-third recover fully.

2° infections: Otitis media, bronchiectasis, pneumonia (main cause of pertussis-related deaths).

PROGNOSIS   Usually lasts 6–8 weeks; however, a prolonged illness may occur ('100-day cough'). There is significant morbidity and mortality in infants <6 months in whom apnoea associated with paroxysms may cause sudden death.

Taking a History in Paediatrics

WHAT IS THE DIFFERENCE BETWEEN ADULT AND PAEDIATRIC CONSULTATIONS?

1. History is often given mainly by third party and may be modified by parental perception or interpretation.
2. Extra components to history: pregnancy and birth, feeding history in infancy, immunisations, growth, developmental milestones, behaviour and schooling.
3. History and examination are modified according to the child's age and development.

IMPORTANT POINTS TO NOTE BEFORE TAKING A HISTORY

1. Check that you know the child's name, age and gender.
2. Is there a need for an interpreter?
3. Introduce yourself; explain who you are and your role in the child's care.
4. Remember to address questions to the child if appropriate.
5. Establish a good rapport and use the empathic approach with the child and family.
6. Make toys available. Observe how the child interacts with parents and siblings.

PRESENTING COMPLAINT

1. It is important to find out what prompted referral to a doctor.
2. What do the parents think or fear may be wrong?
3. Use open questions such as 'What is worrying you about Tom?'.
4. Let the parent tell the story of the presenting problem without interruptions.
5. Was the child completely well beforehand? Has there been any foreign travel/sick contacts? Have there been any similar episodes in the past?
6. How has the illness affected the family? Has it prevented the child from attending nursery/school?
7. Avoid using medical terminology. Use the child's and parents' own words, and clarify the meaning of terms used, e.g. wheeze.

GENERAL ENQUIRY

1. Is the child active and lively as usual? Any recent change in behaviour or personality?
2. Does the child have the same appetite as usual: eating and drinking usual amounts? Changes in feeding cycle (infants)?
3. Normal bowel movements/wet nappies or passing urine?
4. Is the child growing/gaining weight at a normal rate?
5. Any fevers, rashes, lumps, pruritus?

SYSTEMS REVIEW IF INDICATED

1. **Cardiovascular:** Cyanosis, exercise tolerance, bleeding disorders.
2. **Respiratory:** Grunting, wheeze, cough (nocturnal/chronic), sputum production.
3. **GI:** Jaundice (duration/onset), diarrhoea, vomiting, stool frequency, abdominal pain.
4. **GU:** How often is the nappy wet? Haematuria, dysuria (older child), sexual development.
5. **Neuromuscular:** Feeding ability, abnormal movements, seizures, headaches, hearing/vision ability.
6. **ENT:** Noisy breathing, ear discharge, sore throat, teething.

PAST MEDICAL HISTORY

1. *In utero:* How was the pregnancy? Any maternal problems? Use of medication, alcohol intake, smoking in pregnancy. Rh disease, maternal rubella, other viral infections *in utero*.
2. **At birth:** Gestation at birth, type of delivery, use of forceps/caesarean, birthweight, condition of infant at birth (APGAR scores), need for medical intervention, admission to SCBU, ventilation.

Taking a History in Paediatrics (continued)

3. **As a neonate:** Jaundice, fits, fevers, feeding problems, weight gain.
4. **Childhood:** Operations, illnesses, hospital admission, accidents, injuries.

IMMUNISATIONS   Take time to go through what has been administered and compare this to the recommended schedule.

GROWTH AND DEVELOPMENT

1. Plot growth measurements on appropriate length/height, weight and head circumference charts.
2. Find out usual daily pattern of food intake (breastfeeding/types of formula feed, intake pattern later).
3. **Infants and toddlers:** Use 'screening' questions that determine developmental progress at hallmark ages for each of the four major areas of development: gross motor control; fine motor and vision; speech, language and hearing; social behaviour and play.
4. **Older children:** Progress in nursery/school, and parent assessment in comparison with siblings/peers.

DRUG HISTORY

1. Past and present medications plus OTC medication and alternative therapies.
2. Drug intolerances, adverse reactions, true allergies.
3. In older children, the use of recreational drugs or solvent use.

FAMILY HISTORY

1. Draw a family tree over three generations, age of parent and siblings, medical problems in the family.
2. Is there a history of consanguinity?
3. Positive family history for atopy, DM, HT, seizures, jaundice, renal disease, TB, congenital malformations, previous miscarriages or stillbirths.

EDUCATIONAL/EMOTIONAL HISTORY

1. Child's experience and attainments at school. Bullying?
2. Specific questions on mood, eating and sleeping habits, interests, hobbies and other activities.

SOCIAL HISTORY

1. Do not make assumptions about the family unit; who is there or 'involved'.
2. Who lives in the household and who provides most of the child's care?
3. Does the child live in more than one household? Marital separation/stresses?
4. Parental occupation? Economic status? Do they receive financial allowances? Housing?
5. Factors that might adversely affect child's health, e.g. household members smoking?
6. Is there childcare if the parents work?
7. Check whether child has a Child Protection Plan.

CLOSING QUESTIONS

1. Is there anything else that is worrying you?
2. Is there anything else I should know or anything I have forgotten to ask you?

Neonatal Resuscitation

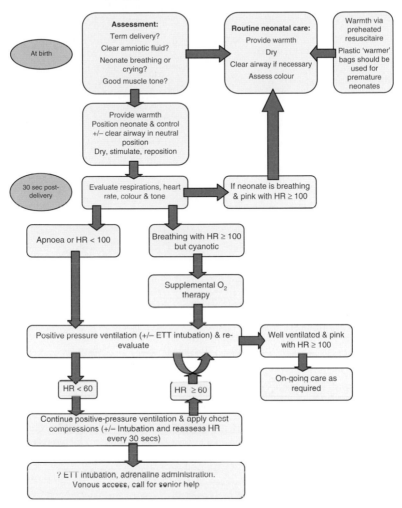

Formal Assessment of the Neonate at Birth

All neonates are graded with an APGAR score at birth. This is a scoring system (out of 10) based on:

A: Activity
P: Pulse
G: Grimacing/reflex irritability on suctioning
A: Appearance
R: Respiratory effort of the baby:

- **7–10** is considered normal
- **4–7** might require some resuscitative measures
- **<3** requires immediate resuscitation

Sign		0 points	1 point	2 points
A	Activity	No movement	Arms and legs flexed	Active movement
P	Pulse	Absent	<100 bpm	>100 bpm
G	Grimacing/reflex irritability	No response	Grimace	Pulls away
A	Appearance	Blue/pale all over	Extremities pale	Normal colour
R	Respiratory effort	Absent	Slow/irregular gasps	Normal rate/effort

APGAR scores are not useful specific predictors of neurodevelopmental outcome except when extremely and persistently low, or when accompanied by deep acidaemia. Even with APGARs as low as 3 at 10 min, 80% of infants of normal birthweight are free of major disability by early school age (National Institute of Health, National Collaborative Perinatal Project).

Fetal scalp/umbilical cord blood:

May be required to identify metabolic acidosis and the necessity for emergency caesarean section (pH <7.25).

APGARs are better predictors than cord pH as some babies are delivered screaming with a pH of 6.9 with nil deficits, whereas the baby who is floppy and unresponsive at 10 min with a normal pH is much more at risk.

Examination of the Newborn

GENERAL

Measurements: Weight, length and head circumference should be recorded on a centile chart.

General observation: Undress infant for the examination.

General neurological state: Can be observed whilst undressing the infant; neuromuscular tone, degree of activity, irritability, lethargy.

Primitive newborn reflexes: Moro (startle) reflex and grasp reflex.

Colour: Jaundice, pallor, plethora, cyanosis.

Dysmorphic features: Pattern recognition for various syndromes.

Limitation of movement: May indicate deep tissue injury, e.g. fractured clavicle or humerus during labour.

SKIN

Vernix: White substance that protects the fetus from overhydration.

Lanugo: Fine downy hair covering the skin of the shoulders, upper arms and thighs.

Petechiae: Small haemorrhagic skin lesions; may be benign on the face but if on the trunk may indicate thrombocytopenia.

Milia: Small sebaceous cysts that occur particularly over the nose.

Vesicles: Uncommon but may be the first signs of infection (e.g. HSV).

Erythema toxicum: Vesiculomacular rash with an erythematous base that is often widespread; the vesicles contain eosinophils.

Pustules: May appear at birth in congenital candidal infection or may appear later with *Staphylococcus aureus* infection.

Birthmarks:

- *Naevus flammeus*: stork bites.
- *Mongolian spots*: pigmented naevus often large and on the lower back.
- *Port-wine stain*: deep vascular naevus may be found in the distribution of a division of the trigeminal nerve (associated Sturge–Weber syndrome).
- *Strawberry naevus*: raised naevus that becomes larger then regresses spontaneously by 3 years.
- *Pigmented naevus*: familial and often large and hairy.

HANDS

Polydactyly: Excessive number of digits/tags.

Lymphoedema: Hands or feet suggestive of Turner syndrome.

Simian creases: Present unilaterally in 5% of the population; if present bilaterally may indicate presence of trisomy 21 (look for other associated features).

LIMBS

Achondroplasia: Short-limbed dwarfism is associated with a reduction in the length of the proximal segment of the limb relative to the distal segment.

Arthrogryposis: Restriction of joint movements; may suggest connective tissue defects.

HEAD

Microcephalus: Head circumference <3rd percentile; associated with trisomy 21, intrauterine infection, symmetrical IUGR.

Macrocephalus: Head circumference >97th percentile; associated with ↑ICP 2° to hydrocephalus, but may be benign 2° to tall stature.

Bradycephalus: Squareness of the head when viewed from above; may indicate trisomy 21.

Plagiocephalus: Elongation of the head; may indicate premature fusion of one of the skull sutures.

Fontanelle: Anterior and posterior, should be palpated for tension and size.

Haematomas: two different types can occur; cephalhaematoma that occurs beneath the periosteum and tissue haematomas that occur spontaneously or as a result of instrumental delivery.

Examination of the Newborn (continued)

Encephalocoele: Caused by the failure of closure of the neural tube and may be present in the midline of the head. Another neural tube defect is spina bifida that results in a lower spine lesion.

FACE

Ears: Size, form and position; patency of the external auditory meatus. Look for pre- or postauricular skin tags.

Eyes: The red reflex should be sought (bright red view though the retina is normal), the pupil is white with congenital cataracts or retinoblastomas.

MOUTH

Cleft lip/palate: Unilateral or bilateral. Elicit by palpation and visualisation of the hard and soft palates.

TONGUE

Macroglossia: Beckwith–Wiedemann syndrome (hypertrophy of limbs and neonatal hypoglycaemia). Trisomy 21, congenital hypothyroidism, triploidy syndrome.

NOSE

Choanal atresia: Abnormal membrane covers the nasopharynx, which causes airways obstruction.

NECK

Lateral masses: May be a cystic hygroma or branchial cyst (soft fluctuant swellings that transluminate).

Midline masses: Most likely to be a goitre.

Lateral fistulas: Remnants of the branchial arch.

THORAX

Respiratory rate: >60/min is tachypnoea.

Signs of respiratory distress: Recession: intercostal/subcostal/sternal/substernal, use of the accessory muscles of respiration, expiratory grunting, nasal flaring.

Asymmetry of the hemithoraces: Pneumothorax or a congenital heart defect with cardiac enlargement.

Breast: Engorgement is common; widely spaced nipples may indicate Turner syndrome.

CARDIOVASCULAR

Pulse rate: Normally 100–160 bpm felt in the antecubital fossa.

Femoral pulses: Weak femoral pulse (COA), strong femoral pulse (PDA).

Auscultation: Innocent flow murmurs (in 30%); usually soft blowing systolic murmur localised to left sternal edge with no radiation and normal heart sounds in an asymptomatic patient. See chapters on congenital cardiac anomalies for details on various pathological murmurs.

ABDOMEN

Shape: Distension may indicate intestinal obstruction; 'scaphoid' (concave) is indicative of a diaphragmatic hernia.

Hepatomegaly: Normal liver may be palpated up to 4 cm below the costal margin. Hepatomegaly may occur in infections (EBV/CMV), malignancy, inborn errors of metabolism or haemolytic anaemia (e.g. sickle cell).

Splenomegaly: Intrauterine infection or underlying haematological condition.

Umbilical cord: Should be clean and contain three vessels.

Hernial orifices: Visual inspection or palpation.

GENITALIA

Females: Prominent labia minora are normal, a mucoid vaginal discharge is common in the first few weeks, and an imperforate hymen may also be present. The site of the anus should be visualised to exclude imperforate anus.

Males: Urethral meatus should be visualised at the tip of the penis, not the underside (hypospadias); physiological phimosis may prevent this. Palpate testes in the scrotum.

HIPS

DDH: Barlow/Ortolani test. Abduction may be limited and a displaced hip relocates with an audible 'clunk'. 'Clicky' hips are usually normal; reflecting cartilaginous/ligamentous involvement.

FEET

Positional talipes: Feet often remain in the *in utero* position but can be dorsiflexed to touch the front of the lower leg (requires physiotherapy input).

Talipes equinovarus (clubfoot): Entire foot is inverted and supinated and the forefoot is adducted. This position is fixed and needs to be corrected surgically.

Toes: May be supernumerary or absent.

Breastfeeding Versus Bottlefeeding

Advantages of breastfeeding vs bottlefeeding	Disadvantages of breastfeeding vs bottlefeeding

Nutritional

(1) Protein, lipid, iron and other vitamins/minerals, e.g. vitamin D; right quantity and better bio-availability.

(2) Appropriate electrolyte content (e.g. sodium) important $2°$ to immaturity of renal concentrating system.

(3) Colostrum (first few days): protein and Ig, important for establishment of lactobacilli in the gut.

(4) Polyunsaturated fatty acids are beneficial in neuronal and retinal development.

(5) Ensures right concentration of nutrients; formula feeds may be too concentrated/dilute.

Humoral immunological transmission

(1) Secretory IgA contributes to mucosal immune barrier.

(2) Bifidus factor promotes growth of *Lactobacillus bifidus* that inhibits growth of GI pathogens.

(3) Lysozyme lyses bacterial cell walls.

(4) Lactoferrin binds iron necessary for replication of *Escherichia coli* and other bacteria.

(5) Interferon is an antiviral agent.

Cellular immunological transmission: macrophages, T and B lymphocytes, polymorphs.

Sterility of breast milk: reduced GI infections, especially in developing countries.

↓**Risk and severity of disease:** GORD, IBD, NEC, SIDS (not proven).

Total sensory experience (all 5 senses).

Bonding with mother.

Psychological: helps mother to establish an intimate, loving relationship with her baby.

Contraindications

(1) Maternal active untreated TB, brucellosis or recently acquired syphilis.

(2) HIV-positive mothers (UK guidelines); in developing countries HIV-positive mothers are still encouraged to breastfeed as the protection from life-threatening gastroenteritis outweighs risk of ↑ transmisson rate of HIV.

(3) Metabolic disorders in the baby, e.g. maple syrup urine disease.

(4) Maternal drugs: antithyroid (carbimazole), antimetabolic (methotrexate), chemotherapy, lithium and tetracycline.

Nutritional

Low in vitamin K; required to prevent haemorrhagic disease of the newborn.

Preventable negative aspects

(1) Prolonged exclusive breastfeeding to >6 months may result in poor weight gain.

(2) Maternal transmission of hepatitis B; mothers can breastfeed once the child is immunised.

(3) Potential transmission of maternal substance: smoking, alcohol, illicit drugs.

(4) Difficulty initialising breastfeeding and failure to fix can cause emotional upset for the mother.

(5) Local infection due to poor management: painful, cracked nipples, mastitis or breast abscesses.

Advantages of breastfeeding vs bottlefeeding	Disadvantages of breastfeeding vs bottlefeeding
Practicalities: (1) Breast milk is sterile and free. (2) Is at the correct temperature. (3) Avoids preparation needed for formula feed. **Reduction in postpartum haemorrhage:** oxytocin released contracts uterine vessels. **Reduction in disease:** (1) Premenopausal breast cancer. (2) Ovarian cancer. (3) Osteoporosis. **Faster return to pre-pregnant weight.** **Contraceptive, especially in developing countries.**	**Work environment:** there may be no convenient place to breastfeed.

Infant Feeding
There is no better nutrition for infants than breastfeeding.

1989 WHO/UNICEF TEN STEPS TO SUCCESSFUL BREASTFEEDING

1. Written breastfeeding policy that is routinely communicated to all healthcare professionals.
2. Train all healthcare staff in skills necessary to implement this policy.
3. Inform all pregnant mothers about the benefits and management of breastfeeding.
4. Help mothers initiate breastfeeding within 1/2 h of delivery.
5. Show mothers how to breastfeed, and how to maintain lactation even if separated from their infants.
6. Give newborn infants no food or drink other than breast milk unless medically indicated.
7. Practise 'rooming-in' (allow mothers and infants to remain together), 24 h a day.
8. Encourage unrestricted breastfeeding.
9. Give no artificial teats or pacifiers (dummies) to breastfeeding infants.
10. Foster the establishment of breastfeeding support groups and refer mothers to them on discharge from hospital or clinic.

LAPSE IN BREASTFEEDING 71% of mothers in the UK start breastfeeding (UK Infant Feeding 2000); however, this reduces to 52% at 2/52 and 39% at 6/52 postpartum. Reasons why mothers give up include:

1. Pain and discomfort from mastitis, breast abscess, cracked nipples, breast candida
2. Concerns that they are not producing enough milk and stressed by 'test' weighing
3. Returning to work, inadequate facilities for breastfeeding, and attitudes in the work environment.

MATERNAL SUPPORT Mothers need to be encouraged to continue breastfeeding by education about the benefits both mother and child will receive. They need to have access to appropriate support such as midwives and healthcare professionals, especially during the initial establishment of breastfeeding, and there needs to be better provision for breastfeeding in the work environment. Do not test weigh.

FORMULA FEEDS Alternative to breast milk where it is contraindicated or decided against, based on modified cow's milk. Unmodified cow's milk contains too much protein, sodium, potassium, calcium and phosphorus, inadequate iron, vitamins and essential fatty acids.
Properties of standard formula feed:

- *Protein*: contains cow's protein modified by addition of whey to modify whey:casein ratio
- *Fats*: from vegetable oils with saturated and unsaturated fatty acids in similar ratio to breast milk
- *Carbohydrates*: from lactose
- *Vitamins and minerals:* supplementation.

Principles of bottlefeeding:

- The infant's appetite should determine the volume and number of feeds, initially ($\approx$150 ml/kg/d)
- Use safe water, sterilised utensils and equipment
- Ensure correct preparation with accurate measurement of powder for formula reconstitution.

Cow's milk: Full-fat cow's milk can be introduced as the main milk source from 12 months of age. Prior to this it may cause microscopic GI blood loss. Reduced fat milk can be introduced after 5 years.
Soya milk formulas: Commonly and inappropriately used:

- *for suspected cow's milk protein allergy under 6 months.*

- *for lactose intolerance*: best to use lactose-modified formulas
- *to prevent allergies*: no evidence of protection with soya.

Risks: Soy formulas have a higher aluminium content and phytates that inhibit absorption of minerals, especially calcium. Phyto-oestrogen exposure (in the form of isoflavones) may exert tissue-specific effects and bind to oestrogen receptors.

Indications: Soy formula is indicated children with galactosaemia and in vegan families who will not use cow's milk.

WEANING

Between 4 and 6/12, infants have the muscle tone and maturity of the digestive system to begin eating solid foods; however, the WHO advises exclusive breastfeeding till 6/12. It also recommends breastfeeding alongside supplementation with solid food until the age of 2. The term 'weaning' can be misleading as it implies the cessation of breastfeeding.

First foods: Soft or puréed food such as iron-fortified cereal foods followed by fruits and vegetables. Previously parents have been advised to delay the introduction of allergenic foods such as wheat, egg, fish and nuts. This is no longer the case. These foods should be introduced from 6 months of age.

Paediatric Resuscitation

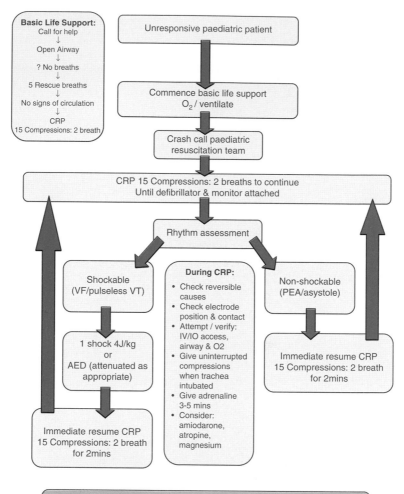

Basic Life Support:
Call for help
↓
Open Airway
↓
? No breaths
↓
5 Rescue breaths
↓
No signs of circulation
↓
CRP
15 Compressions: 2 breath

Unresponsive paediatric patient

Commence basic life support
O₂ / ventilate

Crash call paediatric
resuscitation team

CRP 15 Compressions: 2 breaths to continue
Until defibrillator & monitor attached

Rhythm assessment

Shockable
(VF/pulseless VT)

During CRP:
- Check reversible causes
- Check electrode position & contact
- Attempt / verify: IV/IO access, airway & O2
- Give uninterrupted compressions when trachea intubated
- Give adrenaline 3-5 mins
- Consider: amiodarone, atropine, magnesium

Non-shockable
(PEA/asystole)

1 shock 4J/kg
or
AED (attenuated as
appropriate)

Immediate resume CRP
15 Compressions: 2 breath
for 2mins

Immediate resume CRP
15 Compressions: 2 breath
for 2mins

Reversible causes (4Hs & 4Ts): Hypoxia; Hypovolaemia;
Hypo/hyperkalaemia/metabolic derangement; Hypothermia; Tension pneumothorax;
Tamponade, cardiac; Toxins, Thromboembolism.

Developmental Stages in Children

Developmental abilities and warning signs* at ages often used in assessment. Remember to correct for prematurity until 24 months

Normal ranges	Gross motor control	Fine motor and vision	Speech, language and hearing	Social behaviour and play
2–4 months	*Asymmetry/absence of primitive reflexes.* Moro, grasp, stepping atonic neck reflex. Lifts head briefly when sitting up.	*Persistent squint.* Stares intently Follows moving object or face by turning the head in 90° arc.	*No response to loud noises.* Stills to mother's voice. Startles to loud noise. Squeals with pleasure.	*Not smiling.* Smiles and coos responsively.
6–9 months	*Persistent primitive reflexes.* Lifts head up from prone with weight on hands, can roll over. Sits without support. Crawls, can pull to stand, can weight bear on legs when standing.	*Persistent hand preference at <6/12.* Palmar grasp (6/12). Index approach (9/12). Transfers from hand to hand/ mouth (7/12). Pincer grip (9/12). Fixes and can follow small objects.	*Reduced response.* *Absence of babble.* Responds to name. 'Ma, Da' at 6/12. Uses sounds indiscriminately. Understands 'No'. Turns to soft sounds out of sight.	*Absent or slow social responses.* Puts food in mouth. Chews biscuit. Plays peak-a-boo. Shows object to mother at 9/12. Pats mirror image. Interest in people. Awareness of strangers.
10–12 months	*Immature grasp/asymmetry of grasp.* *No sitting or weight bearing.* Reaches behind. Cruises round furniture. Walks alone but unsteadily with broad gait and hands apart.	*Holds objects close up to eyes.* Throws objects. Watches them fall. Picks up crumbs from carpet. Bangs bricks together.	*No frequent babble by 13/12.* Understands some words. Uses 'Mama, Dada' discriminately. Uses 2–3 other words. Shakes head for 'No'.	*Constant mouthing.* Comes when called. Lets go on request. Finds hidden objects. Waves bye-bye. Drinks from cup.

Developmental Stages in Children (continued)

Normal ranges	Gross motor control	Fine motor and vision	Speech, language and hearing	Social behaviour and play
13–18 months	*Not walking: consider muscular dystrophy.* Walks well, carries toys, climbs stairs, climbs into chair.	*Absent pincer grip.* Neat pincer grip: picks up threads, pins. Scribbles using fist. Builds tower of 3–4 × 1″ (2.5 cm) cubes. Turns 2 pages at a time.	*Drools. No words. Not understanding commands.* Points to parts of body on request. Obeys single commands. Echoes speech: 6 words, jargons.	*Not interacting appropriately.* Lifts cups, drinks and puts down safely, spoon-feeds self. Pulls at dirty nappy. Domestic mimicry, finger-feeding. Proto-declarative pointing, symbolic play.
2–2.5 years	*Unsteady on feet.* Runs, kicks ball, jumps on the spot, and walks down stairs 2 feet per tread.	*Parental concerns.* Turns 1 page at a time. Imitates a straight vertical and horizontal line and a circle. Unscrews lids. Builds tower of 6–8 × 1″ cubes.	*Lack of understanding of speech. No phrases by 2.5 years.* Phrases of 2–3 words, gives names, naming games, 50 + words.	*Parental concerns.* Plays alone. Tantrums, demanding. Dry by day. Puts on shoes and pants. Turns door-handles. Uses spoon and fork. Interested in other children.
3–3.5 years	*Clumsy (motor cause).* Stands on one leg for a few seconds. Peddles tricycle. Adult ascent of stairs. Jumps off bottom step.	*Clumsy (visual cause).* Mature pen grasp, copies + and O. Correctly matches 2 + colours. Tower of 9 × 1″ cubes.	*No phrases. Echolalia.* Gives full name, sex. Counts to 10 by rote. Uses plurals. Understands prepositions. 3 to 5-word sentences.	*Persistent daytime wetting/ soiling.* Uses toilet unassisted except wiping bottom. Dresses and undresses with minimum assistance. 'Why' questions. Nursery rhymes. Uses knife and fork. Plays with peers.

4–5 years

Any parental concerns.
4 years: climbs trees and ladders.
Enjoys ball games.
5 years: hops, skips, jumps 3 steps, catches a ball.

*Any parental concerns.**
Matches 4 colours.
5 years: copies cross, square, triangle.
4 years: 3 steps with 6 cubes.
5 years: 4 steps with 10 cubes
Draws a recognisable man.

*Unintelligible/ungram-
matical speech.**
*Unable to give name/
address.**
4 years: counts to 10.
5 years: counts to 20.
Transient stammer from urgency to speak is common.
Asks meaning of abstract words.

*Socially isolated/bullied.**
Wipes own bottom.
Eats using knife and fork.
Dresses unsupervised except for tie, laces.
Imaginative play.
Separates from mother.

Immunisation Schedule

The single most useful thing that doctors can do to improve child health...

(UK National Immunisation Programme 2000)

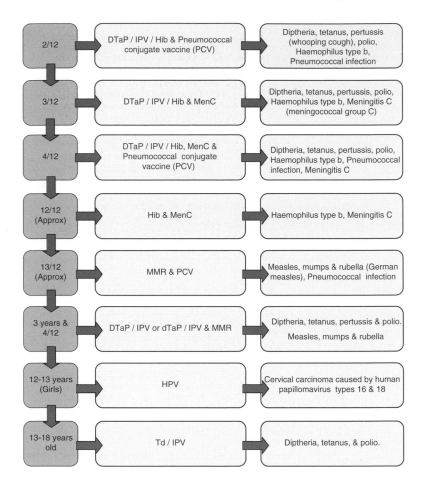

2/12	DTaP / IPV / Hib & Pneumococcal conjugate vaccine (PCV)	Diptheria, tetanus, pertussis (whooping cough), polio, Haemophilus type b, Pneumococcal infection
3/12	DTaP / IPV / Hib & MenC	Diptheria, tetanus, pertussis, polio, Haemophilus type b, Meningitis C (meningococcal group C)
4/12	DTaP / IPV / Hib, MenC & Pneumococcal conjugate vaccine (PCV)	Diptheria, tetanus, pertussis, polio, Haemophilus type b, Pneumococcal infection, Meningitis C
12/12 (Approx)	Hib & MenC	Haemophilus type b, Meningitis C
13/12 (Approx)	MMR & PCV	Measles, mumps & rubella (German measles), Pneumococcal infection
3 years & 4/12	DTaP / IPV or dTaP / IPV & MMR	Diptheria, tetanus, pertussis & polio. Measles, mumps & rubella
12-13 years (Girls)	HPV	Cervical carcinoma caused by human papillomavirus types 16 & 18
13-18 years old	Td / IPV	Diptheria, tetanus, & polio.

Child Health Promotion Programme

Aims: High levels of immunisations of all children; vaccinations in high-risk groups; education on SIDS (e.g. 'back to sleep' campaign, avoiding smoky environments, overheating); education on inadvertent injury (including poisoning). Parental personal child health records: parents hold this main record of their child's health and development so as to encourage a partnership between health care professionals and parents.

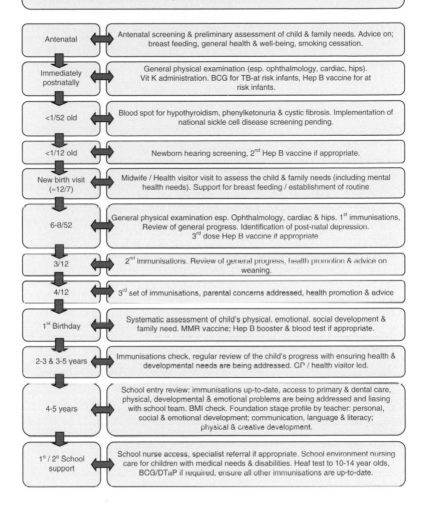

Antenatal	Antenatal screening & preliminary assessment of child & family needs. Advice on; breast feeding, general health & well-being, smoking cessation.
Immediately postnatally	General physical examination (esp. ophthalmology, cardiac, hips). Vit K administration. BCG for TB-at risk infants, Hep B vaccine for at risk infants.
<1/52 old	Blood spot for hypothyroidism, phenylketonuria & cystic fibrosis. Implementation of national sickle cell disease screening pending.
<1/12 old	Newborn hearing screening, 2nd Hep B vaccine if appropriate.
New birth visit (≈12/7)	Midwife / Health visitor visit to assess the child & family needs (including mental health needs). Support for breast feeding / establishment of routine
6-8/52	General physical examination esp. Ophthalmology, cardiac & hips. 1st immunisations, Review of general progress. Identification of post-natal depression. 3rd dose Hep B vaccine if appropriate.
3/12	2nd immunisations. Review of general progress, health promotion & advice on weaning.
4/12	3rd set of immunisations, parental concerns addressed, health promotion & advice
1st Birthday	Systematic assessment of child's physical, emotional, social development & family need. MMR vaccine; Hep B booster & blood test if appropriate.
2-3 & 3-5 years	Immunisations check, regular review of the child's progress with ensuring health & developmental needs are being addressed. GP / health visitor led.
4-5 years	School entry review: immunisations up-to-date, access to primary & dental care, physical, developmental & emotional problems are being addressed and liasing with school team. BMI check. Foundation stage profile by teacher: personal, social & emotional development; communication, language & literacy; physical & creative development.
1° / 2° School support	School nurse access, specialist referral if appropriate. School environment nursing care for children with medical needs & disabilities. Heaf test to 10-14 year olds, BCG/DTaP if required, ensure all other immunisations are up-to-date.

Status Epilepticus

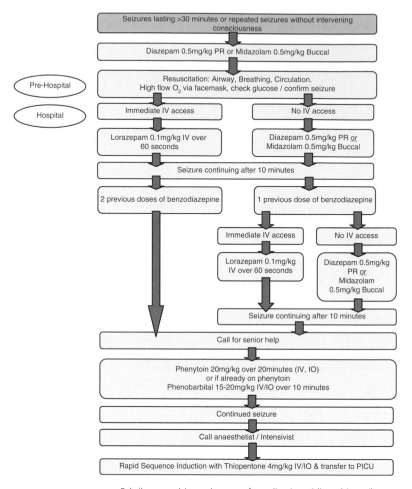

THINK OF A CAUSE Febrile convulsion, change of medication, idiopathic epilepsy, encephalitis, meningitis, poisoning, metabolic disorder, hypoxia, acute cerebral trauma.

MANDATORY INVESTIGATIONS Blood glucose, calcium, phosphate, magnesium, FBC, U&E, ABG, ECG.

Optional investigations
Toxicology, septic screen (beware of raised ICP and consider carefully if LP is necessary), LFTs, metabolic screen, coagulation, CXR, cranial imaging.

Modified from BPNA 2000 guidelines.

ACNE VULGARIS
Haedersdal M, Togsverd-bo K, Wulf HC. Evidence-based review of lasers, light sources and photodynamic therapy in the treatment of acne vulgaris. J Eur Acad Dermatol Venereol 2008;3:267–78.

Strauss JS, Krowchuk DP, Leyden JJ, et al. Guidelines of care for acne vulgaris management. J Am Acad Dermatol 2007;56(4):651–63.

ALLERGIC RHINITIS
Bousquet J, Khaltaev N, Cruz AA, et al. Allergic Rhinitis and its Impact on Asthma (ARIA) 2008 update (in collaboration with the World Health Organization, GA(2)LEN and AllerGen). Allergy 2008;63:(Suppl 86):8–160.

EAACI, Position Paper Consensus statement on the treatment of allergic rhinitis. Allergy 2000;55:116–34.

ANAEMIA, APLASTIC
Guinan EC. Aplastic anemia: management of pediatric patients. Hematol Am Soc Hematol Educ Program 2005:104–9.

ANAEMIA, IRON DEFICIENCY
Harris RJ. Nutrition in the 21st century: what is going wrong. Arch Dis Child 2004;89(2):154–8.

ANAEMIA OF PREMATURITY
Kirpalani H, Whyte RK, Andersen C, et al. The Premature Infants in Need of Transfusion (PINT) study: a randomized, controlled trial of a restrictive (low) versus liberal (high) transfusion threshold for extremely low birth weight infants. J Pediatr. Sep 2006;149(3):301–7.

Ohlsson A, Aher SM. Early erythropoietin for preventing red blood cell transfusion in preterm and/or low birth weight infants. Cochrane Database Syst Rev 2006;3: CD004863.

ANORECTAL MALFORMATIONS
Levitt MA, Pena A. Anorectal malformations. Orphanet J Rare Dis 2007;26;2:33.

APPENDICITIS, ACUTE
IPEG Standards Safety Committee IPEG guidelines for appendectomy. J Laparoendosc Adv Surg Tech A 2009;19(1):vii–ix.

Rothrock SG, Pagane J. Acute appendicitis in children: emergency department diagnosis and management. Ann Emerg Med 2000;36(1):39–51.

ASTHMA
Douglas G, Higgins B, Barnes N, C et al. British guideline on the management of asthma: a national clinical guideline. Thorax 2008;S4:iv1–iv121.

ATOPIC ECZEMA
National Collaborating Centre for Women's and Children's Health. *Atopic eczema in children. Management of atopic eczema in children from birth up to the age of 12 years.* London: RCOG Press, 2007.

ATTENTION DEFICIT HYPERACTIVITY DISORDER (ADHD)
National Institute for Clinical Excellence. *Attention deficit hyperactivity disorder: diagnosis and management of ADHD in children, young people and adults.* London: NICE, 2008.

National Institute for Clinical Excellence. *Methylphenidate, atomoxetine and dexamfetamine for attention deficit hyperactivity disorder (ADHD) in children and adolescents. Review of Technology Appraisal 13.* London: NICE, 2009.

BRONCHIOLITIS, ACUTE

Connor EM. Palivizumab, a humanized respiratory syncytial virus monoclonal antibody, reduces hospitalization from respiratory syncytial virus infection in high-risk infants. Pediatrics 1998;3I:531–7.

Deshpande SA, Northern V. The clinical and health economic burden of respiratory syncytial virus disease among children under 2 years of age in a defined geographical area. Arch Dis Child 2003;12:1065–9.

Kneyber MCJ, Steyerberg EW, De GR, Moll HA. Long-term effects of respiratory syncytial virus (RSV) bronchiolitis in infants and young children: a quantitative review. Acta Paediatr 2000;6:654–60.

CEREBRAL HAEMORRHAGE

National Collaborating Centre for Acute Care. *Head injury: triage, assessment, investigation and early management of head injury in infants, children and adults.* London: NICE, 2007.

CHRONIC LUNG DISEASE (CLD) OF PREMATURITY

Henderson-Smart DJ, de Paoli AG, Clark RH, Bhuta T. High frequency oscillatory ventilation versus conventional ventilation for infants with severe pulmonary dysfunction born at or near term. Cochrane Database Syst Rev 2009;3:CD002974.

Sekar KC, Corff KE. To tube or not to tube babies with respiratory distress syndrome. J Perinatol 2009;29(Suppl 2):S68–72.

CLEFT LIP (CL) AND PALATE (CLP)

Ciminello FS, Morin R, Nguyen T, Wolfe S. Cleft lip and palate: review. Compr Ther 2009;35(1):37–43.

COARCTATION OF THE AORTA (COA)

Rao PS. Coarctation of the aorta. Curr Cardiol Rep 2005;7(6):425–34.

Valdes-Cruz LM, Cayre RO: *Echocardiographic diagnosis of congenital heart disease.* Philadelphia 1998.

COELIAC DISEASE

Clinical Resource Efficiency Support Team (CREST). Guidelines for the diagnosis and management of coeliac disease in adults. 2006. www.crestni.org.uk.

National Institute for Clinical Excellence. *Coeliac disease: recognition and assessment of coeliac disease.* London: NICE, 2009.

CONDUCT DISORDER

National Institute for Clinical Excellence. *Parent-training/education programmes in the management of children with conduct disorders.* London: NICE, 2006.

Woolfenden SR, Williams K, Peat J.Family and parenting interventions in children and adolescents with conduct disorder and delinquency aged 10–17 (Cochrane review). Cochrane Library, Issue 2, 2003.

CONGENITAL HYPOTHYROIDISM

Beardsall K, Ogilvy-Stuart AL. Congenital hypothyroidism. Curr Paediatr 2004;14(5): 422–9.

CONGENITAL INFECTIONS

Nassetta L, Kimberlin D, Whitley R. Treatment of congenital cytomegalovirus infection: implications for future therapeutic strategies. J Antimicrob Chemother 2009;63(5): 862–7.

CONSTIPATION

Baker SS, Liptak GS, Colletti RB, et al. A medical position statement of the North American Society for Pediatric Gastroenterology and Nutrition. Constipation in infants and children: evaluation and treatment. J Ped Gastroenterol Nutr 1999;29:612–26.

Clarke MC, Chase JW, Gibb S, Hutson JM, Southwell BR. Improvement of quality of life in children with slow transit constipation after treatment with transcutaneous electrical stimulation. J Pediatr Surg 2009;44(6):1268–72; discussion 1272.

COW'S MILK PROTEIN ALLERGY

Vandenplas Y, Brueton M, Dupont C, et al. Guidelines for the diagnosis and management of cow's milk protein allergy in infants. Arch Dis Child 2007;10:902–8.

Muraro A, Dreborg S, Halken S, et al. Dietary prevention of allergic diseases in infants and small children. Part III: Critical review of published peer-reviewed observational and interventional studies and final recommendations. Pediatr Allergy Immunol 2004;4:291–307.

CRYPTORCHIDISM

Tomiyama H, Sasaki Y, Huynh J, et al. Testicular descent, cryptorchidism and inguinal hernia: the Melbourne perspective. J Pediatr Urol 2005;1(1):11–25.

CYSTIC FIBROSIS (CF)

Cystic Fibrosis Trust Clinical Standards and Accreditation Group. *Standards for the clinical care of children and adults with cystic fibrosis in the UK.* Bromley, Kent: Cystic Fibrosis Trust, 2001.

DELAYED PUBERTY

Traggiai C, Stanhope R. Delayed puberty. Best Pract Res Clin Endocrinol Metab 2002; 16(1):139–51.

DEPRESSION

National Collaborating Centre for Mental Health. *Depression in children and young people: identification and management in primary, community and secondary care.* London: National Institute for Clinical Excellence, 2005.

DIABETES MELLITUS (TYPE I) (DM)

Guo T, Hebrok M. Stem cells to pancreatic β-cells: new sources for diabetes cell therapy. Endocr Rev 2009;30(3):214–27.

DUCHENNE/BECKER MUSCULAR DYSTROPHY

Manzur AY, Kuntzer T, Pike M, Swan A. Glucocorticoid corticosteroids for Duchenne muscular dystrophy. Cochrane Database Syst Rev 2008;1:CD003725.

EPIGLOTTITIS, ACUTE

Glynn F, Fenton JE. Diagnosis and management of supraglottitis (epiglottitis). Curr Infect Dis Rep 2008;10(3):200–4.

Guldfred LA, Lyhne D, Becker BC. Acute epiglottitis: epidemiology, clinical presentation, management and outcome. et al. J Laryngol Otol 2008;122(8):818–23.

EPILEPSY IN CHILDHOOD

National Collaborating Centre for Primary Care. *The diagnosis and management of the epilepsies in adults and children in primary and secondary care.* London: National Institute for Clinical Excellence, 2004.

Roger J, Dreifuss FE, Martinez-Lage M, et al. Proposal for revised classification of epilepsies and epileptic syndromes. Epilepsia 1989;30(4):389–99.

EXOMPHALOS AND GASTROSCHISIS
Ledbetter DJ. Gastroschisis and omphalocele. Surg Clin North Am 2006; 86(2):249–60, vii.

FAECAL SOILING (ENCOPRESIS)
Levitt M, Pena A. Update on pediatric faecal incontinence. Eur J Pediatr Surg 2009;19(1):1–9.

FOOD ALLERGY
Muraro A, Roberts G, Clark A, et al. The management of anaphylaxis in childhood: position paper of the European Academy of Allergology and Clinical Immunology. Allergy: Eur J Allergy Clin Immunol 2007;8:857–71.

FUNCTIONAL ABDOMINAL PAIN
Huertas-Ceballos AA, Logan S, Bennett C, Macarthur C. Psychosocial interventions for recurrent abdominal pain (RAP) and irritable bowel syndrome (IBS) in childhood. Cochrane Database Syst Rev 2008;1:CD003014.

Huertas-Ceballos AA, Logan S, Bennett C, Macarthur C. Dietary interventions for recurrent abdominal pain (RAP) and irritable bowel syndrome (IBS) in childhood. Cochrane Database Syst Rev 2009;1:CD003019.

GASTROENTERITIS
Szajewska H, Hoekstra JH, Sandhu B. Management of acute gastroenteritis in Europe and the impact of the new recommendations: a multicenter study. Working Group on Acute Diarrhea of the European Society for Paediatric Gastroenterology, Hepatology, and Nutrition. J Pediatr Gastroenterol Nutr 2000;30(5):522–7.

GASTRO-OESOPHAGEAL REFLUX DISEASE (GORD)
Rudolph CD, Mazur L, Liptak G. Guidelines for evaluation and treatment of gastroesophageal reflux in infants and children: recommendations of the North American Society for Pediatric Gastroenterology and Nutrition. J Pediatr Gastroenterol Nutr 2001;32:S1–S22.

GROUP B STREPTOCOCCAL (GBS) INFECTION
Ohlsson A, Shah VS. Intrapartum antibiotics for known maternal Group B streptococcal colonization. Cochrane Database Syst Rev 2009;3:CD007467.

HEART FAILURE
Rosenthal D, Chrisant MRK, Edens E, et al. International Society for Heart and Lung Transplantation: practice guidelines for management of heart failure in children. J Heart Lung Transplant 2004;12:1313–33.

HERNIA, CONGENITAL DIAPHRAGMATIC (CDH)
Downard C, Wilson J. Current therapy of infants with congenital diaphragmatic hernia. Semin Neonatol 2003;8(3):215–21.

HERNIAS, INGUINAL
Brandt ML. Pediatric hernias. Surg Clin North Am 2008;88(1):27–43, vii–viii.

Ron O, Eaton S, Pierro A. Systematic review of the risk of developing a metachronous contralateral inguinal hernia in children. Br J Surg 2007;94(7):804–11.

HERPES SIMPLEX
Jones CA, Walker KS, Badawi N. Antiviral agents for treatment of herpes simplex virus infection in neonates. Cochrane Database Syst Rev 2009;3:CD004206.

HIRSCHSPRUNG DISEASE

Georgeson KE, Robertson DJ. Laparoscopic-assisted approached for the definitive surgery for Hirschsprung's disease. Semin Pediatr Surg 2004;13(4):256–62.

HUMAN IMMUNODEFICIENCY VIRUS (HIV)

British HIV Association, British Association of Sexual Health and HIV British Infection Society. *UK national guidelines for HIV testing.* London: British HIV Association, 2008.

HYPOGLYCAEMIA IN NEONATES

Al-Shanafey S. Laparoscopic vs open pancreatectomy for persistent hyperinsulinemic hypoglycemia of infancy. J Pediatr Surg 2009;44(5):957–61.

Kapoor RR, Flanagan SE, James C, et al. Hyperinsulinaemic hypoglycaemia. Arch Dis Child 2009;94(6):450–7.

HYPOSPADIAS

Baskin LS. Hypospadias and urethral development. J Urol 2000;163(3):951–6.

Snodgrass W. Tubularized, incised plate urethroplasty for distal hypospadias. J Urol 1994;151(2):464–5.

HYPOXIC-ISCHAEMIC ENCEPHALOPATHY (HIE)

Jacobs S, Hunt R, Tarnow-Mordi W, Inder T, Davis P. Cooling for newborns with hypoxic ischaemic encephalopathy. Cochrane Database Syst Rev 2007;4:CD003311.

INFLAMMATORY BOWEL DISEASE

Sandhu BK, Fell JME, Beattie RM, Mitton SG.BSPGHAN IBD guidelines. 2008. www.bspghan.org.uk.

Sawczenko A, Sandhu B. Presenting features of inflammatory bowel disease in Great Britain and Ireland. Arch Dis Child 2003;88:995–1000.

INTUSSUSCEPTION

Applegate KE. Intussusceptions in children: evidence-based diagnosis and treatment. Pediatr Radiol 2009;39:(Suppl 2):S140–3.

Bonnard A, Demarche M, Dimitriu C, et al. Indications for laparoscopy in the management of intussusceptions: a multicenter retrospective study conducted by the French Study Group for Pediatric Laparoscopy (GECI). J Pediatr Surg 2008;43(7):1249–53.

JUVENILE IDIOPATHIC ARTHRITIS

Foster HE, Kay LJ, Friswell M, Coady D, Myers A. Musculoskeletal screening examination (pGALS) for school-age children based on the adult GALS screen. Arthritis Care Res 2006;5:709–16.

Petty RE, Southwood TR, Manners P, et al. International League of Associations for Rheumatology Classification of Juvenile Idiopathic Arthritis: Second Revision, Edmonton, 2001. J Rheumatol 2004;2:390–2.

KAWASAKI DISEASE

Ayusawa M, Sonobe T, Uemura S, et al. Revision of diagnostic guidelines for Kawasaki disease (the 5th revised edition). Pediatr Int 2005;2:232–4.

Newburger JW, Takahashi M, Gerber MA, et al. Diagnosis, treatment, and long-term management of Kawasaki disease: a statement for health professionals from the Committee on Rheumatic Fever, Endocarditis, and Kawasaki Disease, Council on Cardiovascular Disease in the Young. American Heart Association. Pediatrics 2004;6:1708–33.

KLINEFELTER SYNDROME
Lanfranco F, Kaminschke A, Zitzmann M, Nieschlag E. Klinefelter's syndrome. Lancet 2004;364(9430):273–83.

LACTOSE INTOLERANCE
Lomer MCE, Parkes GC, Sanderson JD. Review article: lactose intolerance in clinical practice – myths and realities. Aliment Pharmacol Therapeut 2008;2:93–103.

LEGG-CALVÉ-PERTHES DISEASE (LCPD)
Hunter JB. Legg Calvé Perthes' disease. Curr Orthop 2004;18:273–83.

LEUKAEMIA, ACUTE LYMPHOBLASTIC (ALL)
Pui CH, Robison LL, Look AT. Acute lymphoblastic leukaemia. Lancet 2008;371(9617):1030–43.

LEUKAEMIA, ACUTE MYELOID (AML)
Hall GW. Childhood myeloid leukaemias. Best Pract Res Clin Haematol 2001;14(3):573–91.

THE LIMPING HIP
Kermond S, Fink K, Graham K, et al. A randomized clinical trial: should the child with transient synovitis of the hip be treated with nonsteroidal anti-inflammatory drugs? Ann Emerg Med 2002;40(3):294–9.

Kocher MS, Zurakowski D, Kasser JR. Differentiating between septic arthritis and transient synovitis of the hip in children: an evidence-based clinical prediction algorithm. J Bone Joint Surg 1999;81(12):1662–70.

LYMPHOMA, NON-HODGKIN (NHL)
Harris NL, Jaffe ES, Diebold J, et al. The World Health Organization classification of neoplastic diseases of the haematopoietic and lymphoid tissues: report of the Clinical Advisory Committee Meeting, Airlie House, Virginia, November 1997. Histopathology 2000;1:69–87.

MALROTATION OF THE INTESTINE
Draus JM Jr, Foley D, Bond S. Laparoscopic Ladd procedure: a minimally invasive approach to malrotation without midgut volvulus. Am Surg 2007;73(7):693–6.

Ladd WE. Surgical diseases of the alimentary tract in infants. N Engl J Med 1936;215:705–8.

MARFAN SYNDROME
Everitt MD, Pinto N, Hawkins J, et al. Cardiovascular surgery in children with Marfan's syndrome or Loeys-Dietz syndrome. J Thorac Cadiovasc Surg 2009;137(6):1332–3.

Loeys BL, Chen J, Neptune ER, et al. A syndrome of altered cardiovascular, craniofacial, neurocognitive and skeletal development caused by mutations in TGFBR1 or TGFBR2. Nat Genet 2005;37(3):275–81.

MEASLES, MUMPS, RUBELLA (MMR)
Health Technology Advisory Committee. MMR vaccine and autism: no evidence of association. Health Technology Assessment (HTA) Database 2003.

MECKEL DIVERTICULUM
Mendelson KG, Bailey BM, Balint TD, et al. Meckel's diverticulum: review and surgical management. Curr Surg 2001;58(5):455–7.

Menezes M, Tareen F, Saeed A, et al. Symptomatic Meckel's diverticulum in children: a 16 year review. Pediatr Surg Int 2008;24(5):575–7.

MECONIUM ASPIRATION SYNDROME
[2005] American Heart Association (AHA) guidelines for cardiopulmonary resuscitation (CPR) and emergency cardiovascular care (ECC) of pediatric and neonatal patients: neonatal resuscitation guidelines. Pediatrics 2006;117(5):e1029–38.

NECROTISING ENTEROCOLITIS (NEC)
Petrosyan M, Guner Y, Williams M, et al. Current concepts regarding the pathogenesis of necrotizing enterocolitis. Pediatr Surg Int 2009;25(4):309–18.

Rees CM, Eaton S, Kiely E, et al. Peritoneal drainage or laparotomy for neonatal bowel perforation? A randomised controlled trial. Ann Surg 2008;248(1):44–51.

NEONATAL JAUNDICE
American Academy of Paediatrics. Management of hyperbilirubinaemia in the newborn infant 35 or more weeks of gestation. Paediatrics 2004;114:297–316.

NOCTURNAL ENURESIS
Robson WL. Clinical practice. Evaluation and management of enuresis. N Engl J Med 2009;360(14):1429–36.

OBESITY IN CHILDREN
NICE Guideline for Childhood Obesity. www.nice.org.uk/CG043.

OESOPHAGEAL ATRESIA AND TRACHEO-OESOPHAGEAL FISTULA
Spitz L. Oesophageal atresia. Lessons I have learned in a 40 year experience. J Pediatr Surg 2006;41:1635–40.

Spitz L, Kiely EM, Drake DP, et al. Long-gap oesophageal atresia. Pediatr Surg Int 1996;11:462–5.

OTITIS MEDIA, ACUTE AND CHRONIC SECRETORY
Khanna R, Lakhanpaul M, Bull PD. Surgical management of otitis media with effusion in children: summary of NICE guidance. Clin Otolaryngol 2008;6:600–605.

Mattila PS. Antibiotics are effective in acute otitis media in children younger than 2 years with bilateral disease and in children with both otorrhea and acute otitis media. J Pediatr 2007;5:562.

Teele DW, Klein JO, Rosner B. Epidemiology of otitis media during the first seven years of life in children in greater Boston: a prospective, cohort study. J Infect Dis 1989;1:83–94.

PATENT DUCTUS ARTERIOSUS (PDA)
Madan JC, Kendrick D, Hagadorn JI, Frantz ID 3rd. Patent ductus arteriosus therapy: impact on neonatal and 18-month outcome. Pediatrics 2009;23(2):674–81.

Ohlsson A, Walia R, Shah S. Ibuprofen for the treatment of patent ductus arteriosus in preterm and/or low birth weight infants. Cochrane Database Syst Rev 2008;1: CD003481.

PHIMOSIS AND FORESKIN DISORDERS
Gairdner DA. The fate of the foreskin: a study of circumcision. BMJ 1949;2:1433–7.

Gray RH, Kigozi G, Serwadda D. Male circumcision for HIV prevention in men in Rakai. Uganda: a randomised trial. Lancet 2007;369(9562):657–66.

Siegfried N, Muller M, Deeks JJ, Volmink J. Male circumcision for prevention of heterosexual acquisition of HIV in men. Cochrane Database Syst Rev 2009;2: CD003362.

PNEUMONIA
British Thoracic Society. BTS guidelines for the management of community acquired pneumonia in children. 2002. www.brit-thoracic.org.uk.

PRECOCIOUS PUBERTY (COMPLETE)
Kaplowitz PB, Oberfield SE. Reexamination of the age limit for defining when puberty is precocious in girls in the United States: implications for evaluation and treatment. Pediatrics 1999;4I:936–41.

PSORIASIS
Menter A, Korman NJ, Elmets CA, et al. Guidelines of care for the management of psoriasis and psoriatic arthritis. Section 3. Guidelines of care for the management and treatment of psoriasis with topical therapies. J Am Acad Dermatol 2009;4:643–59.

PULMONARY VALVE STENOSIS
Karagoz T, Asoh K, Hickey E, et al. Balloon dilation of pulmonary valve stenosis in infants less than 3 kg: a 20-year experience. Catheter Cardiovasc Interv 2009;74(5):753–61.

PYLORIC STENOSIS
Hall NJ, Pacilli M, Eaton S, et al. Recovery after open versus laparoscopic pyloromyotomy for pyloric stenosis: a double-blind multicentre randomised controlled trial. Lancet 2009;373(9661):390–8.

Kim SS, Lau ST, Lee SL. Pyloromyotomy: a comparison of laparoscopic, circumumbilical, and right upper quadrant operative techniques. J Am Coll Surg 2005;201(1):66–70.

Rogers IM. The true cause of pyloric stenosis is hyperacidity. Acta Paediatr 2006;95(2):132–6.

RESPIRATORY DISTRESS SYNDROME (RDS)
Verder H, Bohlin K, Kamper J, et al. Nasal CPAP and surfactant for treatment of respiratory distress syndrome and prevention of bronchopulmonary dysplasia. Acta Paediatr 2009;98(9):1400–8.

RETINOPATHY OF PREMATURITY (ROP)
Clark D, Mandal K. Treatment of retinopathy of prematurity. Early Hum Dev 2008;84(2):95–9.

RHEUMATIC FEVER
Dajani AS, Ayoub E, Bierman FZ, et al. Guidelines for the diagnosis of rheumatic fever: Jones Criteria, 1992 update. JAMA 1992;15:2069–73.

SAFEGUARDING CHILDREN
National Collaborating Centre for Women's and Children's Health. *When to suspect child maltreatment*. London: NICE, 2009.

Department of Health, Home Office, Department for Education and Employment. *Working together to safeguard children. A guide to inter-agency working to safeguard and promote the welfare of children*. London: Stationery Office, 2006.

SCABIES
Strong M, Johnstone PW. Interventions for treating scabies. Cochrane Database Syst Rev 2007;3:CD000320.

SEPTICAEMIA
National Collaborating Centre for Women's and Children's Health. *Feverish illness in children – assessment and initial management in children younger than 5 years*. London: NICE, 2007.

SICKLE CELL ANAEMIA

Ballas SK. Complications of sickle cell anemia in adults: guidelines for effective management. Cleve Clin J Med 1999;66(1):48–58.

Bunn HF. Pathogenesis and treatment of sickle cell disease. N Engl J Med 1997;337(11):762–9.

SMALL BOWEL ATRESIA

Louw JH, Barnard CN. Congenital intestinal atresia: observations on its origin. Lancet 1955;269(6899):1065–7.

SUDDEN INFANT DEATH SYNDROME (SIDS)

Royal College of Pathologists and Royal College of Paediatrics and Child Health Working Group. *Sudden unexpected death in infancy: a multi-agency protocol for care and investigation*. London: Royal College of Pathologists and Royal College of Paediatrics and Child Health, 2004.

SUPRAVENTRICULAR TACHYCARDIA (SVT)

Maok JP. Supraventricular tachycardia in the neonate and infant. Prog Pediatr Cardiol 2000;11(1):25–38.

TESTICULAR TORSION

Kapoor S. Testiclar torsion: a race against time. Int J Clin Pract 2008;62(5):821–7.

Ringdahl E, Teague L. Testicular torsion. Am Fam Physician 2006;74(10):1739–43.

TRANSIENT TACHYPNOEA OF THE NEWBORN (TTN)

Liem JJ, Huq SI, Ekuma O, et al. Transient tachypnea of the newborn may be an early clinical manifestation of wheezing symptoms. J Pediatr 2007;151:1;29–33.

TRANSPOSITION OF THE GREAT ARTERIES (TGA)

Martins P, Castela E. Transposition of the great arteries. Orphanet J Rare Dis 2008;13(3):27.

UPPER RESPIRATORY TRACT INFECTION (URTI)

National Collaborating Centre for Women's and Children's Health. *Feverish illness in children – assessment and initial management in children younger than 5 years*. London: NICE, 2007.

URINARY TRACT ANOMALIES

Sanna-Cherchi S, Ravani P, Corbani V, et al. Renal outcome in patients with congenital anomalies of the kidney and urinary tract. Kidney Int 2009;76(5):528–33.

URINARY TRACT INFECTION (UTI)

National Institute for Health and Clinical Excellence Guidelines. UTI in children. www.nice.org.uk.

VENTRICULAR SEPTAL DEFECT (VSD)

Kenny D, Morgan G, Bajwa A, et al. Evolution of transcatheter closure of perimembranous ventricular septal defects in a single centre. Catheter Cardiovasc Interv 2009;73(4):568–75.

VITAMIN D DEFICIENCY

No authors listed, Primary vitamin D deficiency in children. Drug Therapeut Bull 2006;2:12–16.

Shaw NJ, Pal BR. Vitamin D deficiency in UK Asian families: activating a new concern. Arch Dis Child 2002;86(3):147–9.